Recent Results in Cancer Research 121

Managing Editors
Ch. Herfarth, Heidelberg · H.-J. Senn, St. Gallen

Associate Editors
M. Baum, London · V. Diehl, Köln
E. Grundmann, Münster · F. Gutzwiller, Zürich
W. Hitzig, Zürich · M.F. Rajewsky, Essen
M. Wannenmacher, Heidelberg

Founding Editor
P. Rentchnick, Geneva

D0267835

Recent Results in Cancer Research

Volume 111
H. Scheurlen, R. Kay, M. Baum (Eds.):
Cancer Clinical Trials: A Critical Appraisal
1988. 37 figures, 53 tables. IX, 272. ISBN 3-540-19098-8

Volume 112
L. Schmid, H.-J. Senn (Eds.): AIDS-Related Neoplasias
1988. 23 figures, 35 tables. IX, 97. ISBN 3-540-19227-1

Volume 113
U. Eppenberger, A. Goldhirsch (Eds.):
Endocrine Therapy and Growth Regulation of Breast Cancer
1989. 26 figures, 17 tables. IX, 92. ISBN 3-540-50456-7

Volume 114
P. Boyle, C.S. Muir, E. Grundmann (Eds.): Cancer Mapping
1989. 97 figures, 64 tables. IX, 277. ISBN 3-540-50490-7

Volume 115
H.-J. Senn, A. Goldhirsch, R.D. Gelber, B. Osterwalder (Eds.):
Adjuvant Therapy of Primary Breast Cancer
1989. 64 figures, 94 tables. XVI, 296. ISBN 3-540-18810-X

Volume 116
K.W. Brunner, H. Fleisch, H.-J. Senn (Eds.):
Bisphosphonates and Tumor Osteolysis
1989. 22 figures, 6 tables. IX, 78. ISBN 3-540-50560-1

Volume 117
V. Diehl, M. Pfreundschuh, M. Loeffler (Eds.):
New Aspects in the Diagnosis and Treatment of Hodgkin's Disease
1989. 71 figures, 91 tables. XIV, 283. ISBN 3-540-51124-5

Volume 118
L. Beck, E. Grundmann, R. Ackermann, H.-D. Röher (Eds.):
Hormone-Related Malignant Tumors
1990. 83 figures, 91 tables. XI, 269. ISBN 3-540-51258-6

Volume 119
S. Brünner, B. Langfeldt (Eds.):
Advances in Breast Cancer Detection
1990. 53 figures, 51 tables. XI, 195. ISBN 3-540-52089-9

Volume 120
P. Band (Ed.): Occupational Cancer Epidemiology
1990. 23 figures, 59 tables. IX, 193. ISBN 3-540-52090-2

H.-J. Senn A. Glaus (Eds.)

Supportive Care in Cancer Patients II

With 49 Figures and 94 Tables

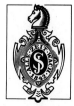

Springer-Verlag

Berlin Heidelberg New York
London Paris Tokyo
Hong Kong Barcelona

Professor Dr. Hans-Jörg Senn
Oberschwester Agnes Glaus

Medizinische Klinik C, Kantonsspital St. Gallen
9007 St. Gallen, Switzerland

ISBN 3-540-52346-4 Springer-Verlag Berlin Heidelberg New York
ISBN 0-387-52346-4 Springer-Verlag New York Berlin Heidelberg

Library of Congress Cataloging-in-Publication Data
Supportive care in cancer patients/H.-J. Senn, A. Glaus (eds.).
p.cm. – (Recent results in cancer research; 121)
Includes bibliographical references and index.
ISBN 3-540-52346-4 (alk. paper). – ISBN 0-387-52346-4 (alk. paper)
1. Cancer-Palliative treatment. 2. Cancer pain-Treatment. I. Senn,
Hansjörg. II. Glaus, Agnes. III. Series
[DNLM: 1. Neoplasms-therapy. 2. Palliative Treatment. 3. Social
Support.   W1   RE106P   v. 121/QZ   266   S9588]
RC261.R35   vol. 121   [RC271.P33]   616.99'406-dc20   DNLM/DLC
90-10404

© Springer-Verlag Berlin Heidelberg 1991
Printed in Germany

The use of registered names, trademarks, etc. in this publication does not imply, even in the absence of a specific statement, that such names are exempt from the relevant protective laws and regulations and therefore free for general use.

Product Liability: The publisher can give no guarantee for information about drug dosage and application thereof contained in the book. In every individual case the respective user must check its accuracy by consulting other pharmaceutical literature.

Typesetting: Macmillan India Ltd., Bangalore-25, India
25/3130-543210-Printed on acid-free paper.

Preface

The second international symposium on "Supportive Care in Cancer Patients" took place March 1–3, 1990 – again in St. Gallen in eastern Switzerland. It was an honor once more to welcome dozens of internationally recognized experts in the field and more than 800 participants from over 30 countries around the world: Australia, Canada, China, USSR, USA and many countries in Europe. The international nature of the grade facilitated lively and exciting contributions and critical discussions, aimed at fostering professional knowledge and skills and rethinking our personal attitudes toward cancer patients in all stages of their disease.

Cancer patients need various types of tailored support, whether during active initial (curative) therapies, in phases of worrying relapsing disease, or during the demanding terminal stage of their illness. The symposium tried to bridge the strange "gap" between "curative" and "palliative" cancer care: it must be our aim to be and remain "supportive" for our patients during both curative and palliative treatment strategies! This requires extended knowledge and even more and flexible professional skills. The symposium was designed to promote improved approaches that are helpful and supportive for all our oncology patients, not just for a selected disease- or stage-dependent minority.

Exactly 3 years ago, the first such multiprofessional symposium also took place in St. Gallen. Many doctors and nurses encouraged us to repeat this experiment. However, in preparing this second symposium we made a slight, but probably significant change, since we purposely composed only one scientific program for all participants, whether nurses, physicians, psychologists social workers etc. Speakers, moderators, and participants come from each of these different groups. We were fully aware of the fact that this might constitute a risky venture, but we hoped to create a comprehensive teaching atmosphere, favoring an efficient team approach.

Looking back over the symposium – and taking into consideration many enthusiastic verbal and written comments – it looks as if this goal has been at least partially achieved. The symposium presented an opportunity to exercise truly interdisciplinary, multiprofessional teamwork. This does not at all mean taking over somebody else's job; it rather means learning to listen to other disciplines, to respect them, and to integrate their knowledge and perspective into a truly holistic approach care to – a lesson to be tested and exercised back home at the regular working place!

We can only hope that the "seeds" of this symposium fell on receptive ground and will grow despite the various structural, professional, and economic adversities which limit our efforts to develop optimal supportive care in cancer patients – inside as well as outside our hospital, cancer centers, and palliative care units. It may be that the historic "fluidum" of the city of St. Gallen, which has been a center of spiritual, ethical, and medical interest since the foundation of its famous monastry in the early middle ages, contributed toward this goal.

St. Gallen, Switzerland, in August 1990   Agnes Glaus
                                                 Hans-Jörg Senn

Contents

B. Roos
Opening Remarks   1

News in Managing Cancer Pain   2

B. Dicks
News in Managing Cancer Pain: An Overview   2

M. Zimmermann
Cancer Pain: Pathogenesis, Therapy, and Assessment . .   8

N. MacDonald
Opiate-Resistant Pain: A Therapeutic Dilemma   24

H.R. Stoll
Effective Pain Control in Cancer Patients
in the Home Care Setting   36

M. Zenz and J. Sorge
Is the Therapeutic Use of Opioids
Adversely Affected by Prejudice and Law?   43

A.H. Lang, K. Abbrederis, A. Dzien, and H. Drexel
Treatment of Severe Cancer Pain by Continuous
Infusion of Subcutaneous Opioids   51

H. Seemann and H. Lang
Coping with Cancer Pain   58

Antiemetics and Cancer Chemotherapy   68

R.J. Gralla
Controlling Emesis in Patients
Receiving Cancer Chemotherapy   68

M. Soukop
5-Hydroxytryptamine-3-Antagonists:
A New Class of Potent Antiemetics in Cancer
Therapy   86

M.S. Aapro
Present Role of Corticosteroids as Antiemetics   91

P.H. Cotanch
Use of Nonpharmacologic Techniques to Prevent
Chemotherapy-Related Nausea and Vomiting 101

Managing Visceral Obstructions 108

J. Forbes and H. McA. Foster
Optimizing Palliative Surgical Support of Cancer
Patients with Visceral Obstructions 108

R.J. Wells
Sexuality: An Unknown Word for Patients
with a Stoma? 115

Hematopoietic Growth Factors and Cancer Therapy . . . 121

R. Mertelsmann, F.M. Rosenthal, A. Lindemann,
and F. Herrmann
Cytokines and Hematopoietins: Physiology,
Pathophysiology, and Potential as Therapeutic Agents   121

G. Seipelt, A. Ganser, and D. Hoelzer
Hemopoietic Growth Factors in the Treatment
of Acute Leukemias and Myelodysplastic Syndromes . . 141

H. Anderson, H. Gurney, N. Thatcher, R. Swindell,
J.H. Scarffe, and J. Weiner
Recombinant Human GM-CSF
in Small Cell Lung Cancer: A Phase I/II Study 155

A. Ganser, A. Lindemann, G. Seipelt, O.G. Ottmann,
M. Eder, F. Herrmann, J. Frisch,
G. Schulz, R. Mertelsmann, and D. Hoelzer
Recombinant Human Interleukin-3
in Patients with Hematopoietic Failure   162

L. Schmid, B. Thürlimann, M. Müller, and H.-J. Senn
Recombinant Human Granulocyte-Macrophage
Colony-Stimulating Factor for the Intensification
of Cytostatic Treatment in Advanced Cancer   173

W.P. Peters
The Potential for the Use of Colony-Stimulation Factors
in Autologous Bone Marrow Transplantation   182

Vascular Access Problems and Implantable Devices   189

U. Laffer, M. Dürig, M.R. Bloch, and J. Landmann
Surgical Experiences with 191 Implanted Venous
Port-a-Cath Systems   189

U. Metzger, W. Weder, M. Röthlin, and F. Largiadèr
Phase II Study of Intra-arterial Fluorouracil and
Mitomycin-C for Liver Metastases of Colorectal Cancer   198

N. Nadau
Maintenance and Care of Patients
with Drug Delivery Systems.   205

L. Schmid and A. Feldges
Implantable Devices in Patients
with Haematological Diseases   208

D.N. Williams
Home Intravenous Antibiotic Therapy:
New Technologies.   215

B. Horisberger, M. Sagmeister, and L. Schmid
Socioeconomic Aspects of an Implantable Drug Delivery
Device   223

Nutrition and the Cancer Patient.   233

P. Schlag and C. Decker-Baumann
Strategies and Needs for Nutritional Support
in Cancer Surgery.   233

G. Ollenschläger, B. Viell, W. Thomas, K. Konkol,
and B. Bürger
Tumor Anorexia: Causes, Assessment, Treatment 249

V.F.P. Souchon
Nutritional Support of Patients with Advanced Cancer 260

A. Millard
Food Service Provisions for the Cancer Patient 266

R. Fietkau, H. Iro, D. Sailer, and R. Sauer
Percutaneous Endoscopically Guided Gastrostomy
in Patients with Head and Neck Cancer 269

S. Klimberg
Prevention of Radiogenic Side-Effects
Using Glutamine-Enriched Elemental Diets. 283

W. F. Jungi
Diet to Prevent Gastrointestinal Cancer? 286

M. Hunter
Alternative Dietary Therapies in Cancer Patients. 293

R. Kreibich-Fischer
Psychological Aspects of Malnutrition
in Cancer Patients. 296

Psychosocial Support in Oncology 301

G.H. Christ
A Model for the Development of Psychosocial
Interventions 301

S. Porchet-Munro
Aspects of Nonverbal Communication 313

Infections in Cancer Patients. 321

M.P. Glauser
Alterations of Host Defenses:
The Key to the Multifaceted Spectrum of Infections
in Immunocompromised Patients 321

T. Calandra
Spectrum and Treatment of Bacterial Infections
in Cancer Patients with Granulocytopenia. 329

M. Rozenberg-Arska, A.W. Dekker, and J. Verhoef
Prevention of Infections in Granulocytopenic Patients
by Fluorinated Quinolones   337

M. Arning, B. Dresen, C. Aul, and W. Schneider
Influence of Infusion Time on the Acute Toxicity
of Amphothericin B:
Results of a Randomized Double-Blind Study   347

U. Jehn
New Antiviral Drugs for Treatment of Viral Infections
in Immunocompromised Patients   353

Support in Agonizing Conditions   360

D.K. Mayer
Prevention, Early Detection,
and Management of Oncologic Emergencies   360

P. Drings and I. Günther
Relief from Respiratory Distress
in Advanced Cancer Patients   366

L.M. Lesko and S. Fleishman
Treatment and Support in Confusional States   378

Optimizing Palliative Cancer Care   393

V. Ventafridda
Palliative Care: A New Reality in Medicine   393

N. MacDonald
Cure and Care: Interaction Between Cancer Centers and
Palliative Care Units   399

J. Webber
Optimizing Palliative Nursing Skills by Education   408

J.F. Forbes and D. Allbrook
Education and Palliative Care: A Different Approach .   414

T. Flöter
Palliative Care in a German Hospice: The Medical and
Psychological Concept of the Christophorus-Haus   423

G.H. Christ and K. Siegel
Parental Death: A Preventive Intervention   426

A. Couldrick
Optimising Breavement Outcome:
Reading the Road Ahead . . . .,.   432

D.K. Mayer
Rehabilitation of the Person with Cancer   437

W. Lehmann and H. Krebs
Interdisciplinary Rehabilitation of the Laryngectomee .   442

C. Odier
Spiritual Support and Palliative Cancer Care.   450

Subject Index   454

List of Contributors*

Aapro, M.S. *91*[1]
Abbrederis, K. *51*
Allbrook, D. *414*
Anderson, H. *155*
Arning, M. *347*
Aul, C. *347*
Bloch, M.R. *189*
Bürger, B. *249*
Calandra, T. *329*
Christ, G.H. *301, 426*
Cotanch, P.H. *101*
Couldrick, A. *432*
Decker-Baumann, C. *233*
Dekker, A.W. *337*
Dicks, B. *2*
Dresen, B. *347*
Drexel, H. *51*
Drings, P. *366*
Dürig, M. *189*
Dzien, A. *51*
Eder, M. *162*
Feldges, A. *208*
Fietkau, R. *269*
Fleishman, S. *378*
Flöter, T. *423*
Forbes, J.F. *108, 414*

Foster, H. McA. *108*
Frisch, J. *162*
Ganser, A. *141, 162*
Glauser, M.P. *321*
Gralla, R.J. *68*
Günther, I. *366*
Gurney, H. *155*
Herrmann, F. *121, 162*
Hoelzer, D. *141, 162*
Horisberger, B. *223*
Hunter, M. *293*
Iro, H. *269*
Jehn, U. *353*
Jungi, W.F. *286*
Klimberg, S. *283*
Konkol, K. *249*
Krebs, H. *442*
Kreibich-Fischer, R. *296*
Laffer, U. *189*
Landmann, J. *189*
Lang, A.H. *51*
Lang, H. *58*
Largiadèr, F. *198*
Lehmann, W. *442*
Lesko, L.M. *378*
Lindemann, A. *121, 162*

---

* The address of the principal author is given on the first page of each
  contribution.
[1] Page on which contribution begins.

MacDonald, N. *24, 399*
Mayer, D.K. *360, 437*
Mertelsmann, R. *121, 162*
Metzger, U. *198*
Millard, A. *266*
Müller, M. *173*
Nadau, N. *205*
Odier, C. *450*
Ollenschläger, G. *249*
Ottmann, O.G. *162*
Peters, W.P. *182*
Roos, B. *1*
Porchet-Munro, S. *313*
Rosenthal, F.M. *121*
Röthlin, M. *198*
Rozenberg-Arska, M. *337*
Sagmeister, M. *223*
Sailer, D. *269*
Sauer, R. *269*
Scarffe, J.H. *155*
Schlag, P. *233*
Schmid, L. *173, 208, 223*
Schneider, W. *347*

Schulz, G. *162*
Seemann, H. *58*
Seipelt, G. *141, 162*
Senn, H.-J. *173*
Siegel, K. *426*
Sorge, J. *43*
Souchon, V.F.P. *260*
Soukop, M. *86*
Stoll, H.R. *36*
Swindell, R. *155*
Thatcher, N. *155*
Thomas, W. *249*
Thürlimann, B. *173*
Ventafridda, V. *393*
Verhoef, J. *337*
Viell, B. *249*
Webber, J. *408*
Weder, W. *198*
Weiner, J. *155*
Wells, R.J. *115*
Williams, D.N. *215*
Zenz, M. *43*
Zimmermann, M. *8*

Opening Remarks

B. Roos

Bundesamt für Gesundheitswesen, Bern, Switzerland

Ladies and Gentlemen,

On behalf of the Federal Government of Switzerland I would like to welcome all of you to this year's International Symposium on Supportive Care in Cancer Patients. Professor Senn and Mrs. Agnes Glaus have been known in our country for many years for their initiative in organizing meetings on topics in the field of care for cancer patients. This year, the Symposium is taking place in conjunction with the Swiss Cancer Conference 1990. The Symposia in St. Gall are renowned for their strongly interdisciplinary character. Particular attention is paid at these meetings to important questions such as the psychosocial care of cancer patients.

The Swiss health care system is characterized by a largely decentralized approach, which is due to the federalistic structure of the political system of our country. Switzerland consists of 26 individual states, or "Cantons", which have considerable autonomy in matters of public health. The Cantons are mainly responsible for curative medicine; the Federal Government, on the other hand, is the competent authority for health protection in the broadest sense of the word. That is why it is most important for our country that everybody involved in the care of cancer patients is able to participate in and exchange experiences at meetings like this Symposium. In addition, the participation of experts from other countries allows comparisons to be made between different views and approaches. This year's programme once again covers every possible approach to and aspect of the day-to-day care and treatment of cancer patients.

I hope that the papers presented in this varied programme will contribute to helping all those affected by cancer to a better acceptance of the disease. I also hope that it will provide people caring for cancer patients with the necessary strength to help these patients face an often terminal disease, and to attend to their needs to the very last day. I would like to thank most cordially those people who have been responsible for the organization of the Symposium and who have again and again organized similar meetings. Last but not least, I would like to wish you, ladies and gentlemen, a most successful meeting and a pleasant stay in St. Gallen.

Recent Results in Cancer Research, Vol. 121
© Springer-Verlag Berlin · Heidelberg 1991

News in Managing Cancer Pain: An Overview

B. Dicks

19 Ashdown Way, Upper Tooting Park, London SW17 7TH, United Kingdom

Growth of Palliative Care

In the last twenty years palliative care services have expanded at a rapid rate. The 1988 Directory of Hospice Services in the United Kingdom and Ireland lists over 120 hospices with over 2300 beds and over 250 support teams working in the community or from hospitals. Palliative medicine has also become an accepted speciality within general medicine. The United States of America has over 1500 hospice programmes and Canada over 200. Although services are expanding more slowly in Europe a significant number are in the pipeline [1]. It is therefore somewhat surprising to note that the literature continues to indicate that cancer pain relief is a neglected public health issue in developed and developing countries alike [2].

Prevalence of Cancer Pain

Cancer, as we are well aware, is a major world problem. Every year nearly six million new patients are diagnosed and more than four million die [3].

Because the main characteristic of cancer is that of uncontrolled growth and spread to sites distant from its origin, patients with advanced cancer may present with a complex array of interrelated symptoms which, if left untended, will result in misery and disability before death intervenes [4]. Of the many symptoms which can arise in this situation, pain is the most prominent, occurring in some 60% of patients managed in a general oncology unit and in up to 85% of patients referred for hospice care.

It is becoming increasingly clear that the challenge of cancer pain management lies not in discovering new knowledge but in acting upon what we *already* know. It is therefore not surprising that the World Health Organisation has stated that one of the major reasons for unsatisfactory management of cancer pain is: "A widespread lack of recognition by health care professionals of the fact that established methods *already* exist for satisfactory cancer pain management".

Take, as an example of this, the situation in relation to the use of analgesics in the control of cancer pain. Analgesic drug therapy is, as we all know, an essential component of cancer pain control, and existing knowledge in this respect should mean that correctly used analgesics are capable of controlling pain in more than 90% of patients [3]. However, numerous published reports indicate that cancer pain is often not treated adequately. An analysis of 11 reports covering nearly 2000 patients in developed countries suggests that between 50%–80% of patients did not have satisfactory relief [3].

Frequent Lack of Availability of Essential Pain Relieving Drugs

The fact that in many countries no strong opioid is available for oral use is another major contributory factor to the unsatisfactory management of cancer pain. The proliferation of national laws and administrative measures regulating the prescription and distribution of the drugs necessary for cancer pain relief continues to hinder access by patients to these drugs. Greater flexibility in drug distribution systems is needed to enable a wider variety of professional health care workers to prescribe and/or distribute drugs for pain relief. Rigid professional boundaries between health care professionals need to be challenged. For example, restricting prescribing powers only to doctors will in many countries seriously hinder access by patients to necessary pain relieving drugs. The United Kingdom Department of Health has recently produced a report which made recommendations on the circumstances in which nurses might prescribe or supply some drugs and vary the timing and dosage of pain relieving drugs prescribed by a doctor. Whilst these recommendations are limited in their scope, they certainly are a step in the right direction. However experienced or highly skilled a United Kingdom nurse is, she or he is not at present able even to write a prescription for products that are needed for *nursing* care, or to prescribe simple pain relieving drugs. Skilled nurses working in the community with terminally ill patients have been unable to use their professional judgement on such matters as the timing and dosage of analgesic drugs or even prescribe an aperient for opioid-induced constipation. This has resulted in a lot of time being wasted as nurses wait to see a doctor to "rubber stamp" a prescribing decision which an appropriately trained nurse could easily make. Not only does this constitute inefficient use of professional time, but lack of clarity about professional responsibilities is demeaning to both nurses and doctors. Changes such as this report recommends are a small but significant step in the direction of aligning prescribing powers with professional responsibility.

Fears Concerning Opioid "Addiction"
Both in Cancer Patients and in the Wider Public

Fears concerning addiction still prevail. The incidence of opioid addiction in 40 000 hospitalized medical patients has been monitored in a prospective study [5]. Among nearly 12 000 patients who received at least one strong opioid preparation, there were only four reasonably well documented cases of addiction in patients. These data, from a survey of a general in-patient population, suggest that the medical use of strong opioids is rarely associated with the development of addiction.

There is still in some countries evidence that concern with illicit drug use can curtail the availability of opioid drugs to patients with cancer pain. Education concerning the fact that addiction is just not a problem for patients in pain receiving opioids, and that the development of a cancer pain relief programme should not be in conflict with programmes to control substance abuse and illicit drug trafficking, needs to be encouraged.

A Multi-disciplinary Approach

It is surely true to say that the responsibility of all health care professionals in general is to identify their particular areas of accountability in the care of patients.

Health care professionals working in a palliative care setting usually place a great deal of emphasis upon multi-disciplinary care. Whilst recognising the appropriateness of this emphasis, we should avoid the tendency to assume that any one professional can be all things to all patients. Successful multi-disciplinary care will only occur when the uniqueness of each individual's contribution is recognised, resulting in a truly integrated inter-disciplinary approach to patient care. Inter-disciplinary care does not mean a system in which one professional directs the activity of another. It means a facilitating environment where professional autonomy is respected, and where the most appropriate practitioner is encouraged to utilise his or her unique skills for the optimal benefit of each patient. The responsibility for the control of cancer pain must rest with the *entire* health care team. An example of a practical demonstration of collaborative, inter-disciplinary care could be in the use of multi-disciplinary records. For example, a chart which is designed for the assessment and monitoring of cancer pain and which is used by *everyone* involved in the patient's pain treatment is more likely to give an overall picture of the pain.

A Multi-modality Approach

Even though only one third of the six million new cancer patients who are diagnosed each year can be cured, advances in the treatment of cancer mean that many cancers are controlled for much longer. Radiotherapy, chemotherapy, hormone therapy and even surgery are playing an increasingly important role in palliative cancer care. Although it has always been recognised that there is far more to analgesia than analgesics, possibly now more than ever before cancer pain management needs to be based on multi-modality as well as multi-disciplinary principles.

The extent to which it is possible to adopt a multi-modality or shared care approach to pain management will depend to a large extent on how well integrated the palliative care services are with cancer treatment centres.

In practice, most patients with advanced cancer spend at least some time in an oncology unit or in an ordinary ward in a general hospital, and in the United Kingdom approximately two thirds of all patients die there [6]. Ideally, each cancer unit or district general hospital should have a palliative care support team able to bring the principles and benefits of palliative care to patients at all stages of their disease. If the support team are allowed to function on the basis of shared care with the referring team, the impact of the services will be greatly enhanced.

Palliative Care in the Community

Even though the control of pain in the home has been shown to be less effective than in hospital or hospice, one survey showed that only 3% of relatives of patients who had died at home subsequently wished that the death had occurred in hospital.

Approximately 30% of cancer deaths take place at home. In fact it is interesting to note that, even though specialist community services have expanded significantly over the past twenty years, the percentage of home deaths has not significantly changed. The basis of palliative care in the community is the provision of specialist advice to the primary health care team. If adequate professional supervision is available, even patients with few or no family members can be supported adequately with the help of voluntary helpers and neighbours.

Non-drug Treatments in Palliative Care

In a hierarchy of cancer pain treatments, without a doubt, and possibly with some justification, drug treatment would be at the top. Many non-drug pain relief measures have been branded as "soft" or "unscientific" and have, as a consequence, usually received little more than a mention in many of the definitive symptom control treatises. Although the importance of evaluating unproven treatments should not be underestimated, we should not necessarily allow a lack of proven efficacy to stop us from utilising strategies which at the very least can give the patient greater involvement in his pain relief treatment and possibly provide him with a means of diversion which can be used to place pain at the periphery of his awareness. It is unfortunate that patients are sometimes denied the possible benefits of some strategies because of a lack of proven efficacy. The use of acupuncture (in the United Kingdom) illustrates this point well: whereas a decade ago most doctors would have viewed acupuncture as little more than oriental hocus pocus, a significant number of controlled clinical trials have been undertaken which have substantiated its benefit and it is now viewed as a useful therapy in the management of chronic pain.

The reluctance to exploit the use of many non-drug treatments is particularly strange when one considers that it is generally recognised that pain is very much a dual phenomenon. We are all very familiar with the clinical model which divides pain into two components: the physical stimulus (or cognitive component) and the related emotional response (or affective component). As the affective component is said to predominate in chronic cancer pain, it goes without saying that attention must be paid to both pharmacological and non-pharmacological strategies for pain relief.

Lack of Systematic Education of Health Care Workers About Cancer Pain Management

The final major reason for unsatisfactory management of cancer pain which I would like to briefly focus on relates to a lack of education. Several reports have described the lack of education of professional health care workers. I have already emphasised that it has been shown that even though effective and relatively inexpensive therapy has existed for some time, cancer pain remains a frequent and neglected health problem [7]. The analysis of a questionnaire devised to highlight the current status of cancer pain relief and attitudes of the nursing profession to the relief of cancer pain revealed a dearth of knowledge and time devoted to the teaching of cancer pain management [8]. Consideration will be given later in this conference to optimising education in palliative care. I will therefore merely stress the importance of education as a priority for ensuring the effective implementation of a cancer pain relief programme.

Conclusion

I would like to emphasise two things in concluding. Firstly, the study of pain is really still in its infancy. Before the introduction of the gate control theory in 1965 by Melzak and Wall, very little appeared in the professional literature about pain. Although we have come a long way since then, information about the principles of palliative care need to be more widely disseminated, and professional accountability for the relief of pain needs to improve.

Secondly, we must remember that the health care team is not the authority about the existence and nature of the patient's pain. The most important and most difficult aspect of helping the patient in pain is to accept and appreciate that only the patient can feel the pain. Recognition of this fact has to underpin all our efforts to improve and co-ordinate a successful national and international cancer pain relief programme.

References

1. Higginson I, McCarthy M (1989) Evaluation of palliative care: steps to quality assurance? Palliat Med 3: 267–274
2. Stjernsward J (1985) Cancer pain relief: an important global health issue. Clin J Pain 1: 95–97
3. WHO (1986) Cancer pain relief. WHO, Geneva
4. Hoskin P J, Dicks B (1988) Symptom control, oncology for nurses and health care professionals, vol 2, 2nd edn. Harper and Row, London
5. Porter J, Tick H (1980) Addiction rate in patients treated with narcotics. N Engl J Med 302: 123
6. WHO (1987) Palliative cancer care. WHO, Geneva
7. Swerdlow M, Stjernsward J (1982) Cancer pain relief—an urgent problem. World Health Forum 3: 325–330
8. Pritchard AP (1988) Management of pain and nursing attitudes. Cancer Nurs 11(3): 203–209

Cancer Pain: Pathogenesis, Therapy, and Assessment

M. Zimmermann

Abteilung für Physiologie des Zentralnervensystems, II. Physiologisches Institut der Universität, Im Neuenheimer Feld 326, W-6900 Heidelberg, FRG

Introduction

Pain in the cancer patient holds an exceptional position among the various types of chronic suffering (Zimmermann 1982; Ahles et al. 1983; Cleeland 1984; Bond 1985; Müller-Busch 1988; Schara 1988). This is because the pain is associated with the prospect of a restricted lifespan, irreversibility of the disease, and the inability of the physicians to cure the disease. In view of these multiple negative functional associations, pain in the cancer patient is particularly destructive. It is, therefore, mandatory to treat the pain by any available measure, be it palliative or symptomatic (Bonica 1984). During the last decade or so, standard forms of pain therapy have emerged from many studies and a committee of experts working on behalf of the World Health Organization (WHO) has condensed these standards into a brochure of practical advice for health professionals (WHO 1986). More recently, progress has been made in solving some controversial issues regarding opioid therapy (Foley 1986; Bruera et al. 1987b; Twycross 1988). However, apart from medical treatment of the pain, care should include psychological support to enhance the patient's abilities to cope with the pain that is the dominant aspect of his or her disease (Cleeland 1987a; Cleeland and Tearnan 1986; Sun 1988; Seemann and Lang, this volume). It is necessary that those who are responsible for the care of the cancer patient have a coherent concept of pain, including its pathogenesis, assessment, and treatment. A survey of these aspects is provided here.

Pathogenesis of Cancer Pain

Various criteria have been used to subdivide pain in cancer patients according to its physiology or pathological anatomy (Zimmermann 1982; Hill 1984; Payne 1987a; Portenoy 1988). Here, I propose a subdivision according to the basic pathogenic mechanisms of the pain that is useful regarding the efficacy of different modalities of pain treatment. Thus, one can discern three basic types of pain depending on the pathogenic mechanism:

- Nociceptor pain
- Neuropathic pain
- Dysregulatory or reactive pain

Nociceptor pain is due to the excitation of specific nociceptive nerve endings, the neural sensors which are abundant everywhere in the body ready to signal potential damage and disease. The pain due to bone metastases or to tension in encapsulated organs (e.g., the pancreas) are typical examples of this kind of pain. In most cases, algesic substances (or pain mediators) such as prostaglandins, bradykinin, or H^+ ions are likely to contribute to the chemical excitation or sensitization of the nociceptors (Zimmermann and Handwerker 1984). It is here that analgesic drugs of the peripheral and anti-inflammatory type have their major site of action, interfering with the biochemistry of pain mediators and the neural excitation of nociceptors. Neuropathic pain is the second class of pain (Devor 1988). Here, damage to sensory nerve fibers results in their firing abnormally and hence in pain. In this case, the nociceptors are bypassed by the stimulus, as the afferent excitation originates at more proximal sites of the sensory fibers. The nerve lesion may be induced by mechanical pressure exerted by a tumor onto the nerve, resulting in prolonged nerve compression, by nerve transection during tumor surgery, or by chemotherapy or irradiation interfering with nerve biochemistry. Any of these influences may result in a painful local or general neuropathy. Usually, analgesic drugs, both of the peripheral (anti-inflammatory) and central (opioid) types, are less effective against neuropathic pain (Arner and Meyerson 1988), although this is a controversial issue (Vecht 1989). Therefore, other drugs interfering with abnormal nerve excitability such as anticonvulsant drugs (e.g., carbamazepine) or tricyclic antidepressant drugs (e.g., imipramine) are preferred. In cases of mechanical nerve compression the corticosteroids can be of great therapeutic benefit (Twycross 1980).

Dysregulatory pain (or reactive pain) is a relatively new term for various types of pain classified according to their pathogenic mechanism. It comprises those types of chronic pain that are due to inappropriate (efferent) nervous control, i.e., in the skeletomotor system (e.g., muscle spasm) or the sympathetic system (e.g., reflex sympathetic dystrophy, lymphedema). Pain caused by these mechanisms is fairly frequent in cancer patients and is sometimes referred to as "pain of paraneoplastic origin." In this case the therapeutic strategy should include attempts to interfere with the dysregulated control signals, e.g., by somatic or sympathetic nerve blocks using local anesthetics or by central myotonolytic drugs. These measures may be combined with peripheral or central analgesic medications.

Table 1. Specific pain syndromes in patients with cancer. (Data from Foley 1979; Hartenstein and Wilmanns 1984; Hill 1984)

Pain syndromes associated with direct tumor infiltration
Tumor infiltration of abdominal hollow organs
   Distension of encapsulated organs (e.g., the liver)
   Tumor-induced necrosis in solid organs (e.g., the pancreas)
   Tumor infiltration and inflammation of serous mucosae

Tumor infiltration of soft tissues
Tumor-induced occlusions of blood vessels
Tumor-induced occlusions of lymphatics

Tumor infiltration of bone
   Base of skull syndromes (e.g., clivus metastases)
   Vertebral body syndromes (e.g., C2 metastases)
   Sacral syndrome

Tumor infiltration of nerve
   Peripheral nerve (e.g., peripheral neuropathy)
   Plexus (brachial plexopathy)
   Spinal root (e.g., leptomeningeal metastases)
   Spinal cord

Compression of central nervous system
   Epidural spinal cord compression
   Intracranial pressure (brain tumor)

Pain syndromes associated with cancer therapy
Postsurgery syndromes
   Postthoracotomy syndrome
   Postmastectomy syndrome
   Postradical neck syndrome
   Phantom limb syndrome
Postchemotherapy syndromes
   Peripheral neuropathy
   Aseptic necrosis of the femoral head
   Steroid pseudorheumatism
   Postherpetic neuralgia
Postirradiation syndromes
   Radiation fibrosis of brachial and lumbar plexus
   Radiation myelopathy
   Radiation-induced second primary tumors
   Radiation necrosis of bone

Pain syndromes not associated with cancer or cancer therapy
   Cervical and lumbar osteoarthritis
   Thoracic and abdominal aneurysms
   Diabetic neuropathy

Determining the Cause of Cancer Pain

In addition to classifying the pain according to the general pathogenic mechanisms, it is essential to establish the etiology in some detail (Table 1) as this will be of practical help to the doctor in determining the best form of therapy (Foley 1979, 1987a,b; Zimmermann and Drings 1984). The following diagnostic questions should therefore be asked:

– Localization of pain: Is it unilateral, midline, over a large diffuse area, in the bone?
– Does the pain depend on movements?
– Is an inflammatory process involved?
– Is a nerve, plexus, or spinal root irritated by a tumor, or by the deformation of vertebrae due to metastases?
– Is there ischemia resulting from arterial occlusion?
– Can a specific nerve conducting pain information be found, e.g., by a diagnostic nerve block with local anesthesia?
– Is the sympathetic efferent system involved?
– Is hypertonus of skeletal muscle involved?
– Is visceral smooth muscle spasm involved?
– Is a nerve lesion or neuropathy, due to surgery, irradiation, or chemotherapy involved?
– Is depression or anxiety a factor enhancing the pain?

The answers will give at least some indications of what may be a rational form of pain therapy. For example, the pain resulting from osseous metastases producing prostaglandins can be effectively treated with anti-inflammatory drugs. Diffuse bone pain, e.g., from widely distributed metastases in the spine, usually cannot be relieved by a cordotomy. However, large-area X-irradiation at a low dose may give long-lasting relief. Pain due to sympathetic disturbances will respond to a sympathetic block. Pain related to muscle spasms can be treated by local anesthesia of trigger points, or by physical therapy.

Thus, systematic assessment of etiological factors and a rational approach to therapy are preferable to a purely empirical approach, which runs the risk of attempted treatment being ineffective. However, both under and over treatment should be avoided as both are a burden on the patient and give rise to doubts about the doctor's skill and competence.

Treatment of Cancer Pain

Who should treat pain in the cancer patient? The best treatment of pain is achieved by an alliance between the physicians, the family, and the patient himself. The physician most responsible for the control of pain and other symptoms should be the family doctor, as he accompanies the patient for most of the duration of the disease. Therefore, it is essential for family doctors to acquire sufficient knowledge on how to treat the patients' pain effectively at home (Ferrell and Schneider 1988). The basic and comprehensive set of guidelines for pain therapy published by the WHO (1986) provides the necessary advice to physicians. Unfortunately, both physicians and patients have mental barriers against the appropriate use of analgesic drugs, resulting in a tendency to undertreat pain (Marks and Sachar 1973; Cleeland 1987b). In countries where prescription is controlled by governmental agencies, the majority of doctors do not prescribe opiates (Gostomzyk and Heller 1986; Sorge and Zenz 1990).

The other physician who is concerned with the cancer patient for a limited period of time is the oncologist. Apart from his interest in curative treatment, the oncologist should accept that pain is a major problem for the patient and therefore also concentrate on concomitant treatment of the pain (Dorrepaal et al. 1989). Thus, the ideal would be for the oncologist to keep his eyes on both the primary disease and the pain, and to find an appropriate balance between controlling both in his therapeutic strategies.

An experienced specialist in pain diagnosis and therapy from any of the disciplines commonly involved in oncology should be available at each cancer center and should have the following tasks:

– To advise the oncologist on how to incorporate prevention and therapy of pain into the design of cancer therapy
– To analyse the likely pathogenesis of the pain
– To provide the symptomatic or palliative treatment of the pain which is least burdensome to the patient but maximally efficacious
– To coordinate specialist treatment of the pain if required, e.g., neurolytic nerve or spinal root blocks, peridural opiates, radiotherapy, general surgery, neurosurgery, hormone therapy, chemotherapy
– To provide advice about pain treatment for the family doctor during home care of the patient

The family and friends of the patient can have a beneficial influence on the patient's pain by giving him emotional support and not allowing him to be in a state of distress and social isolation. The security provided by a friendly, communicative, but not overreacting family environment greatly improves the benefit a patient gains from any symptomatic pain therapy. Unfortunately, a maladapted family often results in neurotic behavior, greatly aggravating the pain.

Drug Therapy for Cancer Pain

Guidelines for the treatment of pain in the cancer patient were developed under the auspices of the WHO (1986). Since then, translations into many languages, including a German version (WHO 1988) have been provided. Field studies in Japan (Takeda 1986), Italy (Ventafridda et al. 1987a, b), Federal Republic of

Germany (Grond et al. 1990b), and the United Kingdom (Walker et al. 1988) have shown that, by following the WHO guidelines in a straightforward manner, sufficient pain relief can be obtained in at least 85% of patients with analgesic and adjuvant drug medication. The remaining patients require some specialist pain treatment, particularly invasive interventions (Lipton 1987). Among these, the neurolytic block of the celiac plexus is of great value in pain due to pancreatic cancer (Saltzburg and Foley 1989). Neurolytic blocks of the spinal dorsal roots and surgical transection or coagulation of the spinal pain pathways (cordotomy) are, by contrast, not in general use nowadays, as epidural administration of morphine has become a highly appreciated alternative treatment at the spinal level (Zenz 1981; Martin et al. 1982; Müller et al. 1988; Payne 1987b). Palliative irradiation and the use of radioisotopes (Kutzner et al. 1981; Kuttig 1984; Hüttner 1988; Markwardt 1988) can result in almost complete pain relief for months. For these invasive procedures a ladder of consecutive use has recently been proposed (Ferrer-Brechner 1989). Palliative chemotherapy or hormone therapy can provide significant pain relief, particularly in patients with hormone-dependent breast or prostate cancer (Reimers 1985; Gürtler and Quadt 1988). Textbooks and handbooks on pain treatment which include both specialist and standard methods are available (Bonica and Ventafridda 1979; Twycross and Ventafridda 1980; Zenz 1981; Twycross and Lack 1983; Zimmermann and Handwerker 1984; Zimmermann et al. 1984; Hackenthal and Wörz 1985; Kossmann et al. 1986; Tontschev 1988; Zech et al. 1988; Hankemeier et al. 1989).

The mainstay of the WHO guidelines is a three-step ladder of analgesic and adjuvant drug use, with administration of the drugs by mouth; by the clock, i.e., at regular intervals; and at the right dose, determined individually. Following these principles the medical practitioner can essentially provide pain relief in the majority of his cancer patients.

The three steps of the WHO analgesic ladder are shown in Table 2. Any pain treatment should start with level I drugs, which comprise analgesic drugs of the peripheral type, i.e., anti-inflammatory and antipyretic analgesic drugs (Beaver 1980). In this group, the prototype drugs of the WHO recommendations are acetylsalicylic acid and paracetamol as these are commonly available worldwide. Of course, other drugs of this type should be used, if available. For example, in the Federal Republic of Germany a first-choice drug is metamizol (dipyrone), which has a higher analgesic potency than acetylsalicylic acid or paracetamol. In addition, metamizol has an antispastic component and therefore has some advantages for treating visceral pain when intestinal smooth muscle contractions are involved. Novel anti-inflammatory drugs available in many countries include the propionic acid derivatives such as ibuprofen and flurbiprofen. Slow-release preparations of diclofenac and ibuprofen became available recently, increasing the interval between administrations to 8 h. A specific indication for anti-inflammatory-type analgesic drugs is bone pain due to bone metastases.

Level II of the WHO analgesic ladder uses a combination of analgesic drugs of the peripheral type (as for level I) with analgesic drugs that have predominantly central effects, namely a weak opioid drug such as dextropropoxyphene or

Table 2. Analgesic medication for cancer pain according to the WHO Analgesic Ladder (modified)

WHO classification	Examples
Level I: analgesic drugs with predominantly peripheral effects	– Ibuprofen (slow release) – Paracetamol (Acetaminophene) – Acetylsalicylic acid – Dipyrone (Metamizol) – Diclofenac (slow release) – Flurbiprofen
Level II: as level I plus analgesic drugs with predominantly central effects	– Nefopam – Flupirtin – Codeine, dihydrocodeine (slow release) – Dextropropoxyphene (slow release) – Tramadol – Tilidine (plus naloxone)
Level III: as level I plus strong opioids	– Buprenorphine – Morphine (slow release) – Methadone – Pethidine – Hydromorphone – Levorphanol

codeine (Table 2). For both drugs, slow-release preparations are available in the Federal Republic of Germany. If a stronger opioid is required, tramadol or tilidine (plus naloxone) may be considered. These opioids are available in the Federal Republic of Germany and do not require special narcotic drug prescription forms. The rationale for the level II regimen is that using drugs whose analgesic effects occur at different sites, i.e., at the nociceptor, the site of origin of the neuronal pain signals, and in the central nervous system, will result in them having additive analgesic effect. Such additive effects of two types of analgesic drugs have been well documented in controlled studies (e.g., Cooper et al. 1982).

If medication of level II does not provide sufficient pain relief at the maximum possible dosage, the level III regimen is required (Table 2). The drug of first choice is morphine, given orally (Mount 1980; Twycross 1983, 1988; Inturrisi and Foley 1984; Ventafridda 1984; Zenz 1984), either as an aqueous solution of morphine sulfate or, preferably, as a slow-release tablet if this is available (Hanks 1987; Zenz et al. 1989). Slow-release morphine is available in many countries. Due to the slow release into the gastrointestinal tract, constant and fairly low plasma levels can be obtained for fairly long periods of time, with analgesia lasting up to 12 h after medication. Such long-duration analgesic effects are highly desirable for the patient's comfort, as two or at most three medications per day are sufficient, and it is not necessary to interrupt sleep during the night. In addition, the low plasma levels of the drug increase safety with regard to toxic effects such as respiratory depression, which is never a problem in patients on oral opiate medication.

An alternative strategy for increasing the time between drug dóses is to use a drug such as methadone which is eliminated slowly and has a very long plasma half-life. However, because of the slow elimination, such types of drugs are difficult to handle as a slow increase in plasma levels might result, with the ensuing risk of overdose. Therefore, particularly in the elderly patient, methadone should not be used.

In addition to the three levels of analgesic treatment, adjuvant medication (Table 3) may be required (Twycross 1980; Foley 1985a, b; Magni et al. 1987), particularly when the pain includes a neuropathic component. If, for instance, compression of a nerve or the spinal cord by a tumor is involved, corticosteroids are of considerable value in reducing the pain (Ettinger and Portenoy 1988). Other types of neuropathic pain, e.g., postherpetic neuralgia or polyneuropathy induced by cancer chemotherapy, may well respond to an antidepressant drug such as imipramine or amitriptyline. If the neuropathic pain has a shooting or lancinating component, anticonvulsant drugs such as carbamazepine or clonazepam should be used (Swerdlow 1984).

Table 3. Adjuvant medication for cancer pain according to the WHO Analgesic Ladder (modified)

Adjuvant drugs	Symptoms	Examples
Antidepressants	Neuropathic pain Depression	Imipramine Amitriptyline Doxepine
Anticonvulsants	Shooting or lancinating neuropathic pain	Carbamazepine Clonazepam
Corticosteroids	Nerve compression Intracranial pressure	Dexamethasone Prednisolone
Calcitonin Biphosphonates	Bone pain	
Myotonolytics	Spasms of skeletal muscles	Baclofen Tizanidine Chlormezanone
Neuroleptics	Agitation Emesis	Chlorpromazine Levomepromazine
Laxatives	Constipation	

If osteolysis due to bone metastases is involved, calcitonin or biphosphonates may provide considerable pain relief (Ziegler 1984; Ringe 1989). These adjuvant drugs, selected according to the specific pathogenesis of a patient's pain, can be combined with analgesic drugs according to the WHO's three-step ladder. The rationale for such a complex combination is the observation that most patients have several types of pain (Twycross and Fairfield 1982; Miser et al. 1987; Portenoy 1988), including both nociceptor and neuropathic pain components.

Nonoral Opiate Administration

Usually, opiates can be given orally for the duration of pain treatment, right up to the time of death. However, there are a few exceptions to this rule: parenteral or spinal administration may be preferred in some cases of far advanced cancer, i.e., when uptake of the drug from the alimentary tract is no longer reliable or when systemic opiates are no longer very effective and the dose would have to be increased dramatically. If there is gastrointestinal dysfunction, subcutaneous administration is a practical solution and automatic infusion systems with an electrical or pneumatic syringe driver or a constant-flow pump are being increasingly used, even in outpatients (Jones and Hanks 1985; Bruera et al. 1987a; Dennis and DeWitty 1987). The infusion techniques for this new route of opiate administration are essentially the same as those used for modern antidiabetic therapy. Equally, intravenous instead of subcutaneous infusion (Portenoy et al. 1986) or an implanted device may be used for opiate delivery (Dennis and DeWitty 1987).

When oral or parenteral systemic opiate administration gives insufficient pain relief even at very high doses, or when sedation or dysphoria is excessive, the peridural route may be an appropriate alternative in some selected patients (Greenberg 1986; Ventafridda et al. 1986; Sjöstrand and Rawal 1986; Payne 1987b; Müller et al. 1988).

Tolerance, Dependence, and Addiction

Tolerance, dependence, and addiction are different phenomena sometimes associated with the repeated use of opioids in humans and experimental animals. Tolerance refers to a decreasing analgesic efficacy of a certain dosage of an opioid which can be compensated for by an increasing dosage. However, in chronic use of opioids tolerance has rarely been seen and in many patients the dosage remains constant or may even be reduced during prolonged treatment. The increase in the analgesic dosage found in some patients may well be due to progress of the disease with concomitant increase in nociceptive stimulation (Kanner and Foley 1981; Twycross and Lack 1983). In a few cases clear signs of tolerance resulting in dose escalations up to several grams of morphine per day have been found. However, as the side effects (e.g., respiratory depression, nausea) develop tolerance faster than the analgesia, these high doses do not usually pose specific problems.

Physical dependence develops during chronic use of opioids in many patients. However, the symptoms of dependence do not appear unless opioid treatment is discontinued, when the patient may suffer from opioid withdrawal symptoms. These can be prevented by continuing the opioid treatment. In cases where opioid treatment is no longer required because of other methods of pain relief (e.g., neurolytic nerve block, radiotherapy), withdrawal symptoms can be kept to a minimum by slowly reducing the opioid dosage.

The third and most severe phenomenon is addiction to opioids. However, many experts have reported that addiction never occurred in patients who used the opioid orally at a regular time schedule (Taub 1982; Portenoy and Foley 1986), and this may be explained by the absence of euphoria when nearly constant levels of the opioid are established by this regimen. It is obvious that for an addicted person to gain the feeling of euphoria, fast intravenous injection of the opioid, resulting in a fast rise of concentration in the brain is required.

Thus, addiction does not occur and dependence and tolerance are not problems in chronic pain treatment with opioids.

Is Cancer Pain Intractable?

Several publications state that between 1% and 10% of cases of pain in cancer patients are most difficult to treat (Sykes 1987) and therefore, presumably, may be termed "intractable." However, there are indications that the proportion of patients suffering from truly intractable pain is rather small and could be virtually zero.

Grond and his colleagues (1990b) analyzed a total of 1140 patients who were referred to their unit for cancer pain treatment by other departments of the hospital or by practitioners because the pain could not be managed. All these patients obtained considerable pain relief in this special unit, although 86% of the patients rated their pain at a severe or excruciating intensity on admission. The major reasons for the inadequacy of previous pain treatment were the following:

- No analgesic drugs prescribed (10%)
- Schedule of medication irregular or intervals too long (66%)
- Underdosage of nonopioid drugs (27%)
- Underdosage of opioid drugs (42%)

Thus, the persistence of pain in these patients was due to inadequate use of analgesic drugs rather than the type or level of the pain involved.

Another situation where periods of intractable pain are believed to occur frequently is the terminal phase of the disease. However, this is not true, as Grond et al. (1990a, b) showed in a retrospective study on 160 terminal cancer patients. None of 114 patients who provided a rating of their pain on a five-step categorial rating scale had "very strong" or "maximum imaginable" pain; only six patients in this group rated their pain as "strong." A total of 46 patients (28% of the sample of 160) were unable to provide a pain rating in the terminal situation, because of general weakness and reduced consciousness. However, according to the judgement of physicians and nurses, probably none of these patients suffered from strong pain.

As to the modalities of treatment in this group of 160 terminal cancer patients, 10% obtained sufficient pain relief from analgesic medication according to WHO level I, 15% were in WHO II, and the majority of 68% were in WHO III. Analgesic medication was not required by 8% of the patients because their pain could be managed by other methods such as neurolytic nerve block. In 53% of the patients the oral route could be maintained up to death, whereas in 39% the parenteral and in 4% the peridural route had to be used in the course of the terminal period. The total duration of pain treatment in these 160 terminal patients was 7840 days. On 80% of these days, oral medication was used, whereas on 9% parenteral and on 5% peridural administration was required. Thus, although the mainstay of pain therapy was via the oral route, the proportion of nonoral treatment was higher than in the average population of cancer patients with pain.

A Pain Diary for the Assessment of Pain

Apart from the diagnosis by the physician, self-evaluation of the pain should be carried out by the patient (Twycross and Lack 1983; Wallenstein 1984; Cleeland 1985; Cleeland et al. 1988). A standardized assessment can be obtained with a pain questionnaire, which should be shorter and more straightforward than those used for detailed analysis in scientific studies of pain. The questions asked should relate to the intensity, quality, localization, history, and daily prevalence of pain as well as to the resulting stress and restricted quality of life for the patient (Ferrell et al. 1989). The questionnaire should contain a simple schematic drawing of the body on which the patient can draw the area(s) in which the pain occurs.

A simple and useful method for subjective rating of the pain intensity level is the visual analog scale (VAS). Most patients can indicate their current pain intensity on this VAS between the reference points "no pain" and "maximum imaginable pain" (Schülin et al. 1989). A pain diary consists of repeated daily records of the patient's pain ratings. These ratings can be arranged into a graphic display of the time course of pain intensity, showing temporal variations of the pain level including the effects of therapy.

Most patients agree to work with the pain diary, since they realize that their problems are taken seriously by the doctor, and that communication with the doctor about their problems is intensified (Schülin et al. 1989). Patients can thus expect improvement in therapy from their efforts with the pain diary.

References

Ahles TA, Blanchard EB, Ruckdeschel JC (1983) The multi-dimensional nature of cancer-related pain. Pain 17: 277–288

Arner S, Meyerson B (1988) Lack of analgesic effect of opioids on neuropathic and idiopathic forms of pain. Pain 33: 11–23

Beaver WT (1980) Management of cancer pain with parenteral medication. JAMA 244: 2653–2657

Bond MR (1985) Cancer pain: psychological substrates and therapy. In: Fields HL, Dubner R, Cervero F (eds) Advances in pain research and therapy, vol 9. Raven, New York, pp 559–567

Bonica J, Ventafridda V (eds) (1979) International symposium on pain of advanced cancer. Raven, New York (Advances in pain research and therpay, vol 2)

Bonica JJ (1984) Management of cancer pain. In: Zimmermann M, Drings P, Wagner G (eds) Pain in the cancer patient. Springer, Berlin Heidelberg New York, pp 13–27 (Recent results in cancer research, vol 89)

Bruera E, Brenneis C, Michaud M, Chadwick S, MacDonald RN (1987a) Continuous s.c. infusion of narcotics using a portable disposable device in patients with advanced cancer. Cancer Treat Rev 71: 635–637

Bruera E, Fox R, Chadwick S, Brenneis C, MacDonald RN (1987b) Changing pattern in the treatment of pain and other symptoms in advanced cancer patients. J Pain Sympt Management 2: 139–144

Cleeland CS (1984) The impact of pain on the patient with cancer. Cancer 54: 2635–2641

Cleeland CS (1985) Measurement and prevalence of pain in cancer. Semin Oncol Nursing 1: 87–92

Cleeland CS (1987a) Nonpharmacological management of cancer pain. J Pain Sympt Management 2: S23–S28

Cleeland CS (1987b) Barriers to the management of cancer pain. Oncology (Suppl): 19–26

Cleeland CS, Tearnan BH (1986) Behavioral control of cancer pain. In: Holzman AD, Turk DC (eds) Pain management. A handbook of psychological treatment approaches. Pergamon, New York. pp 193–212

Cleeland CS, Ladinsky JL, Serlin RC, Thuy NC (1988) Multidimensional measurement of cancer pain: comparisons of US and Vietnamese patients. J Pain Sympt Management 3: 23–27

Cooper KE, Veale WL, Kasting NW (1982) Temperature regulation, fever and antipyretics. In: Barnett HJM, Hirsh J, Mustard JF (eds) Acetylsalicylic acid: new uses for an old drug. Raven, New York, pp. 153–163

Dennis GC, DeWitty R (1987) Management of intractable pain in cancer patients by implantable morphine infusion systems. J Natl Med Assoc 79: 939–944

Devor M (1988) Central changes mediating neuropathic pain. In: Dubner R, Gebhart GF, Bond MR (eds) Proceedings of the Vth world congress on pain. Elsevier, Amsterdam, pp 114–128 (Pain research and clinical management, vol 3)

Dorrepaal KL, Aaronson NK, van Dam FSAM (1989) Pain experience and pain management among hospitalized cancer patients. Cancer 63: 593–598

Ettinger AB, Portenoy RK (1988) The use of corticosteroids in the treatment of symptoms associated with cancer. J Pain Sympt Management 3: 99–103

Ferrell BR, Schneider C (1988) Experience and management of cancer pain at home. Cancer Nursing 11: 84–90

Ferrell BR, Wisdom C, Wenzl C (1989) Quality of life as an outcome variable in the management of cancer pain. Cancer 63: 2321–2327

Ferrer-Brechner T (1989) Anesthetic techniques for the management of cancer pain. Cancer 63: 2343–2347

Foley KM (1979) Pain syndromes in patients with cancer. In: Bonica JJ, Ventafridda V (eds) Advances in pain research and therapy, vol 2. Raven, New York, pp 59–75

Foley KM (1985a) The treatment of cancer pain. N Engl J Med 313: 84–95

Foley KM (1985b) Adjuvant analgesic drugs in cancer pain management.·In: Aronoff GM (ed.) Evaluation and treatment of chronic pain. Urban and Schwarzenberg, Baltimore, pp 425–434

Foley KM (1986) Current controversies in opioid therapy. In: Foley KM, Inturrisi CE (eds) Advances in pain research and therapy, vol 8. Raven, New York, pp 3–11

Foley KM (1987a) Cancer pain syndromes. J Pain Sympt Management 2: S13–S17

Foley KM (1987b) Pain syndromes in patients with cancer. Med Clin North Am 71: 169–184

Gostomzyk JG, Heller W-D (1986) Zur Verschreibung von Betäubungsmitteln durch niedergelassene Ärzte. Dtsch Arzteblatt 83: 3456

Greenberg HS (1986) Continuous spinal opioid infusion for intractable cancer pain. In: Foley KM, Inturrisi CE (eds) Advances in pain research and therapy, vol 8. Raven, New York, pp 351–359

Grond S, Zech D, Horrichs-Haermeyer G, Lehmann KA (1990a) Schmerztherapie in der Finalphase maligner Erkrankungen. Schmerz 4: 22–28

Grond S, Zech D, Dahlmann H, Stobbe B, Lehmann KA (1990b) Therapieresistente Tumorschmerzen: Analyse der Schmerzmechanismen und der medikamentösen Vorbehandlung. Schmerz (in press)

Gürtler R, Quadt C (1988) Die Chemo- und Hormontherapie bei Krebsschmerzen. In: Tontschev G (ed.) Therapie des Krebsschmerzes. Akademie-Verlag, Berlin (DDR), pp 60–74

Hackenthal E, Wörz R (eds) (1985) Medikamentöse Schmerzbehandlung in der Praxis. Fischer, Stuttgart

Hankemeier U, Bowdler I, Zech D (eds) (1989) Tumorschmerztherapie. Springer, Berlin Heidelberg New York

Hanks GW, Twycross RG, Bliss JM (1987) Controlled release morphine tablets: a double-blind trial in patients with advanced cancer. Anaesthesia 42: 840–844

Hartenstein R, Wilmanns W (1984) Clinical pain syndromes in cancer patients and their causes. In: Zimmermann M, Drings P, Wagner G (eds) Pain in the cancer patient. Springer, Berlin Heidelberg New York, pp 72–78 (Recent results in cancer research, vol 89)

Hill K (1984) Pathological anatomy of cancer pain. In: Zimmermann M, Drings P, Wagner G (eds) Pain in the cancer patient. Springer, Berlin Heidelberg New York, pp 33–44 (Recent results in cancer research, vol 89)

Hüttner J (1988) Strahlentherapie bei Krebsschmerzen. In: Tontschev G (ed.) Therapie des Krebsschmerzes. Akademie-Verlag, Berlin (DDR), pp 92–102

Inturrisi CE, Foley KM (1984) Narcotic analgesics in the management of pain. In: Kuhar M, Pasternak GW (eds) Analgesics: neurochemical, behavioural and clinical perspectives. Raven, New York, pp 257–288

Jones VA, Hanks GW (1986) New portable infusion pump for prolonged subcutaneous administration of opioid analgesics in patients with advanced cancer. Br Med J 292: 1496

Kanner RM, Foley KM (1981) Patterns of narcotic drug use in cancer pain clinic. Ann NY Acad Sci 362: 162–172

Kossmann B, Ahnefeld FW, Bowdler I, Zimmermann M (1986) Manual der Schmerztherapie. Kohlhammer, Stuttgart

Kuttig H (1984) Radiotherapy of cancer pain. In: Zimmermann M, Drings P, Wagner G (eds) Pain in the cancer patient. Springer, Berlin Heidelberg New York, pp 190–194 (Recent results in cancer research, vol 89)

Kutzner J, Dähmert W, Schreyer T, Grimm W, Brod KH, Becker M (1981) Yttrium-90 zur Schmerztherapie von Knochenmetastasen. Nuclearmedizin 20: 229–235

Lipton S (1987) Neurodestructive procedures in the management of cancer pain. J Pain Sympt Management 2: 219–228

Magni G, Arsie D, De Leo D (1987) Antidepressants in the treatment of cancer pain. A survey in Italy. Pain 29: 347–353

Marks RM, Sachar EJ (1973) Undertreatment of medical inpatients with narcotic analgesics. Ann Intern Med 78: 173–181

Markwardt J (1988) Radionuklidtherapie bei Krebsschmerzen. In: Tontschev G (ed.) Therapie des Krebsschmerzes. Akademie-Verlag, Berlin (DDR), pp 103–110

Martin R, Salbaing J, Blaise G, Tetrault J-P, Tetreault L (1982) Epidural morphine for postoperative pain relief: a dose-response curve. Anesthesiology 56: 423–426

Miser AW, Dothage JA, Wesley RA, Miser JS (1987) The prevalence of pain in a pediatric and young adult cancer population. Pain 29: 73–83

Mount BM (1980) Narcotic analgesics. In: Twycross RG, Ventafridda V (eds) The continuing care of terminal cancer patients. Pergamon, Oxford, pp 97–116

Müller H, Schnorr C, Zierski J, Hempelmann G (1988) Rückenmarksnahe Medikamenteninfusion bei Schmerzen durch maligne Tumoren oder Spastizität. Medwelt 39: 829–834

Müller-Busch H-C (1988) Zur Bedeutung des Schmerzes bei Krebspatienten. Schmerzther Kolloq 4/4: 6–9

Payne R (1987a) Anatomy, physiology, and neuropharmacology of cancer pain. Med Clin North Am 71: 153–167

Payne R (1987b) Role of epidural and intrathecal narcotics and peptides in the management of cancer pain. Med Clin North Am 71: 313–327

Portenoy RK (1987) Optimal pain control in elderly cancer patients. Geriatrics 42/5: 33–44

Portenoy RK (1988) Practical aspects of pain control in the patient with cancer. CA 38: 327–352

Portenoy RK, Foley KM (1986) Chronic use of opioid analgesics in non-malignant pain: report of 38 cases. Pain 25: 171–186

Portenoy RK, Moulin DE, Rogers A, Inturrisi CE, Foley KM (1986) I.v. infusion of opioids for cancer pain: clinical review and guidelines for use. Cancer Treat Rev 70: 575–581

Reimers HJ (1985) Hormontherapie als palliative Maßnahme bei der Schmerzbekämpfung. In: Friedrich-Thieding-Stiftung (ed) 6. Fortbildungskongreß Krebsnachsorge. Hartmannbund, Bonn, pp 46–52

Ringe JD (1989) Clodronat zur Behandlung von Tumorosteolysen. Arzneimitteltherapie 6: 68–70

Saltzburg D, Foley KM (1989) Management of pain in pancreatic cancer. Surg Clin North Am 69: 629–649

Schara J (1988) Gedanken zur Betreuung terminal Kranker mit Krebsschmerz. Schmerz 2: 151–160

Schülin C, Seemann H, Zimmermann M (1989) Erfahrungen mit der Anwendung von Schmerztagebüchern in der ambulanten Versorgung von Patienten mit chronischen Schmerzen. Schmerz 3: 133–139

Sjöstrand UH, Rawal N (1986) Regional opioids in anesthesiology and pain management. Little, Brown, Boston (International anesthesiology clinics, vol 24 (2)

Sorge J, Zenz M (1990) Analyse des Verschreibungsverhaltens niedergelassener Ärzte für BtM-Analgetika. Schmerz (in press)

Sun Y (1988) The role of traditional Chinese medicine in supportive care of cancer patients. Springer, Berlin Heidelberg New York, pp 327–334 (Recent results in cancer research, vol 105)

Swerdlow M (1984) Anticonvulsant drugs and chronic pain. Clin Neuropharmacol 7: 51–82

Sykes NP (1987) Pain control in terminal cancer. Int Disabil Stud 9: 33–37

Takeda F (1986) Results of field-testing in Japan of the WHO draft interim guidelines on relief of cancer pain. Pain Clin 1: 89–89

Taub A (1982) Opioid analgesics in the treatment of chronic intractable pain of non-neoplastic origin. In: Kitahata LM, Collins JG (eds) Narcotic analgesics in anesthesiology, Williams and Wilkins, Baltimore, pp 199–208

Tontschev G (ed) (1988) Therapie des Krebsschmerzes. Akademie-Verlag, Berlin (DDR)

Twycross RG (1980) Non-narcotic, corticosteroid and psychotropic drugs. In: Twycross RG, Ventafridda V (eds) The continuing care of terminal cancer patients. Pergamon, Oxford, pp 117–134

Twycross RG (1983) Narcotic analgesics in clinical practice. In: Bonica JJ, Lindblom U, Iggo A (eds) Advances in pain research and therapy, vol 5. Raven, New York, pp 435–459

Twycross RG (1988) Opioid analgesics in cancer pain: current practice and controversies. Cancer Surveys 7: 29–53

Twycross RG, Fairfield S (1982) Pain in far advanced cancer. Pain 14: 303–310

Twycross RG, Lack SA (1983) Symptom control in far advanced cancer: pain relief. Pitman, London

Twycross RG, Ventafridda V (eds) (1980) The continuing care of terminal cancer patients. Pergamon, Oxford

Vecht CJ (1989) Nociceptive nerve pain and neuropathic pain. Pain 39: 243–244

Ventafridda V (1984) Use of systemic analgesic drugs in cancer pain. Adv Pain Res Ther 7: 557–574

Ventafridda V, De Conno F, Tamburini M, Pappalettera M (1986) Clinical evaluation of chronic infusion of intrathecal morphine in cancer pain. In: Foley KM, Inturrisi CE (eds) Advances in pain research and therapy, vol 8, Raven, New York, pp 391–405

Ventafridda V, Oliveri E, Caraceni A, Spoldi E, De Conno F, Saita L, Ripamonti C (1987a) A retrospective study on the use of oral morphine in cancer pain. J Pain Sympt Management 2: 77–81

Ventafridda V, Tamburini M, Caraceni A, De Conno F, Naldi F (1987b) A validation study of the WHO method for cancer pain relief. Cancer 59: 850–856

Walker VA, Hoskin PJ, Hanks GW, White ID (1988) Evaluation of WHO analgesic guidelines for cancer pain in a hospital-based palliative care unit. J Pain Sympt Management 3: 145–149

Wallenstein SL (1984) Measurement of pain and analgesia in cancer patients. Cancer 53: 2260–2266

World Health Organization (1986) Cancer pain relief. WHO, Geneva

World Health Organization (1988) Therapie tumorbedingter Schmerzen. AMV AV-Kommunikation- und Medizin-Verlag, München

Zech D, Schug St A, Horsch M (1988) Therapiekompendium Tumorschmerz. Perimed, Erlangen

Zenz M (1981) Peridurale Opiat-Analgesie. Fischer, Stuttgart

Zenz M (1984) Schmerztherapie mit Opiaten. In: Zimmermann M, Handwerker HO (eds) Schmerz: Konzepte und ärztliches Handeln. Springer, Berlin Heidelberg New York, pp 189–213

Zenz M, Strumpf M, Tryba M, Röhrs E, Steffmann B (1989) Retardiertes Morphin zur Langzeittherapie schwerer Tumorschmerzen. Dtsch Med Wochenschr 114: 43–47

Ziegler R (1984) Calcitonin: analgesic effects. In: Zimmermann M, Drings P, Wagner G (eds) Pain in the cancer patient. Springer, Berlin Heidelberg New York, pp 178–184 (Recent results in cancer research, vol 89)

Zimmermann M (1982) Schmerz bei Tumorpatienten—Auslösende Mechanismen, Diagnose, Therapie. Anaesthesist 31: 599–603

Zimmermann M, Drings P (1984) Guidelines for therapy of pain in cancer patients. In: Zimmermann M, Drings P, Wagner G (eds) Pain in the cancer patient. Springer, Berlin Heidelberg New York, pp 1–12 (Recent results in cancer research, vol 89)

Zimmermann M, Handwerker HO (eds) (1984) Schmerz: Konzepte und ärztliches Handeln. Springer, Berlin Heidelberg New York

Zimmermann M, Drings P, Wagner G (eds) (1984) Pain in the cancer patient. Springer, Berlin Heidelberg New York (Recent results in cancer research, vol 89)

Opiate-Resistant Pain: A Therapeutic Dilemma

N. MacDonald

University of Alberta, Palliative Medicine, Edmonton, Alberta, Canada

Pain is opiate-resistant when inadequate analgesia is achieved at levels of opiate therapy which cause intolerable side effects. Opiate resistance is associated with a number of cancer pain syndromes and patient profiles characterized by psychosocial distress, metabolic abnormalities, idiosyncratic reactions to opiate therapy, or the rapid development of tolerance. In the first group nerve damage pain, activity-related (incident) pain, muscle spasm pain, many forms of headache and tenesmoid pain are characteristically difficult to treat with opiates. When cancer occurs against a background of profound psychosocial and emotional distress, opiate and indeed virtually all pharmacological therapies are of little avail—pain only improves with resolution of the emotional-spiritual crisis. Aside from psychological disturbances, factors of inheritance, background metabolic abnormalities, increasing age and/or diminished cognitive status may cause certain cancer patients to be subject to increased side effects of opiates. Less clearly defined is the problem of some cancer patients who develop rapid tolerance and require spiralling doses of opiates to maintain pain control.

Factors Influencing Opiate Response

The analgesia–response ratio is influenced by many factors, some of which are related to patient variability and others to the nature of the pain which dictated the use of the opiate. Table 1 itemizes these critical factors.

Patient Variability

Older patients are more sensitive to opiates (Kaiko et al. 1983). This sensitivity may be manifested when an underlying confusional state (common in cancer patients at the end of life) is present or if the patient is taking other psychoactive drugs. Animals demonstrate genetic differences in opiate response and it is

Recent Results in Cancer Research, Vol. 121
© Springer-Verlag Berlin · Heidelberg 1991

Table 1. Factors influencing the response to opiate
analgesics

Patient factors I
   Age—confusional States
   Genetic predisposition
   Drug bioavailability
   Tolerance
   'Total suffering'

Patient factors II
   Metabolic failure
      liver
      kidney
   Respiratory failure
   Intermittent bowel obstruction
   Intractable nausea

Pain factors
   Neuropathic pain:
      – de-afferentation
      – peripheral neuropathy
      – nerve compression
      – sympathetic mediated
      – central (e.g., thalamic pain)

   Spasm pain:
      – tenesmoid
      – muscle spasms

   Incident pain
   Headache

---

possible that similar changes exist in human populations. Variability may in part
be due to different rates of oral absorption of drugs; the oral bioavailability of
morphine, for example, varies from person to person. The concentration of drug
at opiate receptor sites presumably also varies from person to person, as may the
number of opiate receptors.

Patients demonstrate differing rates of opiate tolerance. Some of the factors
which influence the development of tolerance are clinically apparent: for
example, it is recognized that tolerance develops more rapidly when a patient is
treated with parenteral opiates. Even within a group of patients receiving
subcutaneous morphine, a subset of individuals appear particularly likely to
develop tolerance. In studies on the subcutaneous administration of narcotics,
Bruera and our group noted that 15% of patients developed tolerance at a rate in
excess of 5% per day (Bruera et al. 1988).

One of the most poorly understood but important facets of opiate resistance is noted in patients with severe emotional, spiritual and psychological problems compounding their pain. Early studies from St. Christopher's Hospice in London reported a phenomenal success rate in the management of cancer pain; those patients who did not respond included a group described as the victims of a state of "total suffering", whereby a mélange of psychological and physiological disturbances left the patient in an isolated state of agony. When the emotional aspects of pain can be addressed, response to drug therapy may occur.

Metabolic changes in cancer patients can influence opiate effectiveness. Opiates are primarily metabolized by the liver, but patients with severe hepatic damage may take opiates without difficulty, while the presence of renal impairment dramatically enhances opiate toxicity. Recent recognition that some of the opiates have active metabolites dependent upon renal excretion provides an explanation for this observation (Osborne et al. 1988). In the present author's experience, the side effects of all opiates are increased in the face of renal failure, suggesting that as yet to be discovered active metabolites, similar in pharmacological property to morphine 6-glucuronide, exist with other opiates.

Respiratory failure has been overestimated as a problem limiting opiate use in cancer patients. One must be careful in the face of existing CO_2 retention, but the presence of dyspnoea should encourage opiate use rather than limit it, since opiates have been shown to increase the effective work of breathing and reduce discomfort (Light et al. 1989).

Altered bowel motility produces the most common distressing side effects of opiates. Nausea at the onset of opiate therapy can normally be controlled by low-dose antinauseants, but the occasional patient may develop intractable nausea, possibly secondary to the added effects of incoordinate peristaltic action produced by opiates (Manara and Bianchetti 1985) and autonomic disturbances in gastric emptying which are common in patients with advanced cancer (Bruera et al. 1987). Patients with intra-abdominal tumours and intermittent bowel obstruction represent another difficult management group.

Pain Syndromes with Reduced Opiate Sensitivity

Cancer pain secondary to nerve damage, either in the peripheral nervous system, the spinal cord, or within the brain itself, is often described as "opiate-resistant". The cascade of events following either peripheral or central nerve damage is poorly understood. Although accorded the single rubric of "neuropathic pain", it is likely that nerve damage does not elicit a solitary response in a "hard-wired" system. In any given situation, multiple factors probably come into play.

Following damage to a peripheral nerve, regenerating nerve sprouts are uniquely sensitive to pain stimuli; they may also serve as a source of ectopic pain-inducing activity. The regenerating nerves also may develop enhanced sensitivity to the action of neurotransmitters released at sympathetic nerve endings. A related phenomenon is the aberrant sympathetic activity sometimes observed in areas of peripheral nerve damage and pain (changes in temperature, vasculariz-ation, sweating, hair growth, etc.). It has also been proposed that nerves that previously only mediated non-painful stimuli may, in a field where other nerves are damaged, take on autonomous pain-transmitting functions, and may be particularly sensitized to sympathetic stimulation (see review by Portenoy 1989b).

Even more poorly understood are the central pathophysiological changes which occur following peripheral (or central) neuron damage. In keeping with the Gate Theory, the loss of large myelinated neurons in the periphery may reduce their tonic inhibition of pain-transmitting neurons in the dorsal horn. Other postulated mechanisms include the loss of opioid inhibition following damage to the peripheral sensory fibre on which opioids act, with consequent change in the discharge characteristics of second order neurons (Wall 1988). It is known that populations of these spinal cord neurons have a "wide dynamic range", meaning that they do not simply function in a hard-wired system but can change their properties following changes in their environment, with consequent development of autonomous pain-transmitting activity. A related mechanism may include the inauguration of spontaneous pain-transmitting activity in previously "silent" reticular spinal cord neuron groups (Portenoy 1989b).

Other types of pain which tend to be less responsive to opiates include incident pain, characterized by the presence of sudden bursts of sharp pain following changes in position. This type of pain is often associated with mechanical skeietal damage. It is not known why opiates often fail to dampen movement-induced pain. Spasm pain, either visceral (tenesmoid pain may serve as an example) or somatic, is also reported by clinicians to be more difficult to treat with opiates. Recent work by Steiner and Siegal (1989) suggest that muscle cramps are most common secondary to either peripheral neuropathy or root and plexus pathology. Therefore, spasm pain may be regarded as another neuro-pathic pain associated with nerve damage. While headache is said to be resistant to opiate management, the wide variety of mechanisms causing headache, the lack of studies on opiate use, and the general caveat that headaches, most commonly occurring in patients with non-malignant disorders, should not be treated with opiates, precludes any conclusions on this point.

Principles of Management of Opiate-Resistant Pain

Six principles to keep in mind when considering the use of opiates in a difficult management situation are listed in Table 2.

Opiates are the mainstay of the treatment of nociceptive cancer pain (pain mediated by an intact and normally functioning peripheral and central nervous system). While neuropathic pain is thought to be relatively opiate-resistant, the mystery and multiplicity of causes of neuropathic pain ordain that an open mind be kept on this topic. Moreover, many patients with cancer-induced nerve damage pain have contributory nociceptive components. Therefore, a rigid

Table 2. Principles for management of opiate-resistant pain

1. Avoid rigid classification of pain
2. Avoid the concept "usually effective dose"
3. Consider alternative opiate
4. Consider alternative route
5. Consider role of adjuvant drugs
     + −(control of side-effects pain)
     − −(enhanced toxicity)
6. Maximize non-pharmacological therapy

classification into "opiate-resistant" and "opiate-responsive" pain should be eschewed.

Nevertheless, as articulated by Arnër and Myerson (1988), many clinicians believe that neuropathic pain syndromes are poorly responsive to opiates. In a thoughtful study recently published in *Pain*, Arnër and his associates conducted a placebo-controlled study demonstrating that patients classified as suffering from neuropathic pain, or who had idiopathic pain, did not show an analgesic response to doses of opiates effective for patients with nociceptive pain. However, they used a "usually effective dose" of an opiate rather than treating patients to the point of intolerable side effects. Therefore, it is possible that some of these patients might have achieved satisfactory analgesia with higher doses of opiates.

In contrast, Portenoy and his colleagues emphasize that there are patients with neuropathic pain syndromes who are opiate-responsive (R. Portenoy, personal communication). They favour the concept of a continuum between no response and good response, the position of a patient on the continuum to be established after an individual opiate trial. He reports that in a study on 28 patients with a predominantly neuropathic cancer pain problem, 21 of the patients experienced greater than 50% pain relief during a titrated opiate infusion. The present author supports the flexible approach advanced by Portenoy.

Nevertheless, there are pain syndromes which appear to be less sensitive to opiates than others. Before foregoing the use of an opiate it is reasonable to switch from one agent to another. While politicians, the lay press, and a few clinicians have made unsubstantiated claims of the inherent superiority of one opiate over another, there is no scientific basis for these statements. However, the side effects of opiates may be mediated by different receptors and the affinity of a given opiate for receptors mediating both analgesia and side effects may vary from individual to individual. Since absolute cross-tolerance does not exist between opiates, it is reasonable to switch from one to another when a satisfactory clinical response has not been obtained. It must not be assumed that a skew of the side effect:analgesia equation towards the left with one opiate obviates the possibility of successful use of another opiate. For example, myoclonus induced by opiate use in high doses or in the presence of renal failure may subside following a switch to an alternative opioid.

As the presence of side effects may be influenced by the route of administration, an improved side effect:analgesia equation may be achieved by altering the delivery port. For example, patients who experience undue sedation followed by increased breakthrough pain on spaced doses of opiates may improve on a continuous infusion.

Portenoy stresses that one cannot say that side effects preclude further use of opiates until a trial of adjuvant drugs designed to control side effects has been carried out. Laxatives, antinauseants and CNS stimulants to control sedation can control the principal side effects of opiates. Conversely, these side effects can be increased by the parallel use of other adjuvant drugs, particularly some of those used in the management of neuropathic pain (antidepressants, benzodiazepines, muscle relaxants, etc.). Concomitant use of psychoactive and bowel-inhibiting drugs with opiates requires judgement, constant assessment, and adjustment.

Treatment of Neuropathic Pain

The pain-controlling action of opiates is enhanced through the uses of co-analgesics with different side effect profiles. Similarly, a variety of non-pharmacological analgesic techniques can complement drug therapy.

Non-pharmacological Techniques

It is axiomatic that patients in pain who are not adequately helped with simple drug therapy should have access to non-drug treatments. A major tenet of the palliative care movement is the enhancement of patient dignity, an objective furthered by ensuring patient control of therapy. Many physical and psychological interventions are particularly attractive because they involve the patient as an active participant rather than a passive recipient of care. The literature on non-drug techniques is not definitive, as there are few blinded randomized trials where end-points are clearly established, follow-up is provided, recognizable patient populations are described, and the sample size is large enough to rule out incorrect conclusions. Because of the specialized nature of many of these procedures, their availability may be limited and the more complex and/or risky techniques are not appropriate for many cancer patients with a pedigree of multiple past therapeutic interventions and a limited comfortable life expectancy.

Based on these considerations the following hierarchy of therapies is proposed for consideration:

Psychological Methods

These range from general techniques aimed at easing the emotional component of suffering to specific procedures (hypnosis and biofeedback) which a patient can learn with professional assistance. The "side effects" are presumably modest, although the inappropriate use of visual imagery has been said to increase some patient's guilt reactions (Holland et al. 1989). Mankind has a strong innate belief that the human mind controls bodily function. While elements of this thesis are extremely controversial and the precise neurophysiological mechanisms are not known, there is evidence that psychosocial interventions reduce the reactive component of pain (Spiegel 1985).

Non-invasive Stimulatory Techniques

Heating pads or cold packs sometimes have a comforting effect on areas of nerve damage. A more sophisticated technique, also in use for centuries, is acupuncture. Filshie and Redman (1985) describe the successful use of acupuncture in cancer patients, some of whom had neuropathic pain, especially those with hyperpathia, dysaesthesia and a subset of patients with post-mastectomy pain. Here we have a therapy whose mechanism of action is not understood assisting patients with pain syndromes which are equally poorly understood. There are no controlled double-blind trials using acupuncture in cancer pain, but there is evidence from the non-cancer pain literature that acupuncture, at least in the short term, offers a higher chance of success than could be achieved through a placebo mechanism (Vincent and Richardson 1986). Transcutaneous nerve stimulation (TENS) is a simple and more readily available form of nerve stimulation. It is thought that acupuncture and low-frequency TENS have similar modes of action. Eriksson et al. (1979) have reported that low-frequency stimulation may be particularly helpful for neuropathic pain. It is the present author's impression that tolerance develops to TENS after a variable time interval. Nevertheless, because of the simplicity of the technique, and its involvement of the patient in active pain management, TENS should be considered for use in neuropathic pain syndromes.

Simple Invasive Procedures

The burning component of nerve damage pain, referred to the skin and often accompanied by hyperpathia and allodynia, is sometimes relieved by interfering with the sympathetic nervous supply to the area of pain (Loh and Nathan 1978). It is not clear whether successful sympathetic block presages a longer term response to oral sympatholytic agents.

Somatic nerve blocks are less favoured because of the difficulty in encompassing the total area of pain, the plasticity of the nervous system, which leads to the return of pain in adjacent areas, and the risk of a more severe de-afferentation syndrome occurring after a brief period of relief. However, as noted with sympathetic blocks, occasionally a local anaesthetic block, which will not further damage the nerve, may provide relief which endures beyond the time of local anaesthetic action. In expert hands, the use of a cryoprobe (which may leave the internal architecture of the nerve intact, permitting orderly nerve regrowth) or of alcohol and phenol may help in select situations, most notably when specific thoracic dermatomes are involved, or in the treatment of cranial nerve syndromes involving the fifth and ninth nerves.

Complex Invasive Procedures

The efficacy of cordotomy is diminished in the face of neuropathic pain (Lahuerta et al. 1985). Other complex invasive procedures with an uncertain predictability of success have little place in the management of advanced cancer patients with a limited life expectancy.

Antidepressants

Antidepressants are a mainstay of management of chronic non-malignant neuropathic pain. They have been demonstrated in a number of double-blind trials to be helpful in post-herpetic neuralgia, diabetic neuropathy and, to a lesser extent, other nerve damage syndromes. No single antidepressant has been demonstrated to be superior to any other; of interest is the fact that the analgesic action of antidepressants is manifested at lower doses than those required to treat depression. Antidepressants, which increase the availability of catecholamines in the central nervous system, are believed to activate a number of descending inhibitory pain modulating pathways. In addition, Ventafridda and his colleagues have demonstrated that the bioavailability of morphine may be increased by antidepressants (Ventafridda et al. 1987). As it is possible that antidepressants impact on other neurotransmitters, a definitive relationship between mode of action and analgesic efficacy has not been established.

With respect to cancer pain, double-blind controlled antidepressant trials have not been published. Because of the delayed response to antidepressants and the difficulty in controlling other factors in patients with advanced cancer, these trials are extremely difficult to mount. At this time the author presumes that the information obtained from non-malignant studies in post-herpetic neuralgia is transferable to the cancer patient. However many antidepressants have anticholinergic actions, additive to the side effects of opiates. They must be used judiciously in the management of cancer pain states.

Anticonvulsants

Neuropathic pain is thought to be associated with abnormal spontaneous discharges from regenerating or damaged nerves or spinal cord neurons. Anticonvulsants which suppress neuron hyperexcitability and the spread of abnormal discharges therefore have a theoretical role in the management of neuropathic pain. Reasonable evidence exists for the efficacy of four anticonvulsants (phenytoin, carbamazepine, valproic acid and clonazepam) in diabetic neuropathy, trigeminal neuralgia and the treatment of the lancinating component of nerve damage pain. Responses are inconsistent and the patients may be helped by one agent when another is ineffective. While these agents are widely used in other forms of neuropathic pain, their efficacy is less clearly established; in particular, there are no studies which delineate their specific use in cancer patients. Therefore, they should be employed when lancinating pain is a prominent cause of suffering. Clonazepam is probably the safest drug to use, as the side effects are those of a benzodiazepine. The other anticonvulsants have a broader range of side effects which sometimes fit awkwardly with the multiple other drugs which may be in the portfolio of an advanced cancer patient. Although not strictly anticonvulsants, some of the muscle relaxants may also relieve lancinating pain. For example, baclofen may be as effective as carbamazepine in the management of trigeminal neuralgia.

Anti-arrythmic Agents (Local Anaesthetics)

Local anaesthetics act primarily on the cell membrane of neurons, preventing the generation and conduction of a nerve impulse by reducing or eliminating sodium flux across the membrane (Gilman et al. 1980). As a result, the inauguration and conduction of a nerve impulse is blocked. Local application of anaesthetic agents proximal to the point of entry have a profound effect on nerve damage pain. However, long-term local use is generally not possible because of pain-inhibition of all nerve function by these agents and the lack of a safe long-acting formulation.

The systemic analgesic effects of these agents were reported in a series of open studies over 40 years ago. More than 30 years later, a number of open-label small studies using intravenous lidocaine in a variety of painful conditions appeared in the literature. Lidocaine appears to be strikingly helpful for the pain associated with a rare disorder, Dercum's disease (Petersen et al. 1984). It has a variable and unpredictable effect on other pain syndromes. An unexplained finding noted in these studies is the prolonged analgesic effect of lidocaine on some patients (up to 1 year) after a single intravenous infusion (the half-life of the drug is in the range of 120 min). The reason for this phenomenon is not known.

Very few double-blind controlled trials have been carried out on these agents. A postoperative continuous infusion trial using lidocaine in a placebo-controlled study reported positive results (Cassutto et al. 1985). Recently, Petersen,

Kastrup and colleagues have carried out two double-blind controlled trials involving 33 patients with diabetic neuropathy. In the study of potentially greatest relevance to cancer patients (as it involved the use of an oral congener of lidocaine, mexiletine taken on a regular basis by mouth) the Copenhagen group reported that 10 out of 16 patients with diabetic neuropathy had a significant drop in pain visual analogue scale scores on mexiletine (Dejgard et al. 1988). This report in the *Lancet* stimulated a letter response from a British hospice unit (Dunlop et al. 1988), reporting in an open-label study extraordinarily good results in cancer-related neuropathic pain following the use of flecainide in a dose of 100 mg twice daily by mouth. Ten patients had complete pain relief, including six in whom the pain relief lasted until the time of their death (1–26 weeks later). An additional five patients noted clinically significant improvement of their pain.

Randomized double-blind trials of anti-arrythmic agents in the management of cancer pain have not been conducted. In view of the report of Dunlop and colleagues, this is an area of extraordinary importance. Because of the sometimes desperate state of patients with neuropathic pain, many hospice programs are embarking on clinical sorties using lidocaine congeners. As these agents have mixed excitatory–inhibitory activity within the central nervous system, and when used by themselves have an appreciable incidence of CNS side effects, it is possible that the concomitant use of anti-arrythmic drugs with the cavalcade of other CNS-active agents used in neuropathic pain syndromes may produce a variety of untoward side effects. Clearly, the role of the anti-arrythmics must soon be clarified.

Corticosteroids

Clinicians often note a dramatic but frequently short-lived response to high-dose corticoid therapy. A simple explanation relates to the role of steroids in reducing inflammation, but the actual mechanism of pain relief is not clear. In addition to their anti-inflammatory action, corticosteroids have been shown to reduce hyperexcitability of neurons (Devor et al. 1985).

Other Drugs

Based on the actions of the sympathetic nervous system in sensitizing peripheral neurons, a few open-label trials of sympatholytic agents have been reported. A controlled trial with propranalol (a β-blocker) in post-traumatic neuralgia was negative (Scadding et al. 1982), but an open-label study of phenoxybenzamine (an α-blocker) on 40 consecutive patients with causalgic pain had a positive outcome (Ghostine et al. 1984). Clonidine, systemically and via a spinal route, has been used successfully in patients with pain. Clonidine, an α_2-agonist, has been said to increase or restore opioid sensitivity, particularly when given spinally. Success following the use of cholinergic agents has also been reported. These studies are interesting, but the role of agents mediating the autonomic nervous system in cancer pain, and their interactions with other drugs required by cancer patients, remains to be determined.

More complete reviews of the drugs used to manage nerve damage pain are contained in three excellent reviews by Maciewicz et al. (1985), McQuay (1988), and Portenoy (1989a).

Conclusion

It is not unusual to encounter a profoundly suffering, metabolically com-promised cancer patient with a neuropathic pain syndrome. Controlled clinical trials in this setting are modest in number and in patient accrual. While waiting for this scenario to change and for further therapeutic guidance to emerge, complex considerations are required to provide the patient and family with a simple therapeutic plan. Oncologists are called upon to be familiar with a literature not usually encountered in their educational grazing, to call upon different disciplines to assist them in patient management and to organize a system for meticulous patient follow-up. Periods of frustration and doubt will be shared by patient and clinician alike. However, a full appreciation of the options available, blended with skill in assessment and application, will pay dividends in this difficult situation requiring the equal application of both the art and the science of medicine.

Acknowledgement. The author acknowledges with gratitude Dr. Russ Portenoy who allowed him to review an unpublished manuscript outlining views on the opiate management of difficult pain syndromes. Any misinterpretation of Dr. Portenoy's approach is the fault of the present author.

References

Arnër S, Myerson BA (1988) Lack of analgesic effect of opioids in neuropathic and idiopathic forms of pain. Pain 33 (1): 11–25

Bruera E, Catz Z, Hooper R, Lentle, MacDonald N (1987) Chronic nausea and anorexia in advanced cancer patients: a possible role for autonomic dysfunction. J Pain Sympt Manag 2 (1): 19–21

Bruera E, Brenneis C, Michaud M, Bacovsky R, Chadwick S, Emeno A, MacDonald N (1988) Use of the subcutaneous route for the administration of narcotics in patients with cancer pain. Cancer 2: 407–411

Cassuto J, Wallin G, Hogstrom S et al. (1985) Inhibition of postoperative pain by continuous low-dose infusion of Lidocaine. Anesta Analg 64: 971–974

Dejgard A, Peterson P, Kastrup J (1988) Mexiletine for treatment of chronic painful diabetic neuropathy. Lancet i: 9–11

Devor M, Govrin-Lippmann R, Raber P (1985) Corticosteroids reduce hyperexcitability. Adv Pain Res Ther 9: 451–455

Dunlop R, Davies R, Vockley J, Turner P (1988) Analgesic effects of oral flecainide. Lancet i: 420–421

Eriksson MBE, Sjölund VH, Nielzen F (1979) Long term results of peripheral conditioning stimulation as an analgesia measure in chronic pain. Pain 6: 335–347

Filshie J, Redman D (1985) Acupuncture and malignant pain problems. Eur J Surg Oncol 11: 389–394

Ghostine SY, Comair YG et al. (1984) Phenoxybenazmine in the treatment of causalgia. J Neurosurg 60: 1263–1268

Gilman AG et al. (eds) (1980) Goodman and Gilman's the pharmacologic basis of therapeutics, 6th edn. Macmillan, New York, p 1307

Holland JC, Geary N, Furman A (1989) Holland JC, Rowland JH (eds) Handbook of psycho-oncology. Oxford University Press, New York

Kaiko R, Wallenstein S et al. (1983) Sources of variation in analgesic responses in cancer patients with chronic pain receiving morphine. Pain 15: 191–200

Lahuerta J, Lipton S, Wells JCD (1985) Percutaneous cervical cordotomy; results and complications in a recent series of 100 patients. Ann R Coll Surg Engl 67: 41–44

Light R, Muro J, Sato R et al. (1989) Effects of oral morphine on breathlessness and exercise tolerance in patients with chronic obstructive pulmonary disease. Am Rev Respir Dis 139: 126–133

Loh L, Nathan PW (1978) Painful peripheral states and sympathetic blocks. J Neurol Neurosurg Psychiatry 41: 664–671

Maciewicz R, Boukoms A, Martin JB (1985) Drug therapy of neuropathic pain. Clin J Pain 1: 39–49

Manara L, Bianchetti A (1985) The central and peripheral influences of opioids on gastro-intestinal obstruction. Annu Rev Pharmacol Toxicol 25: 249–73

McQuay HJ (1988) Pharmacological treatment of neuralgic and neuropathic pain. Cancer Surv 7 (1): 141–159

Osborne RJ, Joel S et al. (1988) The pharmacologic activity and pharmaco-kinetics of intravenous morphine in man. J Pain Sympt Manag S15 (3): 3

Petersen P, Kastrup P, Skagenk et al. (1984) Treating the pain of Dercum's disease. Br Med J 288: 1880

Portenoy RK (1989a) Drug treatment of pain syndromes. Semin Neurol 7: 2 139–149

Portenoy RK (1989b) Mechanisms of clinical pain. Neurol Clin 7 (2): 205–230

Scadding JW, Wall PD et al. (1982) Clinical trial of propranolol in post-traumatic neuralgia. Pain 14: 283–292

Spiegel D (1985) Psychosocial interventions with cancer patients. J Psychosoc Oncol 3: 83–95

Steiner I, Siegal T (1989) Muscle cramps in cancer patients. Cancer 63: 574–577

Ventafridda V, Ripamonti C, Deconno F et al. (1987) Antidepressants increase bioavailability of morphine in cancer patients. Lancet i: 1204

Vincent CA, Richardson PA (1986) Evaluation of therapeutic acupuncture: concepts and methods. Pain 24: 1–13

Wall PD (1988) Neurological mechanisms in cancer pain. Cancer Surv 7 (1): 127–140

Effective Pain Control in Cancer Patients in the Home Care Setting

H.R. Stoll

Spitalexterne Onkologiepflege Basel-Stadt (SEOP), Heuberg 16, 4051 Basel, Switzerland

Introduction

The basis for this article is the fact that, by putting today's knowledge into consistent practice, according to WHO 98% of all cancer patients could be free of pain. In the opinion of nursing staff, cancer and pain go hand in hand: a certain degree of pain is considered normal and untreatable. The goals set by the WHO are widely unknown or are considered utopian. The purpose of this paper is to list several reasons for this attitude, and also to examine the possibilities of controlling pharmacologically treatable cancer pain in the home environment.

The Problem

The principal form of pain control is surely pharmacological therapy, both in the hospital and at home. Further common problems, in and outside hospital, are caused not only by inadequate knowledge but also by inner fears and myths harboured by nursing staff and doctors about potent analgesics. In the case of patients at home, the problem is merely magnified by the fact that patients requiring potent pharmacological therapy are rare; thus, the opportunity for the doctor and nursing staff to acquire positive experience is lacking.

To add to this, pain control is frequently commenced in hospital before the patient is discharged. In such cases a precise pain assessment is seldom made by the doctor and nursing staff, and the pain therapy prescribed is often accordingly imprecise. As a result of this lack of experience with *efficacious* pharmacological therapy regimens, the doctors' and nurses' own conception of pain control takes over.

A Solution

In view of the above, it is not surprising that the principal activity of SEOP (the home care cancer service of Basel) is contributing to pharmacological pain control. This is always carried out in cooperation with the existing resources such as medical and nursing services. Our approach has three steps:

1. Assessment of pain
2. Dialogue
3. Pain medication

Assessment of Pain

On the first home visit, patients are assessed for their risk of developing pain. For patients with inadequate pain control the pain assessment form from the Royal Marsden Hospital in London is used (Fig. 1, see p. 38–40). The accent here is how the *patient* experiences and assesses the pain, *not* the home care staff. It is important for the patient to break down the overall pain into different areas. Then and then only can the pathogenic part of the overall pain be treated with analgesics; all other areas, such as psychogenic pain and suffering of social, religious, or financial origin, are then treated by discussion, if necessary with specialists.

The detailed pain assessment recorded in these forms gives an idea of the subjective pain felt by the patient. For instance, one patient (patient 1) receiving 3×4 mg morphine epidurally and tilidine drops on request described pain alternating throughout the whole body, the main areas being shoulder and sternum. The pains were always very strong in one specific place. The graph on the assessment form was filled in very carefully and meticulously for 10 days. The evaluation with the patient produced the following result:

The main source of pain could be explained by the location of the tumour: the patient had lung cancer. The remaining areas were discussed in the course of conversation. It emerged that the patient had been feeling neglected for years. As a result of his disease, however, he received regular visits from the district nurse, his two children, two neighbours who cooked for him, his doctor, and SEOP. In the evaluating discussion the patient came to realize that, in his isolation, his pain had been bringing him attention and consideration.

On the other hand this patient (patient 2) had pain only in one clearly defined area. He was severely handicapped by this pain, which he described as extremely unpleasant. Pain therapy for this specific pain was instituted, and thereafter the course of the therapy and the quality of the pain became increasingly poorly recorded, since the pain, as a result of the positive effect of the pain therapy, was no longer a problem.

Dialogue

The purpose of the dialogue is to enable the patient to "find" and understand himself. This is the most exhausting but also the most interesting part of pain therapy. It prevents nonpathogenic pain areas from being treated with medication.

PAIN ASSESSMENT CHART

SURNAME: HOSPITAL NO.

FIRST NAME: DATE:

INITIAL ASSESSMENT

Patient's own description of the pain(s):

What helps relieve the pain?

What makes the pain worse?

Do you have pain

i)   at night?   Yes/No   (comment if required).

ii)   at rest?   Yes/No   (comment if required).

iii)   on movement?   Yes/No   (comment if required)

By kind permission of the Royal Marsden Hospital
sponsored by Napp Laboratories

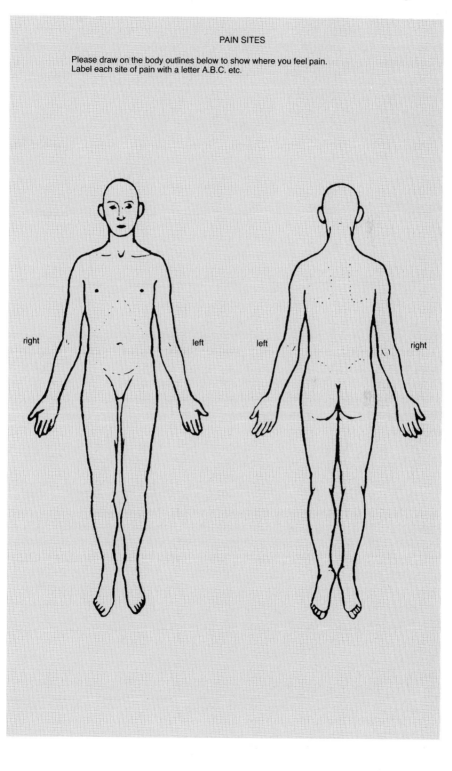

PAIN SITES

Please draw on the body outlines below to show where you feel pain.
Label each site of pain with a letter A.B.C. etc.

PAIN ASSESSMENT CHART

KEY TO PAIN INTENSITY   CONTINUATION NO: _____

0 = no pain
1 = mild pain
2 = moderate pain
3 = severe pain

4 = very severe pain
5 = intolerable/overwhelming pain

s = sleeping

It may be easier to determine the intensity of pain by looking at the pain scale below.

no pain	0		1		2		3		4		5	intolerable/ overwhelming pain

mild pain   moderate pain   severe pain   very severe pain

DATE	TIMES	PAIN SITES								ANALGESIA NAME, ROUTE & DOSE	PATIENT ACTIVITY AND COMMENTS
		A	B	C	D	E	F	G	H		

Analgesics

For the patient under pharmacological pain therapy, rapid, often spectacular success has a decisive effect and frequently creates a suitable climate in which to discuss the remaining ailments. It seems incomprehensible that this is not done more often. SEOP has, for this reason, a large assortment of analgesics permanently in the car, so as to be able to begin therapy immediately after consultation with the doctor in charge. The pain therapies are strictly divided up according to the three principles of the WHO.

Therapy by the Ladder

To put it simply, this means that pain is the sole criterion in the choice and dosage of analgesic. The aim is to achieve freedom from pain day by day, even when the patient is mobile. The initial stage of determining medication and dosage at home is often intensive, as the dose has to be fixed as quickly as possible. Here it is also important that the patient be fully informed, can express his fears, and is made aware of possible or probable side effects. The patient agrees to both choice of medication and dosage.

Therapy by Mouth

Pain therapy with a morphine pump controlled by the patient, although dramatic and interesting, makes the patient dependent on the staff providing the necessary support. Swallowing tablets, which nearly everybody is able to do, is therefore preferable, and since it has been proved that morphine slow-release tablets can be effectively administered via the rectum, the consciousness of the patient ceases to be a criterion for using the pump. Nevertheless, where indicated, we give pain therapy with the necessary backup by implanted epidural catheter systems or by means of a morphine pump.

Therapy by the Clock

Patients with chronic pain always have to have a regular rhythm of therapy, adjusted to the duration of effect of the medication. In addition, every patient has access to effective reserve medication, which he takes as he thinks fit.

Case Studies

The following two examples demonstrate to what extent pain therapy at home is possible. The most important condition for the success of pain therapy is the right approach to the patient. The patient is treated as adult who, though restricted by his disease, remains in possession of his faculties and perhaps needs our support to attain his original autonomy.

Case 1

JL was 80 years old, suffering from carcinoma of the kidney with pelvic metastases, and lived alone on the 2nd floor without a lift. Twelve months before his death he had a total fracture of the pelvis. During these 12 months he lived at home, supported by a home help, district nurse, SEOP, and his doctor, the pain being treated with morphine tablets, anti-rheumatics and paracetamol. This time he spent in preparing for death. After 12 months the femur collapsed after a fall and the patient was admitted to hospital in the understanding and according to his will that he would receive neither a bladder nor a vein catheter. He died within a week, his pain not under control.

Case 2

F. G. is 35 years old, with cancer of the colon, lumbar spine metastases, and local tumour growth in the rectum. He has extensive bed sores, 6×6 cm, after a 6-week Breuss diet of vegetable juices. The pains caused by the lumbar spine metastases are effectively controlled by 2×3 mg morphine administered epidurally via an implanted catheter system. The patient injects himself, and his wife has also been instructed. The pains due to local tumour growth in the rectum require 240–400 mg morphine injected subcutaneously daily. This is done via a pump, controlled by the patient, through a butterfly-needle placed subcutaneously. The patient adjusts the pump according to the pain. Depending on his position, the bed sores cause additional pain. This is checked by Novamin-Sulfon tablets.

These two examples illustrate that, given the appropriate support and correct interaction in the help system, the most large-scale and complicated pain therapies can be carried out at home. In the experience of SEOP, the stumbling block is not primarily the patient and his pain—it is rather the helpers and their inhibitions and fears which appear restrictive in pain therapy with tumour patients. It seems to me that this is a problem which exists both in and outside hospital.

Is the Therapeutic Use of Opioids Adversely Affected by Prejudice and Law?

M. Zenz and J. Sorge

Universitätsklinik für Anaesthesiologie, Intensiv- und Schmerztherapie,
Berufsgenossenschaftliche Krankenanstalt Bergmannsheil Bochum,
Gilsingstraße 14, W-4630 Bochum, FRG

There is no doubt about the severe undertreatment of cancer pain worldwide. Every day 3.5 million people are suffering from cancer pain (WHO 1986). This remains true even though treatment is so easy and effective with non-narcotic analgesics and opioids (Twycross and Lack 1983). Just with these drugs, pain relief can be achieved in as many as 90% of our patients. But opioids are not used enough in chronic pain treatment. The reasons for this deficit are the lack of systematic teaching, lack of curricula for pain treatment, lack of awareness of the problem, fear of side effects from the treatment, prejudices, and legislative restrictions.

On the other side, the example of the English hospices demonstrates all the possibilities available to us in treating cancer pain effectively and without major side effects. The gap between the current situation and what could be is unnecessarily wide and must be closed as soon as possible.

Prejudices

"Opioids are addictive". Fear of dependence is the major concern about opioids. Ask colleagues about morphine and its predominant effects and "addiction" is one of the first answers. The same is true when we ask our patients about the known facts on morphine. But there is no scientific basis for this statement. On the contrary, everything we know indicates that opiods given in the right way are not addictive. The present authors have never seen a patient under proper opioid treatment and in a painfree state who was addicted. The same has been demonstrated in a large survey on nearly 12 000 in-patients: only four (0.03%) were considered to be addicted, and only one had signs of major dependence (Porter and Jick 1980). This is an extremely low figure in face of the figures known about benzodiazepines. There is no doubt that dependence is very common in patients given benzodiazepine, and yet in the Federal Republic of Germany 800 million daily doses of benzodiazepines are given every year without any restrictions. Only 0.7 million daily doses of sustained-release morphine are given in the same time (Schmidt 1989). Among the top ten registered abused drugs in Germany there is only one opioid, representing 6.5% of the cases. Seven of the ten were benzodiazepines, representing 61% of the cases of addiction (Müller-Oerlinghausen 1984).

"Tolerance of opioids is very common." "Once start giving opioids, you inevitably have to increase the dose." This too is one of the common concerns about opioid treatment which prevents effective treatment, but in fact clinical experience cannot show any evidence of true tolerance to opioids. Usually it is the manner of administration that is the cause for concern. Giving opioids at irregular intervals and allowing pain to return again and again is the main reason for increasing doses. Weissman and Haddox (1989) have called this problem "opioid pseudoaddiction" and "an iatrogenic syndrome". In our own figures for opioid treatment in malignant and non-malignant pain there is no evidence of any development of tolerance; most patients could be effectively treated by a stable dose over long periods of time (Table 1). To achieve this, however, it is necessary to give opioids "by the clock" and at an individualized dosage, to prevent pain from re-emerging.

"Opioids induce respiratory depression." Certainly, any painfree volunteer will develop respiratory depression when given a small amount of morphine. By contrast, a patient with cancer pain will tolerate an enormous dose of morphine without any effect on respiratory effort, even if opioid-naive. The only difference between these two situations is the pain, which seems to be a potent respiratory stimulator (Hanks et al. 1980). The same has been demonstrated for the postoperative period, where opioids increase the respiratory force by eliminating the adverse effects of pain on respiratory function (Bromage 1955).

"Opioids induce euphoria." We often extrapolate from heroin addicts to pain patients. But there are huge differences between these two groups. Addicts are taking opioids with a high liposolubility (e.g. heroin), drugs which pass the blood–brain barrier very quickly. Morphine, however, the mother drug of cancer pain treatment, is a highly water-soluble drug. It passes into the brain very slowly and hardly induces effects comparable to heroin. On the other hand,

Table 1. Dose development in cancer patients treated with morphine and buprenorphine. (Adapted from Zenz et al. 1985, 1989)

	Buprenorphine $n=41$	Morphine $n=35$
Increasing dose	16	14
Constant dose	15	4
Decreasing dose	2	17
Changing dose	8	

opioids are given regularly for cancer pain, but there are no peaks and valleys inducing feelings of well-being here. Euphoria is not a typical side effect of a correctly carried out opioid treatment. On the contrary, morphine very often induces depression, sometimes so severe as to require treatment with antidepressants (Twycross and Lack 1983).

"Opioids decrease mental performance." Patients and doctors often believe that opioids decrease vigilance and induce somnolence. On this point too, clinical experience contradicts common belief. The mental and physical performance of patients are not depressed; indeed in most cases the opposite is true. To prove this, we have performed reaction tests with patients before and after instituting opioid treatment. No patient demonstrated impaired reaction: indeed, in all but one patient receiving morphine treatment reaction time and number of correct reactions improved. One patient's reactions did not change after morphine therapy was started. Many of our patients return to their former occupation when morphine therapy has freed them from pain.

These are some of the prejudices which are commonplace in opioid therapy. They are taught by most pharmacological textbooks and most medical teachers, but they need to be replaced by experience with patients and not be reinforced by experiments in volunteers. All these prejudices are perhaps valid for situations in which opioids are given to pain-free volunteers, but not for the clinical situation, in which opioids are given in the correct manner to patients in pain. We have to distinguish between these two very different situations.

Legal Restrictions

In some countries opioids underly certain legal restrictions which were instituted to reduce abuse of opioids. Most of these legal developments go back to a time when the registered drugs were the only means of access to morphine and other drugs from this group. Nowadays, heroin, cocaine, crack are the attractive drugs, and all the registered drugs play a minor role because the market allows sufficient access to psychotropic substances. But the legal restrictions have not changed. In Germany, opioids can only be prescribed on particular prescription forms, in triplicate. Exceptions to this rule are only made for codeine, tramadol, dextropropoxyphene, and tilidine. All other drugs underly the *Betäubungsmittelverschreibungsverordnung* "regulation regarding the prescription of narcotics" BtMVV). The prescriptions have to be ordered from a place called the *Bundesopiumstelle,* the name demonstrates the quiet historic view of opioid treatment in our country. Every prescription has to be written by hand in a particular manner, which is very complicated even for the expert; e.g. buprenorphine sublingual tablets, which contain 0.2 mg of active substance, have to be prescribed as "Temgesic 0.216 mg"—related to buprenorphine hydrochloride. One copy of the prescription has to remain with the doctor for 3 years. Two copies go to the patient. One of these has to be kept at the pharmacy for 3 years as well, to allow for official controls. Every opioid has a certain maximum daily

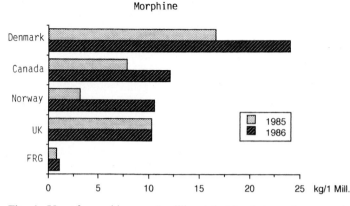

Fig. 1. Use of morphine per 1 million inhabitants in various countries (WHO 1987)

dose. Any opioid can only be prescribed for a maximum of 1 week; after that a new prescription has to be written. There is no official way to prescribe morphine to cover a 2-week holiday. If a patient needs more than 1000 mg of morphine per day, treatment can only be carried out in hospital, not on an outpatient basis. Any mistake in prescribing or handling strong opioids can end in penalties of up to 50 000 DM. The official regulations with commentary on this topic in our country fill a book of 500 pages.

It is obvious that by these regulations restrict the clinical use of strong analgesics to the smallest amount necessary. Consequently, in no other country is the use of morphine as low as in Germany (Fig. 1).

Opioid Prescription Habits in Germany

We investigated the prescription habits in Hannover in 1985 and 1988 to gain information on the current situation regarding treatment with strong analgesics.

The investigation included 325 000 patients and 930 doctors. A total amount of 1 088 148 prescriptions were registered in the first 6 months of 1988. Of these, 1 581 prescriptions were for opioids, i.e. 0.145% (Table 2). From among more

Table 2. Total prescriptions and opioid prescriptions in Hannover, 1985 and 1988. (Adapted from Sorge and Zenz 1989)

	Jan.–June 1985	Jan.–June 1988
Total prescriptions	1 059 787	1 088 148
Opioid prescriptions	994	1 581
	(0.094%)	(0.145%)

Table 3. Proportion of patients prescribed opioids in Hannover, 1985 and 1988. (Adapted from Sorge and Zenz 1989)

	Jan.–June 1985	Jan.–June 1988
Total patients	322 467	325 506
Patients prescribed opioids	184	243
	(0.060%)	(0.075%)

Table 4. Proportion of doctors prescribing opioids in Hannover, 1985 and 1988. (Adapted from Sorge and Zenz 1989)

	Jan.–June 1985	Jan.–June 1988
Total doctors	872	930
Doctors prescribing opioids	142	151
	(16.3%)	(16.2%)

than 325 000 patients, 243 patients received opioids (0.075%; Table 3). But between 1985 and 1988 there was no change in prescribing habits: only 16% of doctors ever prescribed opioids, —only 22% of the internists and only 4% of the gynaecologists (Table 4). Only 4% of the patients received prescriptions for more than 20 weeks in a 26-week period (Fig. 2).

These figures indicate significant undertreatment. The reasons may be on two sides. The doctors may not be making best use of the possibilities for prescribing opioids. On the other hand, it may be that the law is restricting doctors from prescribing as they would do if opioids were regarded like any other medical drug. This became obvious when the two opioids buprenorphine and pentazocine became subject to the BtMVV: there was a 61% drop in prescriptions for buprenorphine and an 84% drop for pentazocine; and, simultaneously, prescriptions for the two nonrestricted opioids tilidine and tramadol went up by 31% and 37%, respectively (Schmidt 1988). From these figures it can be seen that the legal restrictions achieve their immediate goal. However, at the same time the supply of strong analgesics for cancer patients is restricted in a way that prevents effective treatment.

Similar figures were revealed by an investigation in which all doctors prescribing restricted opioids were questioned by their local health department (Gostomzyk and Heller 1986). After this interview the prescription of opioids dropped by over 60% in this area. When the interviews stopped, opioid prescriptions rose again. The authors' conclusion is that our law is effective in preventing illegal use of opioids, but at the same time has severe side effects on the supply to patients in pain. These limitations need to be corrected as soon as possible (Gostomzyk and Heller 1986).

Patients

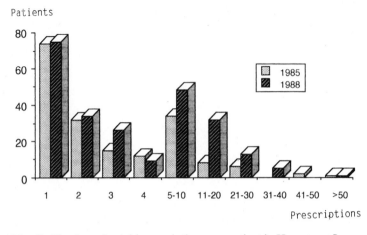

Fig. 2. Number of opioid prescriptions per patient in Hannover, January–July 1985 and 1988. (Adapted from Sorge and Zenz 1989)

Discussion

The triplicate forms, the legal restrictions, the possible penalties and old-fashioned medical teaching about "addictive" drugs prevent necessary pain treatment. As long as we still regard the triplicate forms as *Giftrezepte* —"poison prescriptions"—as they are commonly called, not much will change. Morphine is thus seen more as a poison than a helpful drug. Doctors prescribing morphine are regarded as verging towards illegal practice. Many doctors are reluctant to continue opioid treatment in cancer patients because they fear the legal consequences of mistakes in prescribing, and because they—very naturally—consider morphine to be a special drug for special cases and not for chronic pain treatment. The myths and misconceptions surrounding opioids are increased by handling morphine in a different way to all other drugs. Stratton Hill (1987) called this "painful prescriptions": painful for the patients, because they are not given the drugs they need.

At the same time, the legal restrictions in Germany have by no means achieved the goal of preventing or reducing drug abuse. The abuser is not interested in slow-release morphine with its very limited psychic effects. The abuser is interested in heroin and cocaine, and has no difficulty in gaining access to these drugs. Although we have one of the strongest opioid laws in the world, the figures for abuse and drug deaths rise from year to year. In 1989 there were 980 deaths from illegal drugs, an increase of 40% from 1988. This means that restrictions on the use of legal strong analgesics have no effect on illegal drug use. The legal restrictions only prevent effective treatment, not the illegal use of psychotropic drugs.

On the other hand, nothing is being done to counteract the enormous abuse of benzodiazepines in Germany. The amount prescribed of bromazepam alone is

200 times that of morphine (Schmidt 1989; Lohse and Müller-Oerlinghausen 1989). On the last sale list there were benzodiazepines in places 13, 15 and 16; morphine was in place 1125 (Litsch and Reichelt 1989).

Conclusion

Proper education and teaching may change some of our misconceptions and prejudices. However, nothing can be changed as long as opioids are regarded as special drugs to be prescribed on special forms in a very complicated way. Morphine is one of the most important drugs in palliative therapy. It must be handled like all other drugs. Legal restrictions must be removed, since they achieve no reduction of drug abuse but a considerable reduction in the treatment of pain. Cancer patients are suffering severely from an outdated law. Liberalization of the law is not enough, because the prejudices will be maintained as long as a law exists. There is no alternative to the complete removal of all legal restrictions to analgesic medication for cancer pain. "Morphine is there to be given, not to be withheld."

References

Bromage PR (1955) Spirometry in assessment of analgesia after abdominal surgery: a method of comparing analgesic drugs. Br Med J 2: 589
Gostomzyk JG, Heller WD (1986) Zur Verschreibung von Betäubungsmitteln durch niedergelassene Ärzte. Dtsch Ärztebl 49: 3456
Hanks GW, Twycross RG, Lloyd JW (1980) Unexpected complication of successful nerve block. Br J Anaesth 36: 37–39
Litsch M, Reichelt H (1989) Ergänzende statistische Übersicht. In: Schwabe U, Paffrath D (eds) Arzneimittelverordnungsreport '89. Fischer, Stuttgart, p 449
Lohse MJ, Müller-Oerlinghausen B (1989) Psychopharmaka. In: Schwabe U, Paffrath D (eds) Arzneiverordnungsreport '89. Fischer, Stuttgart, pp 352–367
Müller-Oerlinghausen B (1984) Medikamentenmißbrauch und -abhängigkeit. Münch Med Wochenschr 126 (42): 1210–1213
Porter I, Jick HI (1980) Addication rare in patients treated with narcotics. N Engl J Med 302: 123
Schmidt G (1988) Analgetika, Antirheumatika und Antiphlogistika. In: Schwabe U, Paffrath D (eds) Arzneiverordnungsreport '88. Fischer, Stuttgart
Schmidt G (1989) Analgetika, Antirheumatika und Antiphlogistika. Schwabe U, Paffrath D (eds) Arzneiverordnungsreport '89. Fischer, Stuttgart
Sorge J, Zenz M (1989) Schmerzpatienten unterversorgt. Dtsch Ärztebl 31/32: 1–4
Stratton Hill C MD (1987) Painful prescriptions. JAMA 257 (15): 2081
Twycross RG, Lack SA (1983) Symptom control in far advanced cancer: pain relief. Pitman, London
Weissman DE, Haddox JD (1989) Opioid pseudoaddiction—an iatrogenic syndrome. Pain 36: 363–366
WHO (1986) Cancer pain relief. WHO, Geneva

WHO (1987) Statistics on narcotic drugs for 1986. United Nations, New York

Zenz M, Piepenbrock S, Tryba M, Glocke M, Everlin, Klauke W (1985) Langzeittherapie von Krebsschmerzen—Kontrollierte Studie mit Buprenorphin. Dtsch Med Wochenschr 110: 448–453

Zenz M, Strumpf M, Tryba M, Röhrs E, Steffmann B (1989) Retardiertes Morphin zur Langzeittherapie schwerer Tumorschmerzen. Dtsch Med Wochenschr 114: 43–47

Treatment of Severe Cancer Pain by Continuous Infusion of Subcutaneous Opioids

A.H. Lang, K. Abbrederis, A. Dzien, and H. Drexel

Abteilung für Medizin, Stadtkrankenhaus Dornbirn, Dornbirn, Austria

Pain is a major symptom in about 70% of cancer patients [1]. Cancer pain relief is therefore a ubiquitous concern in public health. The guidelines for a three-step treatment as proposed by the World Health Organisation are widely accepted [2]. With this therapeutic strategy, using the WHO analgesic ladder, cancer pain relief can be achieved in a majority of patients [3].

Nevertheless, there is a group of patients with severe cancer pain who do not obtain adequate pain relief with the preferred oral route of drug administration. Major sources of problems may be the inability to swallow, nausea and vomiting, bowel obstruction, and the need for very high oral dosages, with consequent inadequate control of the chronic pain associated with malignant disease. Also, the conventional pulsatile pattern of oral, subcutaneous and intramuscular opioid administration, with the resulting peaks and troughs of the drug plasma concentration, can be responsible for insufficient pain control. Continuous infusion eliminates these undulations.

Since its first description by Russell in 1979 [4], several publications have reported successful use of continuous subcutaneous opioids in patients with advanced cancer [5–18]. Most of the reports are based on a small number of patients and different routes of drug administration are not compared. In a prospective and intraindividually controlled trial, we have compared the efficacy and safety of continuous morphine infusion with conventional intermittent oral or subcutaneous morphine administration [9, 17].

Materials and Methods

Naturally, all possibilities of causal antitumour therapy had been tried. Patients were included in this study when oral administration of strong opioids had produced severe drowsiness or nausea and/or failed to control pain adequately. After conventional treatment and after the patients had given their informed consent, continuous subcutaneous infusion of morphine was implemented in all

Table 1. Patients' clinical data

Patient	Age	Sex	Primary tumour	Cause of pain
In-patient group				
1	79	M	Pancreatic carcinoma	Liver metastases
2	79	M	Bronchogenic carcinoma	Bone metastases
3	64	F	Bronchogenic carcinoma	Bone metastases
4	75	F	Ovarian carcinoma	Peritoneal carcinosis
5	80	F	Ovarian carcinoma	Peritoneal carcinosis
6	68	M	Bronchogenic carcinoma	Bone metastases
7	44	F	Uterus carcinoma	Tumour infiltration
8	48	F	Uterus carcinoma	Tumour infiltration
9	73	M	Pancreatic carcinoma	Liver metastases
10	47	M	Kidney carcinoma	Bone metastases
11	78	F	Uterus carcinoma	Tumour infiltration
12	62	F	Pancreatic carcinoma	Liver metastases
13	73	F	Pleural mesothelioma	Tumour infiltration
14	72	F	Breast carcinoma	Bone metastases
15	21	F	Glioblastoma	Headache
16	78	F	Breast carcinoma	Liver and bone metastases
17	42	F	Bronchogenic carcinoma	Bone metastases
18	72	F	Non-Hodgkin lymphoma	Liver involvement
19	80	M	Pancreatic carcinoma	Liver metastases
20	78	F	Oesophageal carcinoma	Tumour infiltration
21	39	M	Bronchogenic carcinoma	Pleural carcinosis
22	63	M	Bronchogenic carcinoma	Pleural carcinosis
23	60	M	Bronchogenic carcinoma	Liver and bone metastases
24	59	M	Colon carcinoma	Bone and liver metastases
25	57	F	Breast carcinoma	Pleural carcinosis
26	14	F	Ovarian carcinoma	Peritoneal carcinosis
27	59	M	Rectum carcinoma	Plexus infiltration
28	58	F	Colon carcinoma	Liver metastases
Out-patient group				
1	62	F	Pancreatic carcinoma	Liver metastases
2	73	F	Pleural mesothelioma	Tumour infiltration
3	62	M	Colon carcinoma	Plexus infiltration
4	52	M	Prostatic carcinoma	Bone metastases
5	69	F	Pancreatic carcinoma	Tumour infiltration
6	83	M	Bronchogenic carcinoma	Pleural carcinosis
7	27	M	Hodgkin lymphoma	Bone involvement
8	43	M	Thymoma	Bone and pleural carcinosis

patients. Twenty-eight patients were studied as in-patients, eight were studied as out-patients. The two phases (conventional versus continuous subcutaneous infusion) were compared for each individual patient.

Clinical data on patients including age, sex, type of tumour and cause of pain are shown in Table 1. No changes were made in adjuvant therapy in relation to non-pharmacological interventions and neuroleptics, tranquillizers and steroids were supplemented occasionally, non-opioids were used frequently for skeletal pain.

Technique and Strategy of Continuous Subcutaneous Infusion (CSCI)

With in-patients 3 and 10 a Nordisk Miniinfuser (Nordisk, Gentofte, Denmark) was used. The remaining patients were treated with a programmable infusion pump (AS 6 MP, Travenol Laboratories Inc., Auto Syringe Division, Hooksett, NH, USA). In continuation of the study after publication, 21 further patients received CSCI by means of a CADD-PCA pump (Model 5200, Pharmacia Deltec Inc., St. Paul, Minn., USA). The pump syringes and reservoir (CADD-PCA) were filled with a solution containing 10 mg morphine sulphate and connected to a butterfly catheters. The needle was inserted into the lower half of the abdominal wall, the site was changed every 4–7 days. Initial doses were identical to the prior 24-h subcutaneous or intramuscular opiate dose; dividing the amount by 24 yielded the initial hourly basal rate. Switching from oral application to CSCI, equianalgesic doses of morphine were used [19]. When analgesia was satisfactory, the rate was tapered off to the minimum required for control of pain. Patients were informed of the possibility of receiving an additional bolus of the drug if pain recurred. The bolus dose equalled approximately a 1-h infusion. When bolus administration became repeatedly necessary, the basal infusion rate was increased.

Assessment of Pain Severity

The pain score of Dewi-Rees [20] was used to quantify the patients' subjective intensity of suffering. At daily intervals in the in-patient group, and weekly intervals in the out-patient group, interviews were carried out to describe the average intensity of pain by a number between 0 (best) and 10 (worst). The same information was obtained during the last week of conventional pulsatile administration of opioids.

Statistical Methods

The significance of a difference in scores between conventional administration and CSCI was assessed by the sign test of Dixon and Mood [21]. The χ^2 test was used to compare the incidence of side effects of the two regimens.

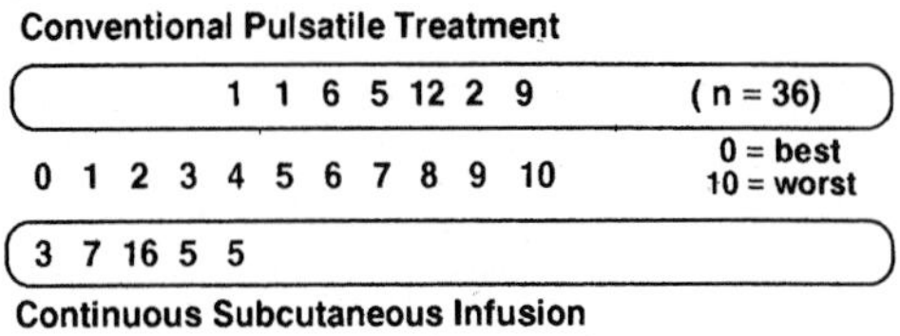

Conventional Pulsatile Treatment

		1	1	6	5	12	2	9		(n = 36)	
0	1	2	3	4	5	6	7	8	9	10	0 = best 10 = worst
3	7	16	5	5							

Continuous Subcutaneous Infusion

Fig. 1. Intensity of pain with conventional pain treatment and CSCI. (Adapted from [21])

Results

Of 327 patients receiving systemic analgesic therapy, 36 patients (28 in- and 8 out-patients) were included in our study because adequate pain relief had not been achieved using conventional analgesic modalities. Figure 1 summarizes the pain severity of all patients in both phases. Every individual patient showed a lower pain score during CSCI; the difference was statistically highly significant ($p < 0.001$). Pain relief was achieved with the first 10 h of CSCI and no patient suffered severe pain. Complete pain relief was rarely achieved, but pain could be kept at a level of about one third under conventional modalities. Comparing conventional treatment with CSCI, untoward side effects were less frequent and milder in CSCI. Constipation, defined as a stool frequency of less than four per week, was observed in 6 patients in CSCI versus 11 with pulsatile administration of morphine. Three of the patients suffering from constipation during both phases had been constipated even before opioid therapy because of peritoneal carcinosis. During conventional therapy 13 patients complained of drowsiness, while none was reported in CSCI ($p < 0.001$). No case of respiratory depression, defined by a respiration rate below eight breaths/min, was observed. Nausea was present in 11 patients in conventional therapy modalities and in one patient in CSCI ($p < 0.001$). Infusion was well tolerated in all patients, including long-term infusion lasting 49–197 days in the home setting. When offered to return to conventional pulsatile treatment, 35 patients wished to continue with the CSCI. Only one patient, who had an indwelling bladder catheter and a colostomy, did not wish an additional permanent device on her body. One other patient at a terminal stage of disease was confused and repeatedly removed his catheter. Conventional therapy was therefore resumed and pain recurred as it had before CSCI; the state of confusion did not recede. In all other patients, the subcutaneous infusion was maintained until death. No signs of tolerance to morphine were seen in the in-patient group, where the duration of CSCI was relatively short. In the out-patient group a rapid dose escalation was necessary in two patients because of pain recurrence at all sites of initial pain. A continuous infusion of methadone, given in a decremental dose, was successfully substituted for morphine for 2 weeks. Thereafter, lower doses of morphine provided pain relief again.

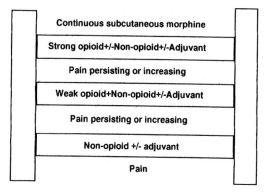

Fig. 2. Treatment sequence for relief from cancer pain. (Adapted from WHO Analgesic Ladder)

Discussion

Pain is a complex somatopsychic symptom that requires a multimodality approach. Pharmacologically, opioid-responsive pain can be treated successfully in the majority (71%) of patients using the WHO sequential ladder only (Fig. 2) [2, 3]. However, for one group of patients the oral route is no longer feasible; possible causes are summarized in Table 2.

In a prospective and intraindividually controlled trial, we compared a regimen of conventional pulsatile (oral or subcutaneous) morphine infusion with continuous subcutaneous infusion. The infusion regimen proved superior in all respects considered, particularly in regard to nausea and sedation, as also reported by other authors [5, 8, 14]. Pain relief, as assessed by the patients themselves with a simple numerical scale, was significantly better with continuous infusion ($p < 0.001$). The strategy of reducing opioid delivery once pain control had been achieved, enabled determination of the lowest fully-operative dose. It was surprising that such low doses as 10–30 mg per 24 h could consistently suppress severe cancer pain. We explain these results by the short duration of morphine pretreatment prior to the implementation of continuous infusion. On the other hand, patients with a progression of disease (for example,

Table 2. Indications for CSCI

Unsatisfactory response to oral administration
Unacceptable nausea, drowsiness or vomiting
Inability to swallow oral medication
Requirement of high oral dosages
Malabsorption syndrome

Table 3. Advantages of CSCI

Avoids peak level toxicity and trough level pain breakthrough
No delay in drug administration
Greater sense of pain control
Less dependence on caregivers
No need for an intravenous route

---

progressive cachexia or liver and renal impairment) needed decremental doses of morphine by CSCI.

Like other authors [3, 12, 14, 15, 18] we saw no opioid toxicity, manifested clinically as respiratory depression. In one study, a respiratory arrest was reported in a patient with significant impairment of his upper respiratory tract, as well as intractable head and neck pain secondary to recurrent oral cancer; this happened within 24 h of initiation of CSCI. In this case there is a questionable connection between the respiratory arrest and CSCI, but the possibility of treatment-related complication was not left out by the authors [16]. In our study, one patient wished to return to conventional treatment because she had a permanent indwelling bladder catheter and a colostomy; all other patients accepted dependence on a pump for pain control. This psychological inability to accept dependence on a "machine" or being unable to manipulate it is one reported reason for the failure of CSCI [16]. Painful chronic focal toxicity has been reported with CSCI [23]; in our series, with the low infused volume, only little local irritation at the site of the subcutaneous needle was seen infrequently.

No signs of tolerance were seen in the short-term treatment in-patient group. In the long-term out-patient group there was a rapid dose escalation in two patients. In both patients CSCI of methadone, given at a decremental dose, was successfully substituted for morphine for 2 weeks. Thereafter, lower doses of morphine again provided adequate pain control. These findings suggest that tolerance is not a clinically relevant problem of CSCI, as noted by Bruera et al. in their updating [22].

As a result of the recent advances in pump technology, CSCI can be offered together with patient-controlled analgesia by additional bolus. However, additional on-demand doses were occasionally needed.

Our data, summarized in Table 3, show the advantages and efficacy of continuous subcutaneous infusion of morphine. Of course, complete pain relief is rarely achieved, but pain can be reduced to a tolerable level. Overall, in our experience, this is a simple, effective and safe treatment for a minority of patients, who do not obtain adequate pain control with oral opioids in hospital or as out-patients.

References

1. Bonica JJ (1985) Treatment of cancer pain: current status and future needs. In: Fields, HL, Dubner R, Cervero F. (eds), Advances in pain research and therapy, vol 9. Raven, New York, pp 589–616
2. Sternswaerd J (1988) WHO cancer pain relief programme. Cancer Surv 7: 195–208
3. Ventafridda V, Tamburini M, Caraceni A, De Conno F, Naldi F. (1987) A validation study of the WHO method for cancer pain relief. Cancer 59: 850
4. Russell P. (1979) Analgesia in terminal malignant disease. (letter) Br Med J 1: 1561.
5. Dickson RJ, Russell PSB (1982) Continuous subcutaneous analgesics for terminal care at home. Lancet i: 165
6. Hutchinson HT, Leedham GD, Knight AM (1981) Continuous subcutaneous analgesics and antiemetics in domiciliary terminal care. Lancet ii: 1279
7. Campbell CF, Mason JB, Weiler JM (1983) Continuous subcutaneous infusion of morphine for the pain of the terminal malignancy. Ann Intern Med 98: 51–52
8. Miser AW, Davis DM, Hughes CS, Mulne AF, Miser JS (1983) Continuous subcutaneous infusion of morphine in children with cancer. Am J Dis Child 137: 383–385
9. Drexel H, Lang AH, Spiegel RW, Abbrederis K. (1985) Pumpengesteuerte kontinuierliche subkutane Opiatinfusion zur Behandlung schwerster Schmerzen. Dtsch Med Wochenschr 110: 1063–1067
10. Bruera E, Chadwick S, Bacovsky R et al. (1985). Continuous subcutaneous infusion of narcotics using a portable disposable pump. J Palliat Care 1: 45–47
11. Jones V, Hanks G. (1986) New portable infusion pump for prolonged subcutaneous administration of opioid analgesics in patients with advanced cancer. Br Med J 1: 1496
12. Coyle N, Mauskop A, Maggard J, Foley K. (1986) Continuous subcutaneous infusions of opiates in cancer patients with pain. Oncol Nurs Forum 13: 53–57
13. Sheehan A, Sauerbier G. (1986) Continuous subcutaneous infusion of morphine. Oncol Nurs Forum 13: 92–93
14. Schoon W, Erdmann H, Kleeberg UR (1987) Kontinuierliche subkutane Opioidinfusion. Med Klin 82: 805–811
15. Bruera E, Brenneis C, Michaud M, MacMillan K, Hanson J, Neil MacDonald R (1988) Patient-controlled subcutaneous hydromorphone versus subcutaneous infusion for the treatment of pain. J Natl Cancer Inst 80: 1152–1154
16. Swanson G, Smith J, Bulich R, New P, Shiffman R (1989) Patient-controlled analgesia for chronic cancer pain on the ambulatory setting: a report of 117 patients. J Clin Oncol 7: 1903–1908
17. Drexel H, Dzien A, Spiegel RW, Lang AH, Breier C, Abbrederis K, Patsch JR, Braunsteiner H (1989) Treatment of severe cancer pain by low-dose continuous subcutaneous morphine. Pain. 36: 169–176
18. Kerr IG, Sone M, DeAngelis C et al. (1988) Continuous narcotic infusion with patient-controlled analgesia for chronic cancer pain in outpatients. Ann Intern Med 108: 554–557
19. Foley KM (1985) The management of cancer pain. N Eng J Med 313: 84–95
20. Dewi-Rees W. (1972) The distress of dying. Br Med J 3: 105–107
21. Dixon WJ, Mood AM (1946) The statistical sign test. J Am Statist Assoc 41: 557–566
22. Bruera E, Brenneis C, Neil MacDonald R. (1987) Continuous sc infusion of narcotics for the treatment of cancer pain: an update. Cancer Treat Rep 71: 953–958
23. Adams F, Cruz L, Deachman MJ, Zamora E. (1989) Focal subdermal toxicity with subcutaneous opioid infusion in patients with cancer pain. J Pain Symptom Manag 4 (1): 31–33

Coping with Cancer Pain*

H. Seemann and H. Lang

Abteilung für Psychotherapie und Medizinische Psychologie der Psychosomatischen Universitätsklinik, Landfriedstraße 12, W-6900 Heidelberg, FRG

With the growing interest in the subject of pain in recent years, the number of publications on cancer pain has risen by leaps and bounds. The vast majority of these publications cite prevalence data to show that cancer pain is a problem that deserves attention (Foley 1979; Bonica 1979; Twycross and Fairfield 1982). They are almost exclusively concerned with (differential) diagnostics (e.g. Foley 1987) and the treatment of cancer pain from the vantage point of the doctor and nursing staff, because to date there have been shown to be enormous problems and deficits of knowledge in this area (e.g. Black 1979; Senn and Glaus 1982; Foley 1985; Ventafridda et al. 1985; WHO 1986; Brigden and Barnett 1987; Portenoy 1987). There can be no doubt that this commitment constitutes an important milestone on the road to improving the situation for cancer patients suffering from pain.

At present many authors, drawing on their practical experiences in caring for cancer patients, point more and more to the mental factors underlying the pain suffered; Portenoy and Foley (1989), for instance, note that "the true scope of the problem is not reflected in prevalence data" (p. 369). In addition, it is broadly accepted that pathophysiological findings can often explain the pain, only in part, or even not at all, and that the assertion of a causal connection between the advance of the cancer and the worsening of the pain is by no means compelling (e.g. Bonica 1979).

Authors who devote their attention to the mental aspects of the pain emphasize the link between acute pain and anxiety, and between chronic pain and depressive states accompanied by autonomic symptoms such as sleep disturbances, loss of appetite and libido, feelings of weakness, inability to concentrate, etc. (Chapman 1979; Stam et al. 1985; Portenoy and Foley 1989). Many of the studies on acute and chronic pain substantiate the finding that each

---

*The research project on which this report is based is funded by the Ministry for Research and Technology (no. 0701501). The responsibility for the contents of this publication lies with the authors.

and every pain is mainly determined by the cognitive and affective approach taken to the pain situation. Here the majority refer to Beecher (1959), who reported that wounded soldiers complained little about pain or required few analgesics when their injury demanded their removal from the battle area. Only a few isolated investigations, however, have considered this in the light of cancer pain, even though precisely here the scope for interpreting pain differs greatly from patient to patient. Thus Spiegel and Bloom (1983), for instance, report that it is easier to determine the degree of pain from its subjective importance than by locating metastases. To this day, however, the individual point of view of the patients suffering pain, their personal pain experiences, and their attempts to cope with them, has remained something of a marginal issue.

As pain research started to get interested in the forms of coping which can prove helpful for both experimentally induced and acute pain (Davidson 1976), it soon became clear that, as a result of the differences in the cognitive and affective means of tackling the situation, ways of coping with pain in artificially created pain situations (e.g. Ahles et al. 1983) cannot be simply transposed to natural pain situations, especially with sustained chronic pain. Recently, effective methods have been found for dealing with chronic pain, especially low back pain, (e.g. Bradley 1983; Rosenstiel and Keefe 1983; Turner and Clancy 1986; Fernandez and Turk 1989), but these also do not seem to be applicable for cancer pain. This is because pain associated with chronic diseases can constitute very differing sorts of burden for the patients, depending on the meaning they are assigned in the course of the disease. In chronic polyarthritis, for instance, the cause of recurring pain can easily be understood by the patient, who will interpret it as relatively unthreatening, and much the same applies to chronic back pain. Usually such patients, who have detailed knowledge about the cause of their pain, either develop coping strategies themselves (see Rosenstiel and Keefe 1983) or can be instructed in helpful pain coping strategies by a therapist. These types of pain are interpreted as limiting but not life threatening, and patients can learn to adjust to their pain and to live with it. Cancer patients, however, interpret pain, if and when it occurs in the course of the disease, as a sign of mortal danger. In many cases pain is the only perceptible warning signal which draws the patient's attention to the disease.

The different types of pain occurring in the course of cancer can, however, evoke such varying interpretations that from a psychological point of view the term "cancer pain" appears to be too general (see Seemann 1989). The subjective significance of pain depends on the timing of its occurrence, and on the way the patient can accept and come to terms with his disease at that point.

We would now like to look at some of the types of cancer pain in detail, analysing them in the light of their impact on the patients' interpretative frameworks and coping. The following remarks represent some of the preliminary findings of an ongoing research project in which cancer patients were interviewed on their subjective feelings about pain and their coping reactions.

Taking a cross-section sample, we questioned 165 out-patients with gynaeco-logical ($n = 74$) and gastro-intestinal tumours ($n = 30$) and malignant haematological diseases ($n = 61$). At the time of the survey 50.3% had pain, 47.3% had no pain and 2.4% (four patients) were free of pain as a result of effective pain treatment being conducted at the time. The two groups with and without pain were matched for age, length of illness and the tumour stage; in the overall sample there were nearly twice as many women as men, because of the greater number of gynaecological tumours. Of the patients with a tumour in the early stage ($n = 58$) 53% suffered from pain, with roughly the same percentage for each type of tumour. Of the patients with a tumour in the middle stage ($n = 66$), 51% suffered from pain but there were noticeable differences depending on the kind of tumour: 70% of gynaecological tumour patients had pain but only 18% of patients with haematological diseases. Of the patients with a tumour in the late stage ($n = 20$), 70% suffered from pain 91% of gynaecological and one-third of haematological cases. Twenty-one patients were still undergoing medical examinations and no data on the tumour stage was available. Of the patients who suffered from pain, 53% reported one type of pain, 31% suffered from two different types of pain and 16% from three or more different types of pain. The absolute intensity of pain is roughly the same in all stages of illness (maximum pain intensity 6.9 cm on a visual analogue scale (VAS) from 0 to 10, average pain intensity 4.3 cm VAS); in later stages of illness the tolerance to pain is reduced, so that the absolute VAS figures reveal a greater intensity of pain.

Pain with Diagnostic Relevance

Cancer starts with pain, often before the cancer is diagnosed, awakening suspicions in the person concerned and making him seek medical examination. Bonica (1985) states that at the time of diagnosis, 20%–50% of all cancer patients report pain. Daut and Cleeland (1982) classify the prevalence of pain according to the different types of tumour.

If pain turns out to have been a warning signal, in retrospect it is often perceived as a saviour, or at least as helpful, despite its role as a "bringer of bad tidings" and the shock of cancer diagnosis. It is therefore not surprising that pain related to diagnosis is described with great exactitude and vigilance, because after all this pain fulfils a function which is generally accepted by all, even if it is connected with considerable fears on the short term.

Post-operative Pain

In the next stage of the disease process, in most cases, comes postoperative pain. Coping with this is usually no problem because it marks an important stage in the treatment which comes as a relief: the tumour has been removed and the pain can be interpreted without reference to cancer, like any post-operative pain. It is noteworthy that patients do not describe post-operative pain with the same precision as the pain at the time of diagnosis. This is due to its lack of diagnostic significance. More important to them seems to be the quality of the pain treatment administered by the doctor and, more particularly, by the nurses, because this gives the patient an indication of how pain will be treated in the hospital if it should occur at a later stage in the disease.

Pain During Diagnostic and Therapeutic Procedures

In terms of its psychological impact, this pain is similar to post-operative pain. It is still easier to attribute causes to it, and it can be understood and accepted as necessary. However, if it is expected that it will recur frequently, anticipatory fears and pain may evolve in to anticipatory vomiting and nausea, these being well-known side effects of chemotherapy (Schwarz et al. 1985). It is known that anticipatory fears may evoke or worsen pain. A typical example here is when a cancer patient's pains intensify just before regular control check-ups.

Coping strategies suitable for pain associated with diagnosis and therapy—for example, relaxation and techniques to distract the imagination—are broadly known to the layman. However, it is one thing to use them for dental treatment, injections or other types of acute pain, quite another to employ them in similar situations during the course of cancer because cancer patients will often not allow themselves to be distracted from pain which is in any way related to their cancer, even if it is an acute pain which is well defined and clearly understandable.

These kinds of coping strategies should be taught early on, e.g. by pain immunization training (Turk and Rennert 1981), before or possibly during therapeutic intervention. This is already done in some institutions, particularly where children have to be subjected to repeated painful bone marrow punctures. The research group around Zeltzer and Le Baron (1982, 1983) and Jay (1985) and Jay et al. (1986), for example, reports very effective diversion techniques, based partly on hypnotic suggestion and partly on behavioural therapy, which often after just one session enable patients to cope effectively with acute pain in frightening situations of this sort. This kind of technique would also be extremely useful for adults because it would strengthen their belief in control, which is very often lost during cancer therapy (Taylor et al. 1984).

The interpretative context is highly important in pain persisting after diagnostic and therapeutic treatment. It makes a difference whether the pain can be seen as the price which has to be paid for improvement—even just temporary improvement— such as breast cancer patients report during breast reconstruction, or as a recurring warning signal of still-present cancer. Here the attending doctor can and must aid the patient's interpretation if effective pain coping is to be possible at all.

Pains During the Course of Cancer

The majority of the patients we interviewed, however, suffered from pain which had arisen at some point during the course of their illness and which now remained, recurred persistently, or had been replaced by some other pain.

When pain of this sort makes its initial appearance, it has at first the character of an appeal, like other acute pains, and demands attention and diagnosis. However, at the same time it arouses serious anxieties that "this could be something new". These anxieties are unendurable in the long term, so patients desperately attempt to attribute the new pain to causes other than cancer, and at the same time fear that they will be unable to maintain this attribution. This leads to constant wavering and constant uncertainty about their interpretations.

The ambivalence about their interpretation in turn leads many of these patients to prefer not to speak to the doctor about the pain, thus avoiding jeopardizing their attribution of a "harmless" cause. However, a basic precondition for the treatment of pain is that its presence is communicated, because obviously one cannot treat pains which one does not know to exist. Among the 87 ambulatory cancer patients in our survey who were currently suffering pain, we found only four who, as a result of effective ongoing pain treatment, were free of pain at the time of asking. They were noticeably younger than the rest and spoke openly about their pain anamnesis and treatment. Although 61% of the remaining 83 patients—a large proportion of whom proved to have considerable levels of pain intensity—allowed their pain to be treated, and although almost all of them followed the regular time table laid down, it was clear that they cut down the prescribed quantities of their medications. For, taken all round, it can be said that almost all of the pain patients asked have an aversion to medications to be taken in addition to the cancer therapy. They want to spare their bodies, offset the cancer therapy, which is felt to be toxic, by a healthy diet and natural remedies, and thus also tend to reject analgesics. The reservations many patients have about morphine, such as the fear of addiction and mental confusion, also add to the difficulties of treating pain in tumour patients.

The fact is that, although almost all of the pain patients questioned expressed the hope that they would receive a good pain therapy from their doctor, they were at the same time hindering their doctor by not talking about their pain, or at least only very late on, and by rejecting pain medication.

What else do we know about patients receiving pain treatment? It is noteworthy that in this group we mainly find patients who have been suffering pain for a long time or who have constant pain: 82% of these patients receive pain treatment. Still, they show a higher intensity of pain (particularly regarding maximum pain) and more psychovegetative complaints, as can be detected by so-called complaint inventories (e.g. von Zerssen 1976). Furthermore, a significantly greater number of "affective" adjectives are used when they describe their pain, especially those indicating suffering such as "wearing", "agonising", "fatiguing", "terrible" etc. (Hoppe 1985). The patient receiving pain treatment also report depression because of the pain more frequently—those in a normal mental state tend to have no pain treatment. The patients suffering continuous pain without being treated report more affective adjectives indicating anxiety, e.g. "alarming", "disquietening", "oppressive" etc. Among patients who report continuous pain, not only do we find that the parameters indicating mental suffering are significantly higher than among those who do not have continuous pain, but also that their pain tolerance, i.e. the pain intensity that is just bearable, is noticeably lower. In earlier stages, only 27% of patients suffer from constant pain. The further the illness progresses, the more frequent is the occurrence of continuous pain (69.2% of patients with late stage disease). In the late stage of gynaecological tumours in particular we often find that constant pain is accompanied by a high level of anxiety.

Pain patients show an increase in pain tolerance if they can share the burden put on them by their disease and pain with their social environment, i.e. by verbalizing it. The parameters of intensity of average and maximum pain (VAS) do not differ from those in patients who do not communicate their pain, but those who communicate seem to cope much better: in their judgement their average pain is "bearable" and they rate their maximum pain as being 1.9 times as strong as their "bearable" pain. For the patients who do not communicate their pain, however, the average pain already exceeds the "bearable" value by 1.4 times, and the maximum pain is 2.6 times as strong. It is also found that those patients who show a high degree of vigilance, i.e. those who look closely at their pain and the disease, are better able to tolerate higher pain intensities than those who do not want to take notice of their cancer or cancer pain. These findings are echoed by the results of Dalton and Feuerstein (1989), who found a connection between the duration and intensity of pain and pronounced alexithymia.

In our research, besides the cancer patients with pain discussed above, we also interviewed 78 cancer patients without pain, matched in terms of age, sex, and duration and stage of illness. The group of patients who had no pain at the time of the survey reported that they either did not think about pain at all, or only rarely; also, as the cancer was diagnosed, other cares had been more important than the fear of pain. This concurs with the findings of Dalton and Feuerstein (1989), but contradicts those of Holland (cited in Seemann et al. 1988) and those of Portenoy and Foley (1989), who report frequent anticipatory fear of pain when the diagnosis is made. When these patients did think about pain, they projected it temporally into the terminal phase of the illness. They expressed the hope that they would then receive good pain therapy, or would die quickly or commit suicide. Those who spoke of the latter were mainly patients who had already had experience of cancer followed by painful death in their immediate family or wider social environment. At the same time they did not show any concern, or only a vague one, about possible pain treatment to come. In our experience it tends to be the relatives who ask us which doctor or institutes might be considered, should the patient later have to undergo pain therapy.

Looking at the way our pain patients deal with pain, it can be seen that they hardly ever use the coping strategies for mastering pain which they otherwise consider to be quite natural for chronic pain, such as headache or backache. With our out-patients it often is merely a matter of just such trivial pain, which is in no way "cancer pain"—. Thus, a few of the patients in the group questioned practices relaxation exercises and cognitive distraction. The most common reactions to pain are lying down, not exerting oneself, waiting until it gets better, or simply putting up with it; a further reaction is being brave and praying (see also Dalton and Feuerstein 1989). A helpful means of distraction is mixing with people; thus, pains are often most severe and hardest to bear during the loneliness of the night or at weekends. To sum up so far: a lot of patients are unable to interpret and cope with the pain which arises during the course of a cancer illness in a similar way to those which arise in the course of a benign illness. The pain, as a signal for disease, is often suppressed and fended off, not only in the person's mind, but also in his social interactions, and thus is often not accessible to the existing possibilities for coping with it. At the same time, the mental and psycho-autonomic stress caused by the pain is considerable.

Psychogenic Pain

The opposite case, as it were, is also to be found: the patient wards off or denies the disease and expresses the anxieties he will not admit to in the form of pain. Here the complaints about pain are at the centre of the interaction, while talking about the cancer itself is not permitted. Pain which arises in this way is the most difficult for doctors and nurses to deal with, especially since there are often no physical findings, or only minor ones, to explain its vehement intensity. The patient does not "understand" his pain either. Because he is unable to accept his anxiety and his feeling of being threatened, and is also unable to communicate and show them to the people around him, he too is unaware that it is his pain which is literally "screaming" his fears, in place of himself. Sometimes resistance to medication and other attempts at treatment is an indication of the presence of this form of pain. It is most easily recognized by the fact that on occasion it can completely disappear, during events or prolonged situations in which the patients are able to forget their illness and the threat it entails. A short case study will hopefully illustrate this.

Mrs. H. (36 years old, married, with two sons) started to have pain under her right shoulder blade in autumn 1988. The pain was treated in various ways but without success, and was experienced by the patient as an increasing hindrance and threat. This was particularly as a result of a dream she had at this time, in which she was lying seriously ill and desolate in hospital, while her husband visited her with another woman. In her dream she said to her husband "But you can see I'm still alive."

Only one of the attempted treatments was briefly successful: a healer treated her shoulder pain by placing his hands on the spot and resting them there for a while. Shortly afterwards, a malignant tumour was discovered in her lung during a further diagnostic examination of the pain. Mrs. H. and her husband were informed of the findings. After the subsequent operation the patient was free of pain for 3 whole weeks. She found the post-operative pain inconsiderable, and she felt well and healthy. Then pain set in on her right-hand side, beneath the costal arch; this was followed by a succession of therapeutic interventions, such as medication, nerve blocks and the like, and then the excision of two ribs. The pain worsened, coming in attacks which descended "out of the blue". The first time I (H. Seemann) met Mrs. H., this state of affairs had already persisted for a good 6 months. With Mrs. H. in a state of relaxation, using hypnotic suggestion, we were able to see clearly that the pains were in fact sudden muscular seizures, a discovery which removed some of their threat.

During our very first meeting Mrs. H. had said, word for word: "If it wasn't for the pain, one would think that there was nothing wrong. It's as if the pain keeps telling me: don't be too sure of yourself!" Although the patient was already in a very poor state, having developed metastases which did not respond to radiotherapy, she behaved as if she just had a slight passing illness, and had simply to wait until it was over and everything was fine again. She also did not want to go home before the pain had been overcome, so that her children would not have to see her "creased up in pain".

On the occasion of a family get-together, which she had greatly looked forward to, she did not have a single attack of pain all day. She related that she had felt healthy and cheerful the whole day long. The next day the pain returned, even stronger. Even when the illness was so advanced that further treatment seemed pointless, her husband still refused to let the doctor talk about it in the presence of his wife. When a doctor—from now on she was in a pain clinic—nevertheless held an open conversation with the couple, it proved to be a great relief for the husband, but landing on deaf ears from his wife. Her pain did not improve, despite appropriate treatment with morphine and psycho-pharmacological drugs. In particular, her pain would interrupt us whenever her husband spoke with me about the hopelessness of further treatment or the deterioration in her condition, screaming out loud and demanding attention. After a pain attack Mrs. H. would at first be exhausted, but afterwards she would be cheerful once more, joking and chatting about trivial everyday matters. I cannot recall her even once mentioning her children of her own accord. While she became physically aged and emaciated, her manner remained playful and slightly cheeky, just as she had always been before her illness. Only about an hour before her death did she for the first time become quiet and serious, and was able to take her leave from her husband. The two children had clearly taken in and internalized their mother's message the whole time; i.e., that they were not to notice the threat her illness posed. They came across as detached and outwardly carefree.

Pain of this sort, which functions as an equivalent of repressed, threatening emotions, can only be overcome indirectly, once the person in question is able to approach his or her anxieties, which are in fact often the fear of death. Here it is particularly clear how closely facing one's illness is connected to overcoming pain.

Terminal Cancer Pain

When it comes to actual "cancer pain", which arises in a late or terminal stage, the main coping strategy of choice is proper pain treatment from a doctor. One should not underestimate the importance of the reassurance that can be given to cancer patients when they are told early on, and as it were in passing, that nowadays even severe cancer pains can be effectively treated.

At present we still do not know what forms of coping are used by terminally ill patients to tackle their pain. However, they certainly benefit from previously learned relaxation techniques and self-hypnosis therapy, as has been impressively shown by Spiegel and Bloom (1983), for instance. For an overview on psychological interventions in cancer pain, see Seemann (1989). In conclusion, one last point should not be left unmentioned; namely, that a supportive social environment, with people willing to talk about problems, is indispensable if cancer patients are to overcome their pain. The English have a special term for this: TLC, meaning "tender loving care".

Acknowledgement. We are grateful to the project workers to the physicians and patients of the polyclinic and departments of gynaecology, obstetrics and internal medicine of the University of Heidelberg for their cooperation.

References

Ahles TA, Blanchard EB, Leventhal H (1983) Cognitive control of pain: attention to the sensory aspects of the cold pressor stimulus. Cogn Ther Res 7: 154–178

Beecher HK (1959) Measurement of subjective responses. Quantitative effects of drugs. Oxford University Press, New York

Black P (1979) Management of cancer pain: an overview. Neurosurgery 5: 507–518

Bonica JJ (1979) Importance of the problem. In: Bonica J, Ventrafridda V (eds) Advances in pain research and therapy, vol 2. Raven, New York, pp 115–130

Bonica JJ (1985) Treatment of cancer pain: current status and future needs. In: Fields HL, Dubner R, Cervero F (eds) Advances in pain research and therapy, vol 9. Raven, New York, pp 589–615

Bradley LA (1983) Coping with chronic pain. In: Burish TG, Bradley LA (eds) Coping with chronic disease. Academic, London, pp 339–379

Brigden ML, Barnett JB (1987) A practical approach to improving pain control in cancer patients. West J Med 146: 580–584

Chapman R (1979) Psychological and behavioral aspects of cancer pain In: Bonica J, Ventafridda V (eds) Advances in pain research and therapy, vol 2. Raven, New York, pp 655–662

Dalton JA, Feuerstein M (1989) Fear, alexithymia and cancer pain. Pain 38: 159–170

Daut RL, Cleeland CS (1982) The prevalence and severity of pain in cancer. Cancer 50: 1913–1918

Davidson PO (1976) The behavioral management of anxiety, depression and pain. Brunner Mazel, New York

Fernandez E, Turk DC (1989) The utility of cognitive coping strategies for altering pain perception: a meta-analysis. Pain 38: 123–136

Foley KM (1979) Pain syndromes in patients with cancer. In Bonica JJ, Ventafridda V (eds) Advances in pain research and therapy, vol 2. Raven, New York, pp 59–75

Foley KM (1985) Pharmacologic approaches to cancer pain management. In: Fields HL, Dubnes R, Cervero F (eds) Advances in pain research and therapy, vol 9. Raven, New York, pp 629–653

Foley KM (1987) Cancer pain syndromes. J Pain Sympt Manag 2: 13–17

Hoppe F (1985) Zur Faktorenstruktur von Schmerzerleben und Schmerzverhalten bei chronischen Schmerzpatienten. Diagnostika 31: 70–78

Jay SM (1985) Behavioral management of children's distress during painful medical procedures. Behav Res Ther 23 (5): 513–520

Jay SM, Elliott CF, Varni JW (1986) Acute and chronic pain in adults and children with cancer. J Consult Clin Psychol 54 (5): 601–607

Portenoy RK (1987) Optimal pain control in elderly cancer patients. Geriatrics 42: 33–44

Portenoy RK, Foley KM (1989) Management of cancer pain. In: Holland JC, Rowland JH (eds) Handbook of psychooncology. Oxford University Press, Oxford, pp 369–382

Rosenstiel A, Keefe F (1983) The use of coping strategies in chronic low back pain patients: relationship to patient characteristics and current adjustment. Pain 17: 33–44

Schwarz R, Michel U, Hornburg E (1985) Chemotherapy and psychological side effects in breast cancer patients. Stress Med 1: 221–224

Seemann H (1989) Aktuelle Trends bei der Schmerzbekämpfung in der Onkologie. In: Verres R, Hasenbring M (eds) Psychosoziale Onkologie: Springer, Berlin Heidelberg New York, Jahrbuch der medizinischen Psychologie, vol (3) pp 193–211

Seemann H, Schug S, Zech D, Zimmermann M (1988) Bericht über den 2nd International Congress on Cancer Pain, 14–17, July 1988, New York. Schmerz 2: 216–224

Senn HJ, Glaus A (1982) Schmerzen und Schmerzbekämpfung bei Tumorkrankheiten. Schweiz Med Wochenschr 112: 1158–1164

Spiegel D, Bloom JR (1983) Group therapy and hypnosis reduce metastatic breast carcinoma pain. Psychosom Med 45 (4): 333–339

Stam H, Goss C, Rosenal L, Ewens S, Urton B (1985) Aspects of psychological distress and pain in cancer patients undergoing radiation therapy. In: Fields HL, Dubner R, Cervero F (eds) Advances in pain research and therapy, vol 9. Raven, New York, pp 589–615

Taylor SE, Lichtman RR, Wood JV (1984) Attributions, beliefs about control, and adjustment to breast cancer. J Pers Soc Psychol 46 (3): 489–502

Turk DC, Rennert KS (1981) Pain and the terminally-ill cancer patient: a cognitive social learning approach. In: Sobel H (ed) Behaviour therapy in terminal care: a humanistic approach. Ballinger, Cambridge

Turner JA, Clancy S (1986) Strategies for coping with chronic low back pain: relationship to pain and disability. Pain 24: 355–364

Twycross RG, Fairfield S (1982) Pain in far advanced cancer. Pain 14: 303–310

Ventafridda V, Tamburini M, De Canno F (1985) Comprehensive treatment in cancer pain. In: Fields HL, Dubner R, Cervero F (eds) Advances in pain research and therapy, vol 9. Raven, New York, pp 617–628

von Zerssen D (1976) Die Beschwerdenliste. Beltz, Weinheim

WHO (1986) Cancer pain relief. WHO Geneva

Zeltzer L, Le Baron S (1982) Hypnosis and nonhypnotic techniques for reduction of pain and anxiety during painful procedures in children and adolescents with cancer. J Pediatr 101: 1032–1035

Zeltzer L, Le Baron S (1983) Behavioral intervention for children and adolescents with cancer. Behav Med 5 (2–3): 17–22

Controlling Emesis in Patients Receiving Cancer Chemotherapy

R.J. Gralla

Ochsner Cancer Institute, Ochsner Medical Institutions, 1516 Jefferson Highway, New Orleans, LA 70121, USA

The decade of the 1980s proved to be an important period for the development of effective methods for controlling chemotherapy-induced emesis. Separate emetic problems were identified, an enhanced understanding of the physiology of emesis came about, effective agents were found, useful doses and schedules for these agents were established, combination regimens of greater efficacy were tested, and the ability to effectively prevent emesis was markedly improved.

With greater use of chemotherapy and with the development of newer cytotoxic agents in which emesis is a major side effect, the need for improved control of nausea and vomiting has become an important consideration in medical oncology and in supportive care. The primary objective of this paper is to provide a practical guide that discusses some of the major issues in the antiemetic approach to the patient receiving chemotherapy. This report will retain the appropriate sections from the 1988 edition [61] and incorporate new information and concepts.

Important areas to discuss include: (1) different types of emesis, (2) patient characteristics that may affect emetic control, (3) the patterns of emesis associated with different chemotherapy drugs, (4) the mode of action of antiemetics, (5) the active available antiemetics, (6) investigational drugs, and (7) antiemetic regimens.

Emetic Problems

In patients receiving chemotherapy, three types of emetic problems have been identified. Careful attention should be paid to which problem it is that requires treatment or prevention, since the causes of and treatments for the problem of emesis may differ significantly. These three emetic syndromes are acute chemotherapy-induced emesis, delayed emesis, and anticipatory emesis. An additional problem is that patients may have emesis for reasons other than their chemotherapy, e.g., it may be induced by pain medications, bronchodilators, other medications, or by tumor-related problems including intestinal obstruction. In these instances, adjustment of medications or treatment of the complications of the tumor may be more important than selection of the proper antiemetic drug. Most antiemetic studies have investigated acute chemotherapy-induced emesis, and this will be the major topic of discussion here, with separate sections concerning the other two emetic problems.

Patient Characteristics and Emesis

Several aspects of a patient's prior experience or characteristics may influence emetic outcome. Studies to date have indicated that the patient's age, alcohol intake history, prior emesis with chemotherapy, and possibly the patient's sex are factors of importance (Table 1).

Age appears not to be of direct concern in the control of emesis. Instead, younger age carries a tendency to acute dystonic reactions to antiemetics with dopamine receptor blocking as a mechanism of action [1]. This category of antiemetics includes such valuable agents as substituted benzamides, butyrophenones, and phenothiazines. In a report summarizing the experience of nearly 500 patients receiving metoclopramide, the incidence of trismus or torticollis was only 2% in those over age 30; a 27% incidence was reported in younger patients [1, 2]. In addition, dystonic reactions are also more common when dopamine blocking antiemetics are given on several consecutive days, [2]. This can be of special significance for younger patients, since several regimens for malignancies of this age group utilize chemotherapy on a daily schedule. Many of the newer antiemetic agents exert their activity by blocking serotonin type 3 (5-HT3) receptors. Agents that are specific for this mechanism do not cause dystonic reactions, so these drugs may prove to be particularly important for younger patients.

Table 1. Factors in chemotherapy-induced emesis

Patient characteristics	– Prior chemotherapy experience
	– Alcohol usage history
	– Age
	– Sex
Chemotherapy	– Emetic potential of the drug
	– Dosage and schedule
	– Route of administration
	– Time of onset of emesis
	– Consideration individually of each drug in combinations
Antiemetics	– Dosage and schedule
	– Route of administration

Three studies have indicated that emesis is more easily controlled in patients with chronic heavy alcohol usage histories (> 100 g/day, or approximately five mixed drinks) than in those without this past experience [3, 4]. In the one prospective evaluation in 52 patients receiving high-dose cisplatin and an appropriate combination antiemetic regimen, 93% of those with the high alcohol history had no emesis, as opposed to 61% ($p < 0.01$) of the other patients [3].

Poor control of emesis in past courses of chemotherapy predisposes a patient to unsatisfactory antiemetic results with subsequent similar chemotherapy. One trial in which patients received their initial treatment with the same antiemetic noted that major control was three times more likely in those who had not previously had chemotherapy [5]. Whether this is due to the development of conditioned anticipatory emesis or to other possible factors is not clear.

Several studies have suggested that it is more difficult to control emesis in women than in men. This is a complicated issue. Women enlisted in antiemetic studies are more likely to be receiving two or more emetic agents given in combination (especially cisplatin plus cyclophosphamide) and are less likely to have had histories of heavy alcohol usage. Thus, it is possible that factors other than sex are of greater importance in affecting the control of emesis. Multivariate analyses of large well-conducted trials will be needed to answer this question. This controversial finding is demonstrated in a recent interesting report [6].

Chemotherapeutic Agents and Emesis

The differences in the likelihood of chemotherapeutic drugs to cause emesis are given in Table 2. In general, the agents most often associated with emesis also induce the greatest severity of this side effect. Differences occur among patients and even among treatment courses in the same patient.

Table 2. Likelihood of chemotherapy agents to induce emesis

High potential	Moderate potential	Low potential
Cisplatin	Carmustine	Etoposide
Dacarbazine	Lomustine	Mitomycin-C
Dactinomycin	Doxorubicin	Methotrexate
Mechlorethamine	Daunorubicin	5-Fluorouracil
Hexamethylmelamine	Cytarabine	Hydroxyurea
Cyclophosphamide[a]	Procarbazine	Bleomycin
	Carboplatin[a]	Vinblastine
		Vincristine
		Vindesine
		Chlorambucil

[a] These agents are associated with a late onset of emesis.

Both the drug dose and the route of administration can affect the incidence of nausea and vomiting (Table 1). With most agents, emesis begins 1–2 h after the start of chemotherapy, in patients who have not previously received chemotherapy. A most important exception to this pattern occurs with cyclophosphamide: when cyclophosphamide is given intravenously in high doses, the onset of emesis is usually delayed until 9–18 h after chemotherapy [7]. Several studies have indicated that carboplatin may also induce a late onset of emesis. Although carboplatin is less emetogenic than cisplatin, it still can cause significant nausea and vomiting. A recent report concluded that a similar degree of good antiemetic control could be achieved for either of these platinum-containing drugs if appropriate antiemetic regimens are utilized [8].

The factor of a late onset of emesis emphasizes two important principles. First, to be effective, an antiemetic regimen must take into account the individual pattern and potential for causing emesis of the particular chemotherapeutic drug being employed. Second, when combination chemotherapy is used, each of the drugs must be individually considered. Thus, a regimen that is effective against cisplatin may not be well designed for the patient receiving cyclophosphamide, in that by the time the late onset of cyclophosphamide-induced emesis is reached, the blood levels of the antiemetic agent may have dropped too low to be effective.

The mechanism by which chemotherapy induces emesis is still not completely understood, although the studies of Borison have been revealing [9]. Studies support the hypothesis that reflex-induced emesis is caused by stimulation of receptors in the central nervous system or in the gastrointestinal tract. Receptor areas have been identified that affect a vomiting center in the lateral reticular formation of the medulla, which then coordinates the act of vomiting. An important area also located in the medulla is the chemoreceptor trigger zone (CTZ), in the area postrema. This receptor region is sensitive to chemical stimuli from both the blood and the cerebrospinal fluid. Chemotherapeutic agents or their metabolites may stimulate receptors in the CTZ. Impulses generated in the CTZ and transmitted to the vomiting center may then lead to the initiation of emesis. Neuroreceptors in the gastrointestinal tract, which was afferents to the vomiting center, may also play a role in chemotherapy-induced nausea and vomiting. These areas have many types of neurotransmitter receptors, including dopamine receptors. As mentioned above, several of the more effective antiemetic drugs bind to dopamine receptors, and are therefore also associated with dystonic reactions.

Of recent interest is the finding that 5-HT3 receptors play an important role [10]. When given in high doses, metoclopramide may effectively block 5-HT3 receptors as well as dopamine receptors. It may be that the antiemetic activity of metoclopramide is exerted through 5-HT3 receptors, while its side effects are the result of interaction with dopamine receptors. The newer antiemetics, to be discussed later, are more specific for 5-HT3 receptors and have a high affinity for these receptors.

Antiemetic agents that block neuroreceptors in the CTZ, the vomiting center, or in the gastrointestinal tract may be useful in preventing or controlling emesis.

Standard Antiemetic Agents

Several antiemetic agents have been shown to be safe and effective (Table 3). Since no agent is ideal, and since appropriate combinations of agents are more effective than single drugs, a familiarity with a few of the more active agents is essential. Among the best studied of the more effective agents are those that exert their activity by blocking dopamine receptors. These include such classes and agents as:

1. Substituted benzamides (metoclopramide, alizapride)
2. Butyrophenones (haloperidol and droperidol)
3. Phenothiazines (prochlorperazine and chlorpromazine).

Additionally, corticosteroids (dexamethasone and methylprednisolone) are effective agents, and benzodiazepines and cannabinoids may also have a role.

Table 3. Dosages and schedules of several standard antiemetic agents

Antiemetic agent	Route	Dose range	Frequency of administration
Substituted benzamide			
Metoclopramide	Intravenous	1–3 mg/kg	Every 2 h
	Oral	1–3 mg/kg	Every 2–4 h
Butyrophenones			
Haloperidol	Intravenous	1–3 mg	Every 2–6 h
	Oral	1–2 mg	Every 3–6 h
Droperidol	Intravenous	0.5–5 mg	Every 4 h
Corticosteroids			
Dexamethasone	I.v./Oral	4–20 mg	Once only, or every 4–6 h
Methylprednisolone	Intravenous	250–500 mg	Once only, or every 4–6 h
Phenothiazines			
Prochlorperazine	Oral	5–10 mg	Every 2–4 h
	Rectal	25 mg	Every 4–6 h
	I.m./i.v.	10–20 mg	Every 3–6 h
Chlorpromazine	Oral	25–50 mg	Every 3–6 h
	I.m./i.v.	25 mg	Every 3–6 h
Benzodiazepine			
Lorazepam	Intravenous	1–2 mg/m^2	Every 4 h
Cannabinoid			
THC	Oral	5–10 mg/m^2	Every 3–4 h

Substituted Benzamides

The most commonly used and most effective drug of this class is metoclopramide. Although some controversy exists, a pharmacologic study demonstrated that efficacy was correlated with high blood levels (>850 ng/ml) of metoclopramide in patients receiving cisplatin [11]. Also of importance is maintenance of an adequate level of this antiemetic at the time of emetic vulnerability through the use of an appropriate dosing schedule. In preventing emesis induced by cisplatin or by cyclophosphamide plus doxorubicin, metoclopramide administration every 2 h (beginning shortly before chemotherapy) appears to be the most effective schedule. Doses and schedules for metoclopramide are outlined in Tables 3 and 4.

Random-assignment studies have shown metoclopramide to be superior, or at least equivalent, to all other antiemetic agents it has been compared with, against cisplatin-induced emesis [12–17]. Several reports have also indicated useful activity against the emesis associated with a number of other chemotherapeutic agents [18–20].

High oral doses of metoclopramide (using 50 mg and 100 mg tablets) can result in therapeutic blood levels and can be highly effective [20–22]. In a comparison trial of similar high doses and schedules of oral versus intravenous metoclopramide (in patients receiving cisplatin 60 mg/m^2), nearly identical results were observed in both arms of the study. Emesis was completely controlled in half of the patients, while two-thirds achieved a major response (two or fewer emetic episodes) [21].

A recent study has explored markedly higher doses of metoclopramide (4 mg/kg to 6 mg/kg) given only once in patients receiving cisplatin [23]. Although the original antiemetic phase I trials did not exceed 3 mg/kg per dose, the total amount administered was as high as 15 mg/kg given over 10 h [5]. The rationale behind the very high single dose study included several points: (a) a single dose of metoclopramide (in this case in combination with dexamethasone plus lorazepam) given prior to chemotherapy would be convenient and economical, with fewer administration charges; (b) a high peak level of the agent would be assured, and a therapeutic level would likely be maintained throughout the period of emetic vulnerability; and (c) such high levels would be likely to saturate 5-HT3 receptors. The results of the trial indicated that these very high dose metoclopramide regimens are as safe and effective as lower dose combinations, and that the single prechemotherapy dose of each of the agents was convenient and cost-effective. The recommended single dose regimen was: lorazepam 1.5 mg/m^2 i.v. given 30 min before chemotherapy, plus dexamethasone 20 mg i.v. (given over 5 min) at 25 min before chemotherapy, followed by a 20-min i.v. infusion of metoclopramide 4 mg/kg immediately before chemotherapy [23].

The side effects commonly associated with metoclopramide include mild sedation, dystonic reactions (age-related, as discussed above), akathisia (restlessness), and diarrhea (which may be an effect of specific chemotherapeutic agents, such as cisplatin) [1, 12, 24]. In general, the side effects are easy to control or prevent. Akathisia is easily prevented or treated with a benzodiazepine; dystonic reactions can be dealt with similarly or with diphenhydramine. As will be discussed in the section on combinations of antiemetics, dexamethasone in addition to metoclopramide both improves efficacy and reduces diarrhea.

Butyrophenones

Haloperidol and droperidol were shown in initial trials to be active antiemetics [25, 26]. No substantial differences have been demonstrated between these two butyrophenones, and most of the comments below will refer to studies conducted with haloperidol. A formal study comparing haloperidol with metoclopramide in patients receiving cisplatin reported that both antiemetics are effective, although a trend toward greater activity was seen with metoclopramide [16]. Doses of 1–3 mg haloperidol given intravenously every 2–6 h have been most commonly used (Table 3); the higher doses and more frequent schedules have more often been associated with better results. Toxicity commonly includes sedation, dystonic reactions, and akathisia, with hypotension occasionally observed.

Phenothiazines

The unsatisfactory results observed with orally and intramuscularly administered phenothiazines encouraged the setting up of new studies to examine other classes of agents, different administration schedules, and higher dosage regimens. Structure–activity studies indicated that variations in the side chain at position 10 of the phenothiazine ring affect the antiemetic properties of these drugs [27]. Agents such as prochlorperazine would be predicted to have greater activity than other commonly used phenothiazines, such as chlorpromazine, but this predicted difference has not been established in patients receiving chemotherapy.

Prochlorperazine given in typical oral and intramuscular doses in random-assignment trials has been found to be less active than metoclopramide [12] or dexamethasone [28], and equivalent to or less active than tetrahydrocannabinol [29–31]. A study using intravenous prochlorperazine in comparison with metoclopramide has indicated more encouraging results [32]. There are two problems with this trial which should be considered: (a) an imbalance in the arms of the study (concerning additional cyclophosphamide with the late onset of emesis), and (b) failure to adequately evaluate the incidence of orthostatic blood pressure changes, an important side effect of phenothiazines with major implications for outpatient usage. Other side effects are similar to those listed for haloperidol.

Corticosteroids

Although several theories exist, the antiemetic mechanism of action of corticosteroids remains unclear. Several open studies and random-assignment trials have confirmed their utility [14, 15, 28, 33–36]. Dexamethasone doses have generally been in the range of 4–20 mg. In the majority of trials in which a corticosteroid is added to an effective agent of another class, improved antiemetic efficacy for the combination has resulted.

Toxicity has generally been mild with short courses of dexamethasone or methylprednisolone. There has been no indication of a lessening of chemotherapeutic effect through the use of steroids as antiemetics. With the low degree of toxicity and with a different mechanism of action than other agents, corticosteroids are ideal candidates for use in combination antiemetic regimens.

Benzodiazepines and Cannabinoids

Recent studies have indicated that benzodiazepines can be useful additions to antiemetic regimens. Trials with lorazepam have shown a high degree of patient acceptance, with a marked decrease in akathisia and in anxiety. Additionally, lorazepam may add a small degree of objective antiemetic efficacy [37]. In a phase I trial only modest major antiemetic activity was observed, but the subjective benefits appeared to make it an agent worth considering for use in combination [38]. A major difficulty in evaluating this agent's true activity is that it produces a dose-related memory loss [37, 38].

Most cannabinoid trials have included δ9-tetra-hydrocannabinol (THC); two synthetic cannabinoids, nabilone and levonantradol, have also been tested clinically [39–42]. THC has been tried at many doses with differing schedules. Doses in the range of 5–10 mg/m^2 given orally every 3–4 h appear to be among the most useful [13, 39, 43]. In general, THC has been found to be superior to placebo, and equivalent to or superior to orally administered prochlorperazine [29, 30]. Similar results have been reported with nabilone [41]. Side effects have been frequent but generally manageable, and have included sedation, dry mouth, orthostatic hypotension, ataxia, dizziness, a "high," and euphoria or dysphoria.

The role of the cannabinoids remains unclear. It is apparent that such agents as metoclopramide and corticosteroids are superior and have fewer side effects [13, 44].

Antiemetic Combinations

Trials of single agents have indicated which are the most effective antiemetics and which are most likely to be compatible with other active drugs. Guidelines for effective combination regimens include the following:

Table 4. Examples of and approach to combination antiemetics in patients receiving some specific chemotherapy regimens

General approach: Neurotransmitter blocking agent

plus

Corticosteroid

plus

Benzodiazepine or antihistamine

Chemotherapeutic agent	Antiemetic regimen	
Cisplatin[a] > 99 mg/m²	Metoclopramide 3 mg/kg i.v.[b] *plus*	30 min before and 90 min after chemotherapy
	dexamethasone 20 mg i.v.[c] *plus*	40 min before chemotherapy
	lorazepam 1.5 mg/m² i.v.	35 min before chemotherapy
40–70 mg/m²	Metoclopramide 2 mg/kg i.v.[b] *plus*	30 min before and 90 min after chemotherapy
	dexamethasone[c] *plus*	(as above)
	lorazepam (as above) *or* diphenhydramine 50 mg i.v.	
< 40 mg/m²	Metoclopramide 1–2 mg/kg i.v.[b] *plus*	35 min before chemotherapy (schedule as above)
	Dexamethasone[c] *plus*	(as above)
	Lorazepam or diphenhydramine	(as above)

Cyclophosphamide + doxorubicin combinations	Metoclopramide 2–3 mg/kg p.o.	every 2 h × 3 doses, then every 4 h × 3 doses
	or	
	metoclopramide 3 mg/kg i.v.	every 2 h × 2 doses, then 40 mg p.o. every 3 h × 4 doses
	or	
	metoclopramide 2 mg/kg i.v.	every 2 h × 3 doses, then 40 mg p.o. every 3 h × 3 doses (as for cisplatin)
	plus	
	dexamethasone 20 mg i.v.[c]	
	plus	
	diphenhydramine 50 mg i.v. or p.o.	with the first and then every other metoclopramide dose
Dacarbazine	(as for cisplatin 40–70 mg/m^2)	

[a] Cisplatin total dose given over 15 to 30 min in these studies. A longer time of cisplatin administration might require more antiemetic doses.

[b] Alternative choice: haloperidol 3 mg i.v.

[c] Alternative choice: methylprednisolone 250–500 mg i.v.

1. Regimens should combine agents that have different mechanisms of activity and do not have overlapping toxicities.
2. The drugs should be active as single agents, with the optimal doses, best route of administration, and proper schedules having been previously established.
3. Agents added to the combination may be useful if they lessen the side effects of the regimen or if they reduce other toxicities of the chemotherapy (Table 4).

Studies have compared the activity of metoclopramide with the combination of metoclopramide plus a corticosteroid. In each of these studies, the combination of the two active antiemetics has been superior to the single agent [6, 36, 45, 46]. In addition to the improved antiemetic efficacy of the steroid plus metoclopramide combination, it was associated with a significantly reduced incidence of diarrhea. An open study combining a butyrophenone with a corticosteroid also reported favorable results [47].

At several institutions the standard regimen for patients receiving high doses of cisplatin (120 mg/m²) is as follows: metoclopramide 3 mg/kg i.v. at 30 min before and at 90 min after the start of the cisplatin treatment, plus dexamethasone 20 mg i.v. at 40 min before cisplatin, plus diphenhydramine 50 mg i.v. at 35 min before cisplatin. The cisplatin, following hydration and mannitol, is administered over 20 min. With the subjective benefits seen with lorazepam, a recent study investigated the combination of metoclopramide plus dexamethasone plus either lorazepam or diphenhydramine, in a random-assignment design. The doses of the agents were as listed above, with the lorazepam given at 1.5 mg/m² i.v. instead of the diphenhydramine. The two arms of the study had similar objective antiemetic efficacy, with over 60% of patients having complete control and nearly 90% having major control. The lorazepam-containing regimen, however, was favored due to improved subjective results, with reduced anxiety and akathisia [37].

Table 4 outlines recommended regimens, and alternatives, for use with a variety of chemotherapeutic drugs. These regimens have all been tested, either in formal comparison studies, or in open trials. It is clear from this table that in nearly all instances, unless an agent is contraindicated for a specific patient, combinations are recommended.

Chemotherapy regimens which involve several consecutive days of treatment present a special problem in controlling emesis, for the antiemetics which block dopamine receptors appear to result in a greater incidence of dystonic reactions when given on multiple consecutive days. Of additional interest is the observation that when agents such as cisplatin or dacarbazine are given over several days, the emesis gradually lessens. An interesting regimen currently· under investigation in patients over age 30 receiving cisplatin at 25–33 mg/m² per day for 3–4 days gives gradually decreasing doses of antiemetics. Patients are given dexamethasone at 20 mg i.v. 30 min before chemotherapy on each day. Metoclopramide 2 mg/kg is also given, at 30 min before cisplatin. On the 1st and 2nd treatment days, the same metoclopramide dose is repeated 90 min after cisplatin; on the 3rd day, the metoclopramide is repeated but at a dose of only at 1 mg/kg, and no repeat dose is given on the 4th day. Diphenhydramine 50 mg i.v. is given with the first metoclopramide dose each day. The study is still in progress, but initial results are encouraging.

New Antiemetic Agents

At the time this paper is being written, several interesting new antiemetics continue to be investigational agents. It is likely that one or more of these will be widely available in the near future. While each of the drugs has unique characteristics, there are some common findings of importance. Each agent is believed to exert its antiemetic efficacy through 5-HT3 receptors. In trials to date, dystonic reactions and akathesia have not occurred. Most importantly, useful activity against cisplatin-induced emesis has been reported for each of the drugs. These agents include the serotonin analogs ondansetron (GR-C 507/75 or GR38032F) [48, 49], granisetron (BRL 43694) [50, 51], ICS 205–930 [52, 53], and MDL 73417. Side effects reported are similar for most of the agents and include mild headache and transient rises in transaminases. A substituted benzamide, batanopride (BMY 25801) [54] also appears to share this mechanism of action and to be free of inducing dystonic reactions.

Factors varying among these agents include short (2–4 h) versus moderate (9–16 h) halflives. This may influence whether single or multiple dose regimens are more likely to be optimal. Most of these drugs have good bioavailability, and studies with oral administration only may prove useful.

Testing continues with all of the drugs; however, there are a few impressions that have emerged from the current progress. First, the major advantage of these agents will likely be fewer side effects (dystonic reactions), which could allow greater ease of use in younger patients. Second, although reports of efficacy vary from ordinary to excellent, it appears that complete control of emesis in previously untreated patients receiving high-dose cisplatin is approximately 40%. This is major activity that is remarkably similar to that observed in well-conducted high-dose metoclopramide studies in this patient population. Thus, the newer agents should allow greater freedom from side effects and the inclusion of groups of patients that are currently difficult to treat. However, emesis will remain a problem for many patients. Optimal results will continue to be obtained by those who apply carefully established regimens in a precise manner.

On the basis of the proposed mechanism of action of the 5-HT3 inhibitors, it can be anticipated that combination regimens will be superior to single agents. The addition of corticosteroids would be a logical choice. Response rates of 60%–70% complete control and 80%–90% major control in patients receiving high-dose cisplatin can be predicted. Again, these are response rates similar to those achieved with metoclopramide plus dexamethasone regimens; the newer agents used in combination would be likely to retain their low side effect characteristics. If these newer agents ultimately have the same efficacy as metoclopramide, it would give credence to the hypothesis that the mechanism of antiemetic action is the same.

Other Emetic Problems

Anticipatory Emesis

This problem is defined as nausea or vomiting, often beginning before the administration of chemotherapy, in patients with poor control of emesis with past chemotherapy. As this is a conditioned response, the hospital environment or other treatment related associations may trigger the onset of emesis. The administration of the chemotherapy itself may bring on this response not only as a chemical stimulus, but also as a psychologic factor. The stronger the likelihood of emesis, and the poorer the control, the greater the likelihood of developing emesis anticipatory [55].

Treatment of this problem is important; however, preventing its arising probably gives better success. The difficulties of anticipatory emesis underscore the importance of giving the most effective antiemetics with the initial course of emesis-producing chemotherapy. Several reports have indicated that behavior therapy can be helpful for patients with anticipatory emesis [56, 57]; however, patients with this problem will need effective control of emesis with the next chemotherapy administration if further anticipatory emesis is to be avoided.

Delayed Emesis

Delayed emesis is defined as nausea or vomiting beginning 24 h or more after chemotherapy administration. This is a particular problem with major sources of emesis such as high-dose cisplatin. A natural history study observed that delayed emesis is less severe than that which occurs acutely, but still causes significant difficulties with hydration and nutrition as well as contributing to a lowered activity level. Although delayed emesis occurs less often in patients who have complete emetic control on the day of chemotherapy, it still can occur in this group.

The majority of patients treated with cisplatin at doses greater than 100 mg/m^2 (with the cisplatin given in a single dose or in consecutive daily doses) experience some degree of delayed emesis. The onset is most frequent 48–72 h after chemotherapy [58]. Two preliminary open trials indicated that steroid plus metoclopramide or prochlorperazine combinations can be useful in controlling this problem [58, 59]. A random-assignment comparison study has now been completed [60]. All patients received cisplatin 120 mg/m^2 as their initial chemotherapy and received a high-dose i.v. metoclopramide plus dexamethasone regimen for acute emesis on the day of cisplatin. Beginning 24 h after chemotherapy, patients were assigned to receive oral placebo, oral dexamethasone for 4

Table 5. Regimen for preventing delayed emesis in patients receiving high cisplatin doses[a]

Days 1 and 2[b]	Dexamethasone 8 mg p.o. twice daily *plus* metoclopramide 0.5 mg/kg p.o. four times a day
Days 3 and 4:	Dexamethasone 4 mg p.o. twice daily (metoclopramide given only if nausea or vomiting occurs)

[a] A modification of the best regimen determined in [60].
[b] Day 0 is defined as the day of cisplatin; therefore day 1 begins 24 h after cisplatin, day 2 48 h after, etc.

days, or the combination of the oral dexamethasone regimen plus oral metoclopramide. Significantly greater complete control over the 4-day period was observed in those receiving the oral combination (52%) over placebo (11%). Side effects were generally mild. The currently recommended regimen for controlling delayed emesis is given in Table 5.

Conclusion

The last 10 years have seen a major improvement in the control of chemotherapy-induced emesis and widespread employment of effective antiemetic regimens. Efforts to control emesis have become an ideal situation for the collaboration of physicians and nurses who are oncology specialists. While new agents are soon to be introduced and are likely to be helpful, better application of the available techniques can result in major improvements in patient care. The newer 5-HT3 inhibitors should widen the groups of patients who can have successful control of emesis. The goal of optimal control of emesis requires a knowledge of the more active drugs, experience with their use in combination, and consideration of the emetic problem of each patient.

It is important that new studies are accurately interpreted. Precision in evaluation techniques is mandatory if accurate results are to be obtained. Additionally, attention to the differing patient characteristics and to the specific emetic patterns associated with individual chemotherapeutic agents must be considered in the design of trials.

The control of emesis is one of many important topics in the supportive care of patients with cancer. The considerable research efforts of the past decade in this area have resulted in improvements; the application of these findings continues to be a responsibility for all of us in clinical oncology.

References

1. Kris MG, Tyson LB, Gralla RJ, et al. (1983) Extrapyramidal reactions with high-dose metoclopramide. N Engl J Med 309: 433
2. Allen JC, Gralla RJ, Reilly C et al. (1985) Metoclopramide: dose-related toxicity and preliminary antiemetic studies in children receiving cancer chemotherapy. J Clin Oncol 3: 1136–1141
3. D'Acquisto RW, Tyson LB, Gralla RJ et al. (1986) The influence of a chronic high alcohol intake on chemotherapy-induced nausea and vomiting. Proc Am Soc Clin Oncol 5: 257
4. Sullivan JR, Leyden MJ, Bell R (1983) Decreased cisplatin induced nausea and vomiting with alcohol ingestion. N Engl J Med 309 (13): 796
5. Gralla RJ, Braun TJ, Squillante A et al. (1981) Metoclopramide: initial clinical studies of high dosage regimens in cisplatin-induced emesis. In: Poster D (ed) The treatment of nausea and vomiting induced by cancer chemotherapy. Masson, New York, pp 167–176
6. Roila F, Tonato M, Basurto C, et al. (1989) Protection from nausea and vomiting in cisplatin-treated patients: high-dose metoclopramide combined with methylprednisolone versus metoclopramide combined with dexamethasone and diphenhydramine: a study of the Italian Oncology Group for Clinical Research. J Clin Oncol 7: 1693–1700
7. Fetting JH, Grochow LB, Folstein MF et al. (1982) The course of nausea and vomiting after high-dose cyclophosphamide. Cancer Treat Rep 66: 1487–1493
8. Mangioni C, Bolis G, Pecorelli et al. (1989) Randomized trial in advanced cancer comparing cisplatin and carboplatin. J Natl Cancer Inst 81: 1464–1471
9. Borison HL, McCarthy LE (1983) Neuropharmacology of chemotherapy induced emesis. Drugs 25: 8–17
10. Fozard JR: (1984) Neuronal 5-HT receptors in the periphery. Neuropharmacology 23: 1473–1486
11. Meyer BR, Lewin M, Dreyer DE et al. (1984) Optimizing metoclopramide control of cisplatin-induced emesis. Ann Intern Med 100: 393–395
12. Gralla RJ, Itri LM, Pisko DE et al. (1981) Antiemetic efficacy of high-dose metoclopramide: randomized trials with placebo and prochlorperazine in patients with chemotherapy-induced nausea and vomiting. N Engl J Med 305: 905–909
13. Gralla RJ, Tyson LB, Borden LB et al. (1984) Antiemetic therapy: a review of recent studies and a report of a random assignment trial comparing metoclopramide with delta-9-tetrahydrocannabinol. Cancer Treat Rep 68: 163–172
14. Frustaci S, Tumolo S, Tirell U et al. (1983) High-dose metoclopramide versus dexamethasone in the prevention of cisplatin induced vomiting. Proc Am Soc Clin Oncol 2: 87
15. Aapro MS, Plezia PM, Alberts DS et al. (1983) Double-blind crossover study of the antiemetic efficacy of high-dose dexamethasone vs high-dose metoclopramide. Proc Am Soc Clin Oncol 2: 93
16. Grunberg SM, Gala KV, Lampenfeld M et al. (1984) Comparison of the antiemetic effect of high-dose intravenous metoclopramide and high-dose intravenous haloperidol in a randomized double-blind crossover study. J Clin Oncol 2: 782–787
17. Richards PD, Flaum MA, Bateman M et al. (1986) The antiemetic efficacy of secobarbital and promazine compared to metoclopramide, diphenhydramine, and dexamethasone. A randomized trial. Cancer 58: 959–962

18. Strum SB, McDermed JE, Opfell RW et al. (1982) Intravenous metoclopramide. An effective antiemetic in cancer chemotherapy. JAMA 247: 2683–2686
19. Tyson LB, Clark RA, Gralla RJ (1982) High-dose metoclopramide; control of dacarbazine-induced emesis in a preliminary trial. Cancer Treat Rep 66: 2108
20. Gralla RJ, Tyson LB, Çlark RA et al. (1985) An all oral combination antiemetic regimen of patients receiving cytoxan + adriamycin + vincristine (CAV). Proc Am Soc Clin Oncol 4: 267
21. Anthony LB, Krozely MG, Woodward NJ et al. (1986) Antiemetic effect of oral versus intravenous metoclopramide in patients receiving cisplatin: a randomized double-blind trial. J Clin Oncol 4: 98–103
22. Garnick MB (1983) Oral metoclopramide and cisplatin chemotherapy. Ann Intern Med 99: 127
23. Clark RA, Gralla RJ, Kris MG, et al. (1989) Exploring very high doses of metoclopramide (4–6 mg/kg): preservation of efficacy and safety with only a single dose in a combination antiemetic regimen. Proc Am Soc Clin Oncol 8: 330
24. Von Hoff DD, Schilsky R, Reichert CM et al. (1979) Toxic effects of cis-dichlorodiamineplatinum (II) in man. Cancer Treat Rep 63: 1527–1531
25. Grossman B, Lessin LS, Cohen P (1979) Droperidol prevents nausea and vomiting from cis-platinum. N Engl J Med 301: 47
26. Neidhart J, Gayden M, Metz E (1980) Haldol is an effective antiemetic for platinum and mustard induced vomiting when other agents fail. Proc Am Soc Clin Oncol 21: 365
27. Wampler G (1983) The pharmacology and clinical effectiveness of phenothiazines and related drugs for managing chemotherapy-induced emesis. Drugs 25: 35–51
28. Markman M, Sheidler V, Ettinger DS et al. (1984) Antiemetic efficacy of dexamethasone. Randomized, double-blind, crossover study with prochlorperazine in patients receiving cancer chemotherapy. N Engl J Med 311: 549–552
29. Frytak S, Moertel CG, O'Fallon J et al. (1979) Delta-9-tetrahydrocannabinol as an antiemetic in patients treated with cancer chemotherapy: a double comparison with prochlorperazine and a placebo. Ann Intern Med 91: 825–830
30. Sallan SE, Cronin CM, Zelen M et al. (1980) Antiemetics in patients receiving chemotherapy for cancer: a randomized comparison of delta-9-tetrahydrocannabinol and prochlorperazine. N Engl J Med 302: 135–138
31. Orr LE, McKerman JF, Bloone B (1980) Antiemetic effect of tetrahydrocannabinol. Arch Intern Med 140: 1431–1433
32. Carr BI, Bertrand M, Browning S et al. (1985) A comparison of the antiemetic efficacy of prochlorperazine and metoclopramide for the treatment of cisplatin-induced emesis: a prospective randomized double-blind study. J Clin Oncol 3: 1127–1132
33. Aapro MS, Alberts DS (1981) High-dose dexamethasone for prevention of cis-platinum induced vomiting. Cancer Chemother Pharmacol 7: 11–14
34. Lee BJ (1981) Methylprednisolone as an antiemetic. N Engl J Med 3034: 486
35. Cassileth PA, Lusk EJ, Torri S et al. (1983) Antiemetic efficacy of dexamethasone therapy in patients receiving cancer chemotherapy. Arch Intern Med 143: 1347–1349
36. Kris MG, Gralla RJ, Tyson LB et al. (1985) Improved control of cisplatin-induced emesis with high-dose metoclopramide and with combinations of metoclopramide, dexamethasone, and diphenhydramine. Results of consecutive trials in 255 patients. Cancer 55: 527–534

37. Kris MG, Gralla RJ, Clark RA et al. (1987) Antiemetic control and prevention of side effects of anti-cancer therapy with lorazepam or diphenhydramine when used in combination with metoclopramide plus dexamethasone. A double-blind, randomized trial. Cancer 60: 2816–2822
38. Laszlo J, Clark RA, Hanson DC et al. (1985) Lorazepam in cancer patients treated with cisplatin: a drug with antiemetic amnestic and anxiolytic effects. J Clin Oncol 3: 864–869
39. Vincent BJ, McQuistion DJ, Einhorn LH et al. (1983) Review of cannabinoids and their antiemetic effectiveness. Drugs 25: 52–62
40. Tyson LB, Gralla RJ, Clark RA et al. (1985) Phase I trial of levonantradol in chemotherapy-induced emesis. Am J Clin Oncol 8: 528–532
41. Herman TS, Einhorn LH, Jones SE (1979) Superiority of nabilone over prochlorperazine as an antiemetic in patients receiving cancer chemotherapy. N Engl J Med 300: 1295–1297
42. Steele N, Gralla RJ, Braun DW Jr (1980) Double-blind comparison of the antiemetic effects of nabilone and prochlorperazine on chemotherapy-induced emesis. Cancer Treat Rep 64: 219–224
43. Chang AE, Shiling DJ, Stillman RC et al. (1979) Delta-9-tetrahydrocannabinol as an antiemetic in patients receiving high-dose methotrexate: a prospective randomized evaluation. Ann Intern Med 91: 819–824
44. Venner P, Bruera E, Drebit D et al. (1986) Intensive treatment of scheduling of nabilone (N) plus dexamethasone (DM) vs. metoclopramide (M) plus DM in cisplatinum (CP)-induced emesis. Proc Am Soc Clin Oncol 5: 253
45. Allan SG, Cornbleet MA, Warrington PS et al. (1984) Dexamethasone and high-dose metoclopramide: efficacy in controlling cisplatin-induced nausea and vomiting. Br Med J 289: 878–879
46. Rosell R, Abad-Esteve A, Ribas-Mundo M et al. (1985) Evaluation of a combination antiemetic regimen including IV high-dose metoclopramide, dexamethasone, and diphenhydramine in cisplatin-based chemotherapy regimens. Cancer Treat Rep 69: 909–910
47. Mason BA, Dambra J, Grossman B et al. (1982) Effective control of cisplatin-induced nausea using high-dose steroids and droperidol. Cancer Treat Rep 66: 243–245
48. Cunningham D, Popic A, Ford I et al. (1987) Prevention of emesis in patients receiving cytotoxic drugs by GR38032F, a selective 5-HT3 receptor antagonist. Lancet: 1461–1462
49. Kris MG, Gralla RJ, Clark RA et al. (1988) Dose-ranging evaluation of the serotonin antagonist GR-C507/75 (GR38032F) when used as an antiemetic in patients receiving anticancer chemotherapy. J Clin Oncol 6: 659–662
50. Addelman M, Erlichman C, Fine S et al. (1990) Phase I/II trial of granisetron: a novel 5-hydroxytryptamine antagonist for the prevention of chemotherapy-induced nausea and vomiting. J Clin Oncol 8: 337–341
51. Joss R, Rohrback D, Pirovino M et al. (1988) BRL 43694: a novel antiemetic to prevent chemotherapy (CT)-induced nausea (N) and vomiting (V). Lung Cancer 4: A181
52. Tyson LR, Gralla RJ, Kris MG et al. (1989) Phase I antiemetic study of the serotonin antagonist ICS 205–930. Proc Am Soc Clin Oncol 8: 331
53. Stamatakis L, Michel J, Van Belle S et al. (1989) ICS 205–930: a dose finding study in the prevention of cisplatin induced nausea and vomiting. Proc Am Soc Clin Oncol 8: 327

54. Smaldone L, Fairchild C, Rozencweig M et al. (1988) Dose-range evaluation of BMY-25801, a non-dopaminergic antiemetic. Proc Am Soc Clin Oncol 7: 280
55. Wilcox PM, Fetting JH, Nettesheim KM et al. (1982) Anticipatory vomiting in women receiving cyclophosphamide, methotrexate and 5-FU (CMF) adjuvant chemotherapy for breast carcinoma. Cancer Treat Rep 66: 1601–1604
56. Morrow GR (1982) Prevalence and correlates of anticipatory nausea and vomiting in chemotherapy patients. J Natl Cancer Inst 68: 585–588
57. Morrow GR, Morrel C (1982) Behavioral treatment for the anticipatory nausea and vomiting induced by cancer chemotherapy. N Engl J Med 307: 1476–1480
58. Kris MG, Gralla RJ, Clark RA et al. (1985) Incidence, course, and severity of delayed nausea and vomiting following the administration of high-dose cisplatin. J Clin Oncol 3: 1379–1384
59. Strum S, McDermed J, Abrahano-Umali R et al. (1985) Management of cisplatin (DDP)-induced delayed-onset nausea (N) and vomiting (V): preliminary results with two drug regimens. Proc Am Soc Clin Oncol 4: 263
60. Kris MG, Gralla RJ, Tyson LB et al. (1989) Controlling delayed vomiting: double-blind randomized trial comparing placebo, dexamethasone alone and metoclopramide plus dexamethasone in patients receiving cisplatin. J Clin Oncol 7: 108–114
61. Gralla RJ, Kris MG, Tyson LB, Clark RA (1988) Controlling emesis in patients receiving cancer chemotherapy. In: Senn HJ, Glaus A, Schmid L (eds) Supportive care in cancer patients. Springer, Berlin Heidelberg New York, pp 89–101

5-Hydroxytryptamine-3 Antagonists:
A New Class of Potent Antiemetics in Cancer Therapy

M. Soukop

Royal Infirmary, Glasgow, G4 OSF, Scotland

For many years nausea and vomiting have been recognized as side-effects of numerous chemotherapeutic regimens. The development of the useful new agent cisplatin, due with its powerful emetic effect, highlighted this patient problem.

The approach by Gralla et al. (1981) in the early 1980s, using intermittent administration of high-dose metoclopramide as an effective antiemetic, seemed an important advance. Experience with the high-dose metoclopramide regimen, however, has shown that even with optimum scheduling, alone, or in combination with other agents, this drug still fails to control emesis in a significant minority of patients (25%–40%). One major disadvantage of high-dose metoclopramide is the relatively high incidence in young patients of extrapyramidal side-effects. At standard doses, metoclopramide (30 mg per day) was found to act as a dopamine receptor antagonist, as well as causing a rise in serum prolactin. It was also recognized that enhancement of gastric emptying was a feature of the drug and that this perhaps occurred via a 5-hydroxytryptamine (serotonin, 5HT) receptor mechanism.

5HT was discovered over 40 years ago by Rapport and colleagues (1948). Recently there has been an explosion of knowledge relating to 5HT, with the development of selective agonists and antagonists for receptor subtypes. There is now good evidence for the presence of three different receptor subtypes, 5HT1–5HT3—possibly all with additional subdivisions.

The M receptor, now designated 5HT3, was first characterised by Gaddum and Picarelli in 1957. Renewed interest and work in the receptor by Fozard et al. (1979) stimulated research teams at Beechams, Merrell Dow, Sandoz and Glaxo, all of whom synthesized novel antagonist drugs with high selectivity and specificity of action. (BRL 43694, MDL 72222, ICS 205–930, GR 38032F). It therefore seems likely that, although the mechanisms of action of high-dose metoclopramide are complex, its improved efficacy at this dosage may be via 5HT3 receptor antagonism.

It rapidly became evident in the ferret model that these selective 5HT3 receptor antagonists were highly effective antiemetic drugs against a variety of chemotherapeutic agents, including cisplatin (Miner and Sanger 1986; Stables et al. 1987). This was true not only prophylactically but also, with BRL 43994, as intervention within 30 s of administration, the ferrets then returning to normal behaviour. In ferrets and in dogs, 5HT3 receptor antagonism does not block apomorphine-induced emesis. These antagonist drugs, therefore, do not exert universal antiemetic function by blocking the final common pathway, e.g. within the vomiting centre. Presumably they act at specific sites where 5HT3 receptors are located. Considerably more information is required on this matter, although 5HT3 receptors have been identified, in animal models, in high densities on afferent vagus nerves, in the area postrema and in the dorsal vagal complex (Kilpatrick et al. 1987, 1989).

Some structural dissimilarities exist between the four 5HT3 receptor antagonists, suggesting either structural differences in 5HT3 receptors or, more likely, variable binding affinities.

Clinical Experience with $5HT_3$ Antagonists

To date, most clinical work has involved either BRL 43694 (granisetron) or GR 38032F (ondansetron). Recent symposia on both these drugs have presented results of several collaborative multicentre studies. The data for each drug can be briefly summarised and features highlighted.

Granisetron

Studies were presented at a symposium on 3 September 1989, London (5th European Conference on Clinical Oncology), reporting collective data on 1229 patients all receiving granisetron with their first course of chemotherapy. I pick out here a number of points from this symposium.

A small placebo-controlled study was reported which clearly demonstrated the antiemetic efficacy of granisetron. In the placebo group emesis usually occurred 3–6 h after chemotherapy. The immediate cessation of emesis in all 13 vomiting subjects was striking and echoed the animal data and the previous ancedotal reports in man.

In two large studies of patients receiving high-dose cisplatin (mean dose 84 mg/m^2), granisetron was able to confer complete protection from emesis in 63%. The level of antiemetic control seemed independent of granisetron dose (40 or 160 μg/kg) and was at least as good as with high-dose metoclopramide and dexamethasone. With other emetogenic but non-cisplatin containing chemotherapy regimens, an even higher level of overall control was established (77%), again irrespective of a four-fold granisetron dose difference. In this study granisetron was being compared to the alternative antiemetic regimen of dexamethasone and chlorpromazine, to which it was superior. The side-effects profile for granisetron in all studies was excellent (Table 1).

Table 1. Incidence of adverse events with granisetron in 982 patients

Headache	13.8%
Constipation	3.5%
Diarrhoea	1.3%
Somnolence	1.6%
Extrapyramidal effects	0%

No significant difference emerged between patients receiving granisetron 40 μg/kg and those receiving 160 μg/kg in these studies. The most common side-effect overall was headache. This was usually mild or moderate and at most required simple analgesia. Pharmacokinetic studies in patients receiving granisetron have demonstrated no major departure from linearity within the dose range 40–160 μg/kg. A broad range in terminal half-life ($t_{1/2}$) has been shown both in patients and normal volunteers, with a mean half-life of 9 h (range 1.5–28.7 h) and 4 h (range 2.5–7.1 h) respectively. The variation in $t_{1/2}$ resulted mainly from variability in clearance values rather than apparent volumes of distribution, (Cassidy et al. 1988).

Ondansetron

A summary of data presented at a symposium on 30 June 1989 in London is presented here with the emphasis on important highlights (Proceedings of Ondansetron Symposium 1989).

Initial pilot studies had suggested that a daily dose of 32 mg ondansetron, given as a continuous infusion or intermittently on a mg/kg basis, gave optimum control of emesis. This was therefore used as the dose in two randomised studies of patients receiving more than 50 mg/m² cisplatin. Complete control of emesis was obtained in 44%, a further 29% receiving significant benefit with 1–2 episodes of vomiting (complete and major control 73%). This level of control was found to be superior to that achieved with high-dose metoclopramide (complete and major control 44%). There was no significant difference between the antiemetic control obtained using continuous and that using intermittent administration of the drug.

The combined results of three trials in patients receiving standard non-platinum treatments, mostly for breast cancer, showed ondansetron to give significantly better complete and major emetic control (74%) than metoclopramide (54%). This superiority over metoclopramide was maintained during follow-up of patients for the 5 days after chemotherapy.

Patients in all studies reported a preference for ondansetron compared to standard antiemetics (Table 2). Headache was mild and did not affect patient acceptance of the drug. Constipation was felt to be a real phenomenon, due to

Table 2. Incidence of adverse events with ondansetron in 773 patients

Headache	19%
Diarrhoea	8%
Constipation	3.8%
Sedation	9%
Abdominal discomfort	5%

effects on 5HT3 receptors in the gut, with consequent slowing of intestinal transit time.

In volunteers, ondansetron has a terminal plasma half-life of 3–3.5 h. The range of $t_{1/2}$ values for this drug, as for granisetron, is variable, especially for the oral formulation, which has a bioavailability of 59%. Data are also accumulating to indicate the value of the 5HT3 antagonists in controlling radiation-induced nausea and emesis.

Conclusion

Clearly the data available to date indicate that the 5HT3 antagonists are a major addition to the field of controlling chemotherapy related emesis. They have very promising efficacy with an excellent side-effect profile. Further work to optimise the use of these compounds is needed, but early evidence already exists that their combination with other antiemetics, e.g. dexamethasone, may be more effective than their use alone (Cunningham et al. 1989, Smith et al. 1990).

References

Cassidy J, Raina V, Lewis C, Adams L, Soukop M, Rappaport WG, Zussman BD, Rankin EM, Kaye SB (1988) Pharmacokinetics and antiemetic efficacy of BRL 43694, a new selective 5HT3 antagonist. Br J Cancer 58: 651–653

Cunningham D, Turner D, Hawthorn J, Rosin D (1989) Ondansetron with and without dexamethasone to threat chemotherapy-induced emesis. Lancet i: 1323

Fozard JR, Mobarok Ali ATM, Newgrosh G (1979) Blockade of serotonin receptors on autonomic neurons by (−)cocaine and some related compounds. Eur J Pharmacol 59: 195–210

Gaddum JH, Picarelli ZP (1957) Two kinds of tryptamine receptor. Br J Pharmacol 12: 323–328

Gralla RJ, Itri LM, Pisko SE, Squillante AE, Kelsen DP, Braun DW, Bordin LA, Braun TJ, Young CW (1981) Antiemetic efficacy of high-dose metoclopramide: randomised trials with placebo and prochlorperazine in patients with chemotherapy-induced nausea and vomiting. N Engl J Med 305: 905–909

Kilpatrick GJ, Jones BJ, Tyers MB (1987) Identification and distribution of 5HT3 receptors in rat brain using radiological binding. Nature 330: 746–748

Kilpatrick GJ, Jones BJ, Tyers MB (1989) Binding of the 5HT3 ligand [^{3}H]GR65630 to rat area postrema, vagus nerve and the brains of several species. Eur J Pharmacol 159: 157–164

Miner WD, Sanger GJ (1986) Inhibition of cisplatin-induced vomiting by selective 5 hydroxytryptamine M-receptor antagonism. Br J Pharmacol 88: 497–499

Proceedings of the Ondansetron Symposium (1989) Eur J Cancer Clin Oncol 25 [Supp 1]

Rapport MM, Green AA, Page IH (1948) Serum vasoconstriction (serotonin): IV. Isolation and characterisation. J Biol Chem 176: 1243–1251

Smith DB, Newlands ES, Spruyt OW, Begent RHJ, Rustin GJS, Mellor B, Bagshawe KD (1990) Ondansetron (GR 38032F) plus dexamethasone: effective antiemetic prophylaxis for patients receiving cytotoxic chemotherapy. Br J Cancer 61: 323–324

Stables R, Andrews PLR, Bailey HE, Costall B, Gunning SJ, Hawthorn J, Naylor RJ, Tyers MB (1987) Antiemetic properties of the 5HT3 receptor antagonist GR 38032F. Cancer Treat Rev 14: 333–336

Present Role of Corticosteroids as Antiemetics

M.S. Aapro

Division d'Onco-Hématologie, Hôpital Cantonal Universitaire,
24, Rue Micheli-du-Crest, 1211 Geneva 4, Switzerland

Many agents used as antiemetics induce severe side-effects. This paradox reduces the rate at which we can control cancer chemotherapy-induced nausea and vomiting. We need more effective agents and combinations thereof in this fight for a major goal in the quality of life of our patients. Indeed, total and not partial control of emesis is considered by most patients as the only clearly significant benefit from antiemetic treatment [1]. Should this goal not be achieved, many patients prefer antiemetic treatment giving minimal side-effects, such as with corticosteroids [2] or the recently developed serotonin (5HT3) receptor antagonists.

Background

The physiology of chemotherapy-induced emesis [3–5] and the relative emetic potency of chemotherapeutic agents or potency of antiemetic agents [6, 7], and the problems related to studies with antiemetics [8–11], have been extensively reviewed. Cisplatin, which invariably induces nausea and vomiting in non-alcohol-dependent patients, has been the main target of antiemetic efforts. Other agents reported to cause severe emesis are less well studied, as their use is infrequent (dacarbazine, actinomycin D, streptozotocin) and few adequately designed studies have investigated agents like cyclophosphamide, which induces delayed emesis. High intravenous doses of agents like droperidol, haloperidol, chlorpromazine or metoclopramide, associated with benzodiazepines and corticosteroids, are the best presently available means for control of chemotherapy-related nausea and vomiting. It may well be that the serotonin antagonists will prove to be just as efficacious, alone or in combination, and to have fewer side-effects (see Soukop, this volume). It should be kept in mind that study of chemotherapy-induced emesis is a new discipline, which has yet to come to an agreed definition of efficacy and treatment-related side-effects. We propose that the only criterion of efficacy is the *absence* of nausea and vomiting, for, as was

Recent Results in Cancer Research, Vol. 121
© Springer-Verlag Berlin · Heidelberg 1991

said in the introduction, this is what the ultimate judge, the patient, feels to be significant.

Pilot Studies

Observers have reported that chemotherapy cycles containing prednisone are better tolerated than those without steroids (as in the original alternation of MOPP/MOP (mustine-oncovin (vincristine)-procarbazine-prednisone/mustineoncovin-procarbazine) for Hodgkin's disease) [12]. Following this lead and other serendipitous observations, pilot studies were conducted using corticosteroids to protect against chemotherapy-induced emesis [13–16]. Most observations of activity were based on patients with a history of severe emesis during previous courses of chemotherapy. The positive results were encouraging, especially because anticipatory nausea and vomiting might have decreased the effectiveness of corticosteroids [17].

Many non-controlled studies have been reported since then and have given similar indications.

Randomized Studies

Corticosteroids Compared to Other Agents or Placebo

In the first of these studies, a double-blind crossover placebo-controlled design [12], 14 out of 20 patients, who received additional antiemetics, were reported to be considerably "helped" by the addition of dexamethasone. Out of 26 studies [2, 18–42], 12 [18–20, 24, 28–31, 33, 35, 36, 42] indicate that corticosteroids are superior to the comparative agent. Furthermore, the result with corticosteroids in "negative" studies is often similar to that with an efficacious but less well tolerated antiemetic. The "positive" studies, however, are limited to patients given chemotherapy involving no or only low-dose (less than $50\ mg/m^2$) cisplatin. It is worth mentioning that even patients who seem to gain no benefit from the antiemetic effect of corticosteroids in double-blind crossover studies indicate a preference for continuing in the study arm which contained these agents [2, 21, 43].

Corticosteroids Added to Other Antiemetic Agents

Controlled studies comprising 22 reports [42–63] can be found in the literature up to December 1989. Overall, 15 reports indicate a minor or major benefit in antiemetic control with the addition of steroids. Some of those considered insufficiently positive [42–44, 56–58, 60] are small studies, in which a difference is easy to miss. It can be concluded that corticosteroid-based antiemetic combinations provide significantly better control of chemotherapy-induced nausea and vomiting than non-steroid-based combinations. This important, sometimes crucial, benefit is observed in patients who are submitted to many types of chemotherapy, from dacarbazine or non-cisplatin combinations to high-dose cisplatin.

Corticosteroids Added to Serotonin (5HT3) Antagonists

Two pilot studies [64, 65] and the first randomized double-blind crossover study evaluating the value of steroids added to those new antiemetics [66] show very clearly that steroids retain a major role in control of cancer chemotherapy-induced nausea and vomiting.

Corticosteroids as Antiemetics in Children

Two pilot studies [67, 68] have shown that it may be possible to use corticosteroids to control emesis in paediatric oncology. There are no controlled studies and one assumes that the efficacy in children is similar to that in adults. As an example of such equivalence, a four-drug regimen including 0.7 mg/kg dexamethasone, metoclopramide, benztropine and lorazepam, has been shown to be superior to chlorpromazine in children aged 4–15 years [69].

Animal Studies

The antiemetic activity of corticosteroids was discovered by a lucky chance. It is only recently that animal study reports confirming these clinical data have appeared. Control of cisplatin-induced emesis has been observed thus in ferrets [64] and dogs [70].

Limitations to the Use of Corticosteroids as Antiemetics

Corticosteroids can decompensate *diabetes* or induce *psychosis*, even when used in single administration. They might reactivate a *duodenal* or *gastric ulcer* [71], but this is unlikely in very short-term use, and anyway, use of active antiulcer agents should allow the use of corticosteroids in the third of chemotherapy patients who need them. The many side-effects due to long-term use of corticosteroids should not be limiting factors in preventing emesis. It is interesting to observe that there may not be significant hypothalamic-pituitary adrenal suppression in cancer patients, even after a 4-week treatment with methylprednisolone [72]. Some concern has been expressed about the immunosuppressive effects of corticosteroids [73, 74], but most antitumour chemotherapies are already highly immunosuppressive in themselves. We have looked for a possible negative interaction between cisplatin and dexamethasone and have been unable to find a decrease of the antitumour activity of cisplatin either in a mouse model or in vitro [75].

Side-Effects of Corticosteroids as Antiemetics

Insomnia, euphoria or anxiety occur with corticosteroids as frequently as with prochlorperazine, an agent which induces significantly more somnolence [23]. Facial flush is often reported with methylprednisolone and several papers have mentioned pharyngeal or perineal itch [2, 19, 44, 76–79] with dexamethasone. It may be that this latter irritation is related to the vehicle for intravenous injection of the substance [76–78]. A single report of a case of acute posterior subcapsular cataracts has been published [80]. ACTH may cause melanodermia in a few patients [81].

Mechanism of Action

We remain without an explanation for the effectiveness of corticosteroids in the control of chemotherapy-induced emesis. The recently developed animal studies mentioned above may provide an explanation, possibly consistent with one of the following hypotheses. It has been proposed that corticosteroids may act on an activated prostaglandin pathway [14], but it has subsequently been reported that no increase in plasma prostaglandins has been observed in patients submitted to cisplatin treatment [82]. Corticosteroids might act on the chemoreceptor trigger zone, either by modifying capillary permeability [83] or by stabilizing some membrane or intracellular components (lysosomes?) It has also been suggested that they may also have a role in endorphin release [84]. Finally, the psychic activity of corticosteroids, the sense of well-being they confer, may play a role in this highly subjective setting.

Dose Schedule of Corticosteroids as Antiemetics

One notices, reading the papers cited in this review, that there is considerable variation in the dose schedules used by different authors. When used as single agent, dexamethasone has been shown to have good efficacy at 8 mg, with no improvement in results when doses were raised to 32 mg [85]. Dose schedule considerations have been addressed recently by one group which found no difference in methylprednisolone given in a single intravenous injection or three times a day [86].

We had speculated that administration of steroids should be started several hours before chemotherapy [87], but this has not been supported by adequate studies. Also, we frequently taper off doses over 2 days, as some patients complain of myalgia or recurrent vomiting after abrupt discontinuation of steroid treatment [16]. These procedures are necessary only for a minority of patients, but may contribute to control of delayed emesis [88, 89].

Conclusion

There are an overwhelming amount of controlled data indicating that corticosteroids decrease the severity of acute and probably delayed chemotherapy-related emesis. Used as suggested—that is, over a day or a few days—they should have no major side-effects, provided care is taken over patients suffering from diabetes or gastrointestinal ulcers, or who have had previous psychotic reactions. Corticosteroids have now been shown to enhance the antiemetic efficacy of serotonin receptor antagonists. It is clear that steroids remain an important part of our antiemetic armamentarium.

References

1. Bennett JM, Byrne P et al. (1985) A randomized multicenter trial of cyclophospham-ide, novantrone and 5-fluorouracil (CNF) versus cyclophosphamide, adriamycin and 5-fluorouracil (CAF) in patients with metastatic breast cancer. Invest New Drugs 3: 179–185
2. Aapro MS, Plezia PM et al. (1984) Double-blind crossover study of the antiemetic efficacy of high-dose dexamethasone versus high-dose metoclopramide. J Clin Oncol 2: 466–471
3. Borison HL, McCarthy LE (1983) Neuropharmacology of chemotherapy-induced emesis. Drugs 25 [Suppl 1]: 8–17
4. Akwari OE (1983) The gastrointestinal tract in chemotherapy-induced emesis. A final common pathway. Drugs 25 [Suppl 1]: 18–34
5. Peroutka SJ, Synder SH (1982) Antiemetics: neurotransmitter receptor binding predicts therapeutic actions. Lancet i: 658
6. Bakowski MT (1984) Advances in anti-emetic therapy. Cancer Treat Rev 11: 237–256
7. Joss R, Galeazzi R et al. (1981) Nausea und Erbrechen bei der Chemotherapie maligner Tumoren. Schweiz Med Wochenschr 111: 1614–1622
8. Pater JL, Willan AR (1984) Methodologic issues in trials of antiemetics. J Clin Oncol 2: 484–487
9. Olver IN, Simon RM, Aisner J (1986) Antiemetic studies: a methodological discussion. Cancer Treat Rep 70: 555–563
10. Morrow GR (1982) Prevalence and correlates of anticipatory nausea and vomiting in chemotherapy patients. J Natl Cancer Inst 68: 585–588
11. Parliament MB, Danjoux CE et al. (1985) Is cancer treatment toxicity accurately reported? Int J Radiat Oncol Biol Phys 11: 603–608
12. Winokur SM, Baker JJ et al. (1981) Dexamethasone in the treatment of nausea and vomiting from cancer chemotherapy. J Med Assoc Ga 70: 263–264
13. Baker JJ, Lockey JL et al. (1979) Nabilone as an antiemetic. N Engl J Med 301: 728

14. Rich NM, Abdulhayoglu G, Disaia PJ (1980) Methylprednisolone as an antiemetic during cancer chemotherapy—a pilot study. Gynecol Oncol 9: 193–198
15. Lee BJ (1981) Methylprednisolone as an antiemetic. N Engl J Med 304: 486 (letter)
16. Aapro MS, Alberts DS (1981) High-dose dexamethasone for prevention of cisplatin-induced vomiting. Cancer Chemother Pharmacol 7: 11–14
17. Morrow GR, Morrel C (1982) Behavioral treatment for the anticipatory nausea and vomiting induced by cancer chemotherapy. N Engl J Med 307: 1476–1480
18. Breau JL, Israel L et al. (1983) Efficacité de la méthylprednisolone dans la prévention des vomissements dus aux chimiothérapies par sels de platine dans un essai randomisé. Presse Med 12: 2058
19. Cassileth PA, Lusk EJ et al. (1983) Antiemetic efficacy of dexamethasone therapy in patients receiving cancer chemotherapy. Arch Intern Med 43: 1347–1349
20. Kolaric K, Roth A (1983) Methylprednisolone as an antiemetic in patients on cis-platinium chemotherapy. Results of a controlled randomized study. Tumori 69: 43–46
21. Cognetti F, Pinnaro P et al. (1984) Randomized open cross-over trial between metoclopramide (MCP) and dexamethasone (DXM) for the prevention of cisplatin-induced nausea and vomiting. Eur J Cancer Clin Oncol 20: 183–187
22. Giaccone G, Donadio M et al. (1984) Comparison of the antiemetic effect of high-dose intravenous metoclopramide in the prophylactic treatment of cis-platin-induced nausea and vomiting. Tumori 70: 237–241
23. Markman M, Sheider V et al. (1984) Antiemetic efficacy of dexamethasone. Randomized, double-blind, crossover study with prochlorperazine in patients receiving cancer chemotherapy. N Engl J Med 311: 549–552
24. Dana BW, Everts EC, Dickison D (1985) Dexamethasone vs placebo for cisplatin-induced emesis. A randomized cross-over trial. Am J Clin Oncol 8: 426–428
25. D'Olimpio JT, Camacho F et al. (1985) Antiemetic efficacy of high-dose dexamethasone versus placebo in patients receiving cisplatin-based chemotherapy: a randomized double-blind controlled clinical trial. J Clin Oncol 3: 1133–1136
26. Frustaci S, Grattoni E et al. (1986) Randomized crossover antiemetic study in cisplatin-treated patients. Comparison between high-dose i.v. metoclopramide and high-dose i.v. dexamethasone. Cancer Chemother Pharmacol 17: 75–79
27. Ibrahim EM, Al-Idrissi HY et al. (1986) Antiemetic efficacy of high-dose dexamethasone: randomized, double-blind, crossover study with high-dose metoclopramide in patients receiving cancer chemotherapy. Eur J Cancer Clin Oncol 39: 619–624
28. Shinkai T, Saijo N et al. (1986) Antiemetic efficacy of high-dose intravenous metoclopramide and dexamethasone in patients receiving cisplatin-based chemotherapy: a randomized controlled trial. Jpn J Clin Oncol 16: 279–287
29. Niijima T, Isurugi K et al. (1986) Randomized cross-over study on the effects of methylprednisolone, metoclopramide and droperidol on the control of nausea and vomiting associated with cis-platinum chemotherapy. Gan To Kagaku Ryoho 13: 2376–2382
30. Chiara S, Scarsi P et al. (1984) Low dose metoclopramide versus methylprednisolone in controlling chemotherapy induced nausea and vomiting. Chemotherapia 3: 333–336
31. Campora E, Chiara S et al. (1985) The antiemetic efficacy of methylprednisolone compared with metoclopramide in outpatients receiving adjuvant CMF chemotherapy for breast cancer: a randomized trial. Tumori 71: 459–462

32. Giaccone G, Donadio M et al. (1984) Comparison of methylprednisolone and metoclopramide in the prophylactic treatment of cis-platin-induced nausea and vomiting. Tumori 70: 237–241

33. Osoba D, Erlichman C et al. (1986) Superiority of methylprednisolone sodium succinate over low dose metoclopramide hydrochloride in the prevention of nausea and vomiting produced by cancer chemotherapy. Clin Invest Med 9: 225–231

34. Metz CA, Freedman RS et al. (1987) Methylprednisolone in cis-platinum induced nausea and emesis: a placebo-controlled trial. Gynecol Oncol 27: 84–89

35. Martin Jimenez M, Diaz-Rubio E (1986) Atlas dosis de metilpredinisolona como tratamiento antiemético adyuvante de la metoclopramida en los vómitos inducidos por cisplatino. Resultados de un estudio controlado. Neoplasia 3: 61–63

36. Cunningham D, Evans C et al. (1987) Comparison of antiemetic efficacy of domperidone, metoclopramide, and dexamethasone in patients receiving outpatient chemotherapy regimens. Br Med J 295: 250

37. Roila F, Tonato M et al. (1987) Double-blind controlled trial of the antiemetic efficacy and toxicity of methylprednisolone (MP), metoclopramide (MTC) and domperidone (DMP) in breast cancer patients treated with i.v. CMF. Eur J Cancer Clin Oncol 23: 615–617

38. Al-Idrissi HY, Ibrahim EM et al. (1988) Antiemetic efficacy of high-dose dexamethasone: randomized, double-blind, crossover study with a combination of dexamethasone, metoclopramide and diphenhydramine. Br J Cancer 57: 308–312

39. Basurto C, Roila F et al. (1988) A double-blind trial comparing antiemetic efficacy and toxicity of metoclopramide versus methylprednisolone versus domperidone in patients receiving doxorubicin chemotherapy alone or in combination with other antiblastic agents. Am J Clin Oncol 11: 594–596

40. Roila F, Basurto C et al. (1988) Methylprednisolone versus metoclopramide for prevention of nausea and vomiting in breast cancer patients treated with intravenous cyclophosphamide methotrexate 5-fluorouracil: a double-blind randomized study. Oncology 45: 346–349

41. Goldstein D, Levi JA, Woods RL et al. (1989) Double-blind randomized cross-over trial of dexamethasone and prochlorperazine as anti-emetics for cancer chemotherapy. Oncology 46: 105–108

42. Pollera CF, Nardi M, Marolla P et al. (1989) Effective control of CMF-related emesis with high-dose dexamethasone: results of a double-blind crossover trail with metoclopramide and placebo. Am J Clin Oncol 12: 524–529

43. Strum SB, Mc Dermed JE et al. (1985) High-dose intravenous metoclopramide versus combination high-dose metoclopramide and intravenous dexamethasone in preventing cisplatin-induced nausea and emesis: a single-blind crossover comparison of antiemetic efficacy. J Clin Oncol 3: 245–251

44. Pollera CF, Nardi M et al. (1987) A randomized trial comparing alizapride alone or with dexamethasone vs a metoclopramide-dexamethasone combination for emesis induced by moderate-dose cisplatin. Cancer Chemother Pharmacol 19: 335–338

45. Gathercole F, Connolly N, Birdsell J (1982) The use of dexamethasone (hexadrol) as an antiemetic in association with chemotherapy for neoplastic disease. Oncol Nurs Forum 9: 17–19

46. Bruera E, Roca E et al. (1986) Improved control of chemotherapy induced emesis by the addition of dexamethasone to metoclopramide in patients resistant to metoclopramide. Cancer Treat Rep 67: 381–383

47. Colbert N, Izrael V et al. (1983) Adrenocorticotropic hormone in the prevention of cisplatin–induced nausea and vomiting. J Clin Oncol 1: 635–639
48. Allan SG, Cornbleet MA et al. (1984) Dexamethasone and high-dose metoclopramide efficacy in controlling cisplatin-induced nausea and vomiting. Br Med J 289: 878–879
49. Donovitz GS, O-Quinn AG et al. (1984) Antiemetic efficacy of high-dose corticosteroids and droperidol and metoclopramide. Gynecol Oncol 18: 320–325
50. Panza N, de Cesare M et al. (1984) Methylprednisolone and chlorpromazine alone or in combination for the control of cisplatin-induced emesis. Cancer Treat Rep 68: 1310–1311
51. Benrubi GI, Norvell M et al. (1985) The use of methylprednisolone and metoclopramide in control of emesis in patients receiving cis-platinum. Gynecol Oncol 21: 306–313
52. Ell C, Konig HJ et al. (1985) Antiemetic efficacy of moderately high-dose metoclopramide in patients receiving varying doses of cisplatin. Controlled comparison with a combination of methylprednisolone and metoclopramide. Oncology 42: 354–357
53. Becouarn Y, Nguyen B et al. (1986) Improved control of cisplatin-induced emesis with a combination of high doses of methylprednisolone and metoclopramide: a single-blind randomized trial. Eur J Cancer Oncol 22: 1421–1424
54. Fujii M, Kiura K et al. (1986) Randomized crossover trial of the antiemetic effects obtained with metoclopramide and droperidol versus those obtained with metoclopramide, droperidol and methylprednisolone in patients receiving cis-platinum chemotherapy. Gan To Kagaku Ryoho 13: 2562–2567
55. Rhinehart SN, Dugan WM et al. (1986) The value of dexamethasone when added to combination drug therapy in the prevention of cisplatin-induced nausea and vomiting, evaluated by time-lapse video technology. Prog Clin Biol Res 216: 407–416
56. Senn HJ, Kohler M et al. (1986) Prevention of nausea and emesis during cytostatic therapy. Antiemetic efficacy of high-dosage oral metoclopramide without and with prednisone. Dtsch Med Wochenschr 11: 129–135
57. Shinkai T, Saijo N et al. (1986) Antiemetic efficacy of high-dose intravenous metoclopramide and dexamethasone in patients receiving cisplatin-based chemotherapy: a randomized controlled trial. Jpn J Clin Oncol 6: 279–287
58. Grunberg SM, Akerley WL et al. (1986) Comparison of metoclopramide and metoclopramide plus dexamethasone for complete protection from cisplatinum-induced emesis. Cancer Invest 4: 379–385
59. Roila F, Tonato M et al. (1987) Antiemetic activity of high doses of metoclopramide combined with methylprednisolone versus metoclopramide alone in cisplatin-treated cancer patients: a randomized double-blind trial of the Italian Oncology Group for Clinical Research. J Clin Oncol 5: 141–149
60. Giaccone G, Bertetto O et al. (1988) High doses of methylprednisolone with or without alizapride in the prevention of cisplatin-induced emesis. A randomized, double-blind, crossover study. Oncology 45: 74–78
61. Martin Jiménez M, Diaz-Rubio E (1986) Actividad antiemetica de las altas dosis de metilprednisolona intravenosa en los vomitos inducicos por quimioterapia antineoplastica. Resultados de un estudio controlado. An Med Intern (Madr) 11: 525–528
62. Gez E, Brufman G, Kaufman B et al. (1989) Methylprednisolone and chlorpromazine in patients receiving cancer chemotherapy: a prospective non-randomized study. J Chemother 1: 140–143

63. Basurto C, Roila F, Tonato M et al. (1989) Antiemetic activity of high-dose metoclopramide combined with methylprednisolone versus metoclopramide alone in dacarbazine-treated cancer patients. A randomized double-blind study of the Italian Oncology Group for Clinical Research. Am J Clin Oncol 12: 235–238
64. Carmichael J, Cantwell BMJ, Edwards CM, Rapeport WG, Harris AL (1988) The serotonin type 3 receptor antagonist BRL 43694 and nausea and vomiting induced by cisplatin. Br Med J 297: 110–111
65. Cunningham D, Turner A, Hawthorn J et al. (1989) Ondansetron with and without dexamethasone to treat chemotherapy-induced emesis. Lancet i: 1323
66. Roila F, Tonato M, Cognetti F et al. (1990) A double-blind multicentre randomized crossover study comparing the antiemetic efficacy and tolerability of ondansetron (OND) vs OND plus dexamethasone (DEX) in cisplatin (CDDP) treated cancer patients (PTS). Presented at the 2nd International Symposium on Supportive Care, St Gallen (this volume)
67. Ise T, Ohira A et al. (1982) Clinical evaluation of antiemetics for vomiting due to cancer chemotherapy in children. Gan To Kagaku Ryoho 9: 1108–1118
68. Mehta P, Gross S et al. (1986) Methylprednisolone for chemotherapy-induced emesis: a double-blind randomized trial in children. J Pediatr 108: 774–776
69. Marshall G, Kerr S, Vowels M et al. (1989) Antiemetic therapy for chemotherapy-induced vomiting: metoclopramide, benzotropine, dexamethasone, and lorazepam regimen compared with chlorpromazine alone. J Pediatr 115: 156–160
70. Matsumoto I, Aikawa T, Kanda T et al. (1989) Amelioration of cisplatin-induced vomiting and anorexia by methylprednisolone. Gan To Kagaku Ryoko 16: 833–838
71. Bloom BS (1989) Risk and cost of gastrointestinal side effects associated with nonsteroidal anti-inflammatory drugs. Arch Intern Med 149: 1019–1022
72. Levitt M, Sharma RN et al. (1979) Normal metyrapone response after 1 month of high-dose methylprednisolone in cancer patients: a phase I study. Cancer Treat Rep 63: 1327–1330
73. Haid M (1981) Steroid antiemesis may be harmful. N Engl J Med 304: 1237
74. Grunewald HW, Rosner F (1984) Dexamethasone as an antiemetic during cancer chemotherapy. Ann Intern Med 101: 398
75. Aapro MS, Alberts DS, Serokman R (1983) Lack of dexamethasone effect on the antitumor activity of cisplatin. Cancer Treat Rep 67: 1013–1017
76. Baharav E, Harpaz D et al. (1986) Dexamethasone-induced perineal irritation. N Engl J Med 314: 515
77. Allan SG, Leonard RCF (1986) Dexamethasone antiemesis and side-effects. Lancet i: 1035
78. Thomas VL (1986) More on dexamethasone-induced perineal irritation. N Engl J Med 314: 1643
79. Palmer MC, Colls BM (1987) Amelioration of cytotoxic-induced emesis with high-dose metoclopramide, dexamethasone and lorazepam. Cancer Chemother Pharmacol 19: 331–334
80. Bluming AZ, Zeegen P (1986) Cataracts induced by intermittent decadron used as an antiemetic. J Clin Oncol 4: 221–223
81. Demuynck B, Gramont A, de Gonzalez-Cavalli G et al. (1989) Randomized trial of sustained-release ACTH versus sustained-release ACTH and metoclopramide for the prevention of emesis induced by cyclophosphamide-adriamycin-5FU chemotherapy (in french). Semin Hôp Paris 65: 1742–1744

82. Stephen LC, Rine J et al. (1981) The role of prostaglandins in the excessive nausea and vomiting after intravascular cis-platinum therapy. Gynecol Oncol 12: 89–91
83. Livera P, Trojano M, Simone IL et al. (1985) Acute changes in blood CSF barrier permselectivity to serum proteins after intrathecal methotrexate and CNS irradiation. J Neurol 231: 336–339
84. Harris AL (1982) Cytotoxic-therapy-induced vomiting is mediated via enkephalin pathways. Lancet i: 714
85. Drapkin RL, Sokl GH et al. (1982) The antiemetic effect and dose response of dexamethasone in patients receiving cis-platinum. Proc Am Soc Clin Oncol 1: 64 (abstr)
86. Chiara S, Campora E et al. (1987) Methylpredinisolonè for the control of CMF-induced emesis. Am J Clin Oncol 10: 264–267
87. Kessler JF, Alberts DS et al. (1986) An effective five-drug antiemetic combination for prevention of chemotherapy-related nausea and vomiting. Experience in eighty-four patients. Cancer Chemother Pharmacol 17: 282–286
88. Kris MG, Richard JG et al. (1985) Improved control of cisplatin-induced emesis with high-dose metoclopramide and with combinations of metoclopramide, dexamethasone, and diphenhydramine. Results of consecutive trials in 255 patients. Cancer 55: 527–534
89. Kris MG, Gralla RJ, Tyson LB et al. (1989) Controlling delayed vomiting: double-blind, randomized trial comparing placebo, dexamethasone alone, and metoclopramide plus dexamethasone in patients receiving cisplatin. J Clin Oncol 7: 108–114

Use of Nonpharmacological Techniques to Prevent Chemotherapy-Related Nausea and Vomiting

P.H. Cotanch

School of Nursing, Georgia State University and School of Medicine, Emory University, Atlanta, GA 30303, USA

Introduction

The use of nonpharmacological techniques as adjuvant antiemetic treatment for oncology patients has gained popularity over the last 10 years at major cancer centers throughout the world. The advantages of these techniques—relaxation therapy, desensitization therapy, guided imagery, and self-hypnosis—extend beyond specific symptom management to potentiating the placebo effect on medication and improving patient–provider relationships. In addition, patient participation in nonpharmacological interventions transforms the role of patient from passive recipient to active participant, thereby improving compliance to chemotherapy regimens (Laszlo 1983).

This paper will present a brief overview of the previously published research on the use of nonpharmacological techniques for cancer patients. Information on the cognitive theories underlying the use of the techniques for specific patients will be explained.

Finally, areas for future research in the application of nonpharmacological techniques as antiemetic therapy emphasizing the potential beneficial psychophysiological effects, will be discussed.

Previous Research

The selected research that has previously been conducted on nonpharmacological techniques as antiemetic therapies is summarized on Table 1. The studies focus on different aspects of chemotherapy-related nausea, vomiting, appetite suppression, and affective responses, such as depression, anxiety, and self-esteem. All of the studies show that nonpharmacological techniques resulted in some degree of benefit for the patients who participated in the experimental group of the clinical trials. Indeed, it has been shown repeatedly in both clinical studies and clinical practice that instituting some type of nonpharmacological,

Table 1. Summary research on nonpharmacological techniques in cancer

Authors	Design	Sample	n	Independent variables	Dependent variables	Instruments	Conclusions
Zeltzer and LeBaron (1982) (1983) Zeltzer et al. 1984	Quasi-experimental	Inpatient and outpatient Age: 6–17 random assignment	<45	Deep breathing, distraction, practice sessions vs. therapist-conducted and self-hypnosis	Pain/anxiety from BM/LP procedures N/V	Self-rating Likert-type anxiety scales	Hypnosis is more effective than nonhypnotic techniques in reducing acute pain and anxiety during BM/LP procedures, and N/V
Frank (1985)	Pre-Post test	Oncology pats. Age: 20–71 with multiple diagnoses and a history of N/V Controlled: chemotherapy antiemetics drug dose	15	Music therapy, Guided mental visual imagery	Anxiety, degree and length of N/V	STAI Nausea/ Vomiting Questionnaire	No significant change in duration/pat. perception of nausea. pat. perceived degree of vomiting reduced ($p < 0.05$), anxiety reduced ($p < 0.001$)
Cotanch (1983)	Pre-Post test	Multiple diagnoses Age: 17–49 yrs. Failed conventional chemotherapy In/out pats. Refractory drug-induced N/V	9	Progressive muscle relaxation (PMR)	N/V Caloric intake Nutritional effects	STAI BP; pulse, Respiration, calorie count Skin fold measurements	N/V improved in some pats. Pulse and respiration decreased after PMR

| Zook and Yasko (1983) | De-scriptive Corre-lational | Oncology pats. Age: 19–78 Initial Tx Chemo Tx > 50% Emetic potential | 26 | Anxiety, hopelessness, & pain | Presence & degree N/V | STAI Beck Hope-lessness Scale McGill–Melzack Pain Question-naire Presence/degree N/V Demographic data | lack of statistical significance between psychological variables and N/V |
| Scott et al. (1986) | Case control | Stae III–IV ovarian cancer Random assign-ment Age: 33–75 yrs. | 17 | Progressive muscle relaxa-tion guided imagery vs. high-dose dopamine antagonist antiemetics | Number of emetic episodes Intensity, amount, duration of vomiting Amount urine Amount diarrhea | Visual Analogue Scale, Emetic Pro-cess Rating Scale | Signif. diff. in frequency of emetic episodes PMR/GI > drug. No diff. in intensities of N/V, retching, or volume of emesis Urine output signif. greater in drug group. No difference in amount of diarrhea |

Table 1 (*continued*)

Authors	Design	Sample	n	Independent variables	Dependent variables	Instruments	Conclusions
Cotanch and Strum (1987)	Randomized 3-group design	Chem Tx > 60% Emetic potential Initial Tx Inpatient	60	PMR vs. music vs. no Intervention	Anxiety, calorie intake N/V	STAI Weight BP, pulse, respiration, calorie intake. Duke Descriptive Scale, Skin fold measurements	PMR effective in reducing frequency and duration of vomiting, general anxiety, physiological arousal, and improving calorie intake.
Cotanch et al. (1985)	Randomized 2-group design	Pediatr. oncology patients (inpatient and outpatient)	20	Hypnosis, guided imagery	N/V, oral intake, antiemetic drugs	Duke Descriptive Scale, Visual Analogue Scale	Hypnosis resulted in improved oral intake and decreased vomiting episodes
Burish and Lyles (1979, 1981) Burrish et al. (1987)	Randomized design	Adult oncology patient with AN/V	30	PMR per study	AN/V, depression, anxiety, P&BP	N/V questionnaire Anxiety Scale	The PMR group had better control over amount and intensity of chem. related AN&V

Abbreviations: AN/V, anticipatory nausea and vomiting; BM/LP bone marrow/lumbar puncture; GI, guided imagery; N/V, nausea and vomiting; P&BP, pulse and blood pressure; STAI, state/trait anxiety inventory; R, respirations; PMR, progressive muscle relaxation.

psychophysiological intervention for patients receiving chemotherapy is better than doing nothing at all.

Underlying Conceptual Framework

Most of the studies summarized on Table 1 used one of the following cognitive conceptual frameworks to explain the effectiveness of nonpharmacological techniques for control of chemotherapy related nausea and vomiting.

Bandura's theory of self-efficacy (1977, 1982) states that patients' expectations of personal efficacy, such as conviction or beliefs that they *can* successfully execute certain behaviors required in a given situation, are likely to produce the desired outcome. The expectations are assumed to influence the initiation of coping behaviors, the amount of effort likely to be expended to maintain coping behavior, and the length of time such behavior will be sustained in the face of external and internal obstacles.

Lazarus and Folkman (1984) describe the threat/appraisal concept to explain the usefulness of nonpharmacological techniques with cancer patients. According to this system-oriented conception of the stress response, subjects' appraisals of environment stimuli will determine whether or not they feel threatened and are aroused to action. Appraisals may be realistic or distorted. Physiological arousal can be very appropriate in some circumstances; at other times it may be totally inappropriate. In this context, relaxation is a response that, when mastered, can neutralize the effects of activation for *fight or flight* and it can also alter the appraisal of a potentially threatening situation. For example, in situations of frustration resulting from a perceived lack of control, relaxation can provide a measure of control and thus change the appraisal of a potentially threatening situation. A change of appraisal generally means a change in response as well.

Unfortunately, most patients confront chemotherapy experiencing a classical "fight or flight" reaction, accompanied by the very different psychological response of dread. These responses put the patient in an anxiety- and depression-producing situation referred to as a "double bind": on the one hand, the feeling develops that it is best to endure the discomfort and, on the other, a desire to escape arises. The dread is thought to be the result of the release of catecholamines; the fight-or-flight response is believed to result from cortisol release (see Fig. 1).

Future Research

Further research in the area of nonpharmacological techniques for oncology patients will focus on issues of improving patient compliance, and tailoring the specific technique to optimize the effect of the intervention. There are many unanswered questions regarding the iatrogenic stressors associated with the

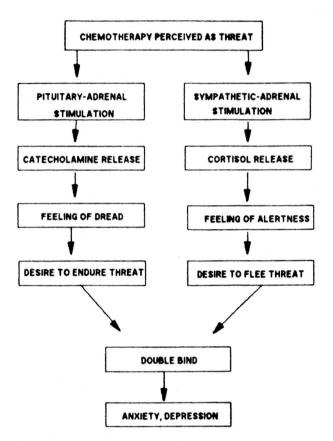

Fig. 1. Psychophysiological pathway leading to anxiety and depression in patients confronting chemotherapy

"double bind trauma" that patients are likely to encounter as they participate in aggressive chemotherapy treatment. The relationship between stress and discomfort of treatment and maladaptive coping behaviors needs to be further investigated. The relationship between stress and concomitant diseases leading to disruption of patients' normal lifestyles is a fertile area for future clinical research in supportive care for oncology patients.

References

Bandura A (1977) Social learning theory. Prentice Hall, Englewood Cliffs

Bandura A (1982) Self-efficacy mechanism in human agency. Am Psychol 37 (2): 122–147

Burish TG, Lyles JN (1979) Effectiveness of relaxation training in reducing the aversiveness of chemotherapy in the treatment of cancer. Behav Ther Exp Psychiatry 10: 357–361

Burish TG, Lyles JN (1981) Effectiveness of relaxation training in reducing adverse reactions to cancer chemotherapy. J Behav Med 4 (1): 65–78

Burish TG, Carey MP, Krozeley MG, Greco FA (1987) Conditioned side effects induced by cancer chemotherapy: prevention through behavioral treatment. J Consult Clin Psychol 55 (1): 42–48

Cotanch PH (1983) Relaxation training for control of nausea and vomiting in patients receiving chemotherapy. Cancer Nurs 6 (4): 277–282

Cotanch PH, Strum S (1987) Progressive muscle relaxation as antiemetic therapy for cancer patients. Oncol Nurs Forum 14 (1): 33–37

Cotanch P, Hockenberry M, Herman S (1985) Self-hypnosis as antiemetic therapy in children receiving chemotherapy. Oncol Nurs Forum 12 (4): 41–46

Frank JM (1985) The effects of music therapy and guided visual imagery on chemotherapy induced nausea and vomiting. Oncol Nurs Forum 12 (5): 47–52

Laszlo J (1983) Antiemetics and cancer chemotherapy. Williams and Wilkins, Baltimore

Lazarus R, Folkman S (1984) Stress, appraisal and coping. Springer, Berlin Heidelberg New York

Scott DW, Donahue DC, Mastrovito RC, Hakes TB (1986) Comparative trials of clinical relaxation and antiemetic drug regimen in reducing chemotherapy-related nausea and vomiting. Cancer Nurs 9 (4): 178–187

Zeltzer L, LeBaron S (1982) Hypnosis and nonhypnotic techniques for reduction of pain and anxiety during painful procedures in children and adolescents with cancer. J Pediatr 101 (6): 1032–1035

Zeltzer L, LeBaron S (1983) Behavioral intervention for children and adolescents with cancer. Behav Med Update 5 (2, 3): 17–21

Zeltzer LK, Kellerman J, Ellenberg L, Dash J (1983) Hypnosis for reduction of vomiting associated with chemotherapy and disease in adolescents with cancer. J Adolesc Health Care 4 (2): 77–84

Zeltzer L, LeBaron S, Zeltzer P (1984) The effectiveness of behavior interventions for reducing nausea and vomiting in children receiving chemotherapy. J Clin Oncol 2 (3): 683–690

Zook D, Yasko J (1983) Psychologic factors: their effect on nausea and vomiting experienced by clients receiving chemotherapy. Oncol Nurs Forum 10 (3): 76–81

Optimizing Palliative Surgical Support of Cancer Patients with Visceral Obstructions

J.F. Forbes and H. McA. Foster

Department of Surgical Oncology, University of Newcastle,
Newcastle Mater Misericordiae Hospital, Waratah, NSW 2298, Australia

Visceral obstruction aggravates surgical problems in cancer patients. It can lead to major organ failure either directly (e.g. hepatic failure from biliary obstruction) or indirectly from complications (e.g. cholecystitis and septicaemia) which in turn can be rapidly fatal. Visceral obstruction often causes a rapid downturn in quality of life (e.g. with pain, distension and vomiting from bowel obstruction); it usually needs rapid and careful reassessment and often equally urgent intervention. The resulting problems and treatment required can dominate a patient's management, making it particularly important to consider principles by which surgical support can be optimized. In particular, good communication, careful assessment and reassessment, meticulous planning and attention to sound surgical techniques are all important.

Not all visceral obstructions are due to cancer, even in a patient with known malignancy. This highlights the need to consider the role of palliative surgery in all cancer patients, even at the outset when cancer seems likely, and also to remember that surgery can palliate by "curing" a benign problem even when a patient's cancer is itself incurable.

Optimizing palliative surgical support for cancer patients requires careful attention to these principles, and pursuing them at all stages, before, during and after surgical intervention.

Extent of the Problem

Visceral obstruction is often encountered in cancer patients and can occur at many sites (Table 1). There are a variety of mechanisms that may be involved, necessitating careful assessment for each individual patient (Table 2).

Recent Results in Cancer Research, Vol. 121
© Springer-Verlag Berlin · Heidelberg 1991

Table 1. Sites of visceral obstruction in cancer patients

Gastrointestinal tract
    Oesophagus
    Stomach
    Small bowel
    Large bowel

Pancreatico-biliary ducts
    Main pancreatic duct
    Common bile duct/hepatic ducts
    Intra-hepatic ducts

Urinary tract
    Renal pelvis
    Ureter
    Bladder neck

Table 2. Mechanisms of visceral obstruction in cancer patients

---

Direct mechanical obstruction	
1. Primary site, e.g.	large bowel
	oesophagus
	pancreatic duct
	prostate
2. Metastases, e.g.	lymph nodes, common bile duct
	small bowel (intussusception)
	retroperitoneal (ureter)
Indirect obstruction	
1. Haemorrhage, e.g.	bladder
	ureter
2. Fibrosis, e.g.	retroperitoneal
	post-radiotherapy
	post-surgery
Non-malignant obstruction	
e.g.	adhesions
	gallstones
	urinary calculi

Pre-Operative Management

Assessment

The surgeon must know the extent and nature of the underlying malignancy and the state of major organ function (especially liver, renal, respiratory and cardiac) to help judge the risks of operation and anaesthesia as well as the type and extent of resuscitation and preparation needed. This can be critically important for fluid, electrolyte and acid–base imbalances in sick patients. Associated infection—commonly present in patients with extra-hepatic biliary obstruction and large bowel obstruction—can alone determine patient survival, and diagnosis of type, extent and sensitivities of organisms is desirable where time permits. The haemostasis profile should be evaluated pre-operatively whenever there is suggestion of abnormality: it can usually be corrected before surgery, and this may allow an otherwise potentially fatal operation to be life saving. Concurrently, the presence, type and degree of anaemia is determined, as marked lowering of haemoglobin levels reduces patients' reserves and puts them at greater risk should they bleed, compromises wound healing, predisposes patients to developing sites of infection, and may reflect underlying bleeding problems or even marrow malfunction due to metastases.

Patients' psychological status and home environment should also be assessed. What after-care is likely to be required can be considered before an operation is undertaken, to ensure that rehabilitation can be continued after discharge from hospital.

Assessment of patients' medical fitness must include their nutritional status. Patients with cancer often have poor oral intake. Bowel obstruction also reduces intake and is often complicated by vomiting; hepatic obstruction compromises digestion and protein production. The assessment must consider current deficiencies, replacements needed (fluids, calories and special supplements) and the optimal delivery system. Due consideration of the planned procedures and postoperative requirements as well as needs for anaesthesia, chemotherapy and pain control can indicate a need for central lines or infusion ports. As mentioned, anaemia is a particular type of nutritional deficiency that may need preoperative correction.

Procedure Planning

Full knowledge of the type and extent of malignancy, as well as the nature, cause of and site of obstruction, allows surgery to be planned. Recognition of the extent of complications and their response to treatment, the overall prognosis, the value of specific therapies and, most importantly, the patient's wishes, can modify this planning process. Full consideration of possible extra requirements, such as for colostomy or drainage tubes, allows proper pre-operative explanations and also specialist nursing input from the outset.

Past treatments, particularly radiotherapy and surgery, should be carefully studied to avoid problems during the operation and with subsequent healing. Operating in an irradiated area can create greater problems than the obstruction, and as radiotherapists may underestimate the extent of damage they have caused caution is needed. Many people involved with treatment may need to have input into a patient's care—including nursing staff, anaesthetist, nutritionist, physiotherapist, social worker and counsellor, treatment specialists, palliative care staff and the surgical oncologist. It is essential that a single clinician takes charge to co-ordinate and plan the involvement of others. When operation is required, this should be the surgical oncologist, at least until the post-operative recovery is complete.

Communication

The patient and key family members should have the details of planned surgery explained, including the extent of illness and complications, what is planned, the potential scope and limitations of the operation, the likely outcome, including likely and possible complications, and details of the anticipated recovery phase. Anxiety can be reduced by proper explanations. A patient and family should learn whether a procedure is planned to be palliative or potentially curative. The patient's wishes must be made known to ensure the surgeon understands them before performing the operation. Careful explanation with a family member and patient together reduces the opportunity for misunderstandings and encourages frankness and trust.

Explanations should also encompass tests and pre-operative procedures, the introduction of new staff involved in care and what their role is, the timing of surgery and why it might be necessary as an emergency. Surgery and hospitals can be frightening to any patient. Sick patients with cancer require special attention.

Timing

Once operation is seen to be necessary and investigations and preoperative resuscitation are complete, further delay must be avoided. Procrastination creates uncertainty and anxiety, and both of these erode patient confidence. Delay can also lead to deterioration in a patient's condition, with, for example, worsening liver failure, perforation of obstructed bowel, or worsening infection. Equally, premature surgery in a patient who has not been sufficiently resuscitated can be fatal. Fine judgement is needed, but it should be apparent if improvement has stopped and no further pre-operative steps are available. This is the time to promptly push on.

Repeated Review and the Decision Not to Operate

A patient's condition can change rapidly, and the need to avoid unnecessary delay when surgery is needed has been stressed. Some patients are clearly not going to be helped by operation and others may be harmed. A patient in stable condition with a known malignancy and severe small bowel obstruction may be helped more by nasogastric suction and correction of fluid and electrolyte deficiencies than by anaesthesia, operation and post-operative recovery. It can be very worthwhile to repair a strangulated hernia even in a cancer patient, but there may be little to gain from laparotomy for recurrent subacute small bowel obstruction due to radiation damage. The key is frequent reassessment, to diagnose at the earliest opportunity the patient whose visceral obstruction is progressing, so that surgery can be completed before progression is too marked.

Optimizing Operative Procedures

Careful surgical technique and attention to detail are the hallmarks of safe surgery in all patients, but no degree of operative skill can compensate for poor preparation of the patient. Disaster and fatal complications have many opportunities to develop and the surgical oncologist must have a heightened awareness of potential hazards. Thorough haemostasis, gentleness in tissue handling—particularly following earlier radiotherapy—careful suturing and meticulous aseptic techniques must all be standard. Incisions require planning to take into account previous surgery, avoidance of irradiated areas, the extent of required surgery, and the possibility of colostomy, drain tube, tissue flap or skin graft.

The procedure undertaken is frequently not decided until the operation has commenced and an operative assessment is completed. The choice is often between a palliative bypass, with the likelihood of major gains in symptom control and a live patient, or a "curative" resection, with its greater operative and post-operative chance of complications. Many patients gain the best palliation from tumour resection, particularly if necrosis, haemorrhage or infection have complicated the tumour. Others, e.g. those with most types of lymphoma, have such a high expectancy of control by other measures that surgery beyond diagnostic laparotomy and simple bypass may be unwise.

Many procedures are best performed in stages. Patients with large bowel obstruction can be dramatically improved by a life saving decompression and live to have a definitive resection later. Others, particularly those with biliary obstruction, might do best to avoid repeated anaesthetics. It can require fine judgement and experience to always achieve optimal surgery, and often it is only with hindsight that the "best decision" becomes apparent.

All surgical wounds require proper suturing. Cancer patients with visceral obstruction heal poorly and delayed healing must be anticipated. Non-absorbable interrupted sutures are ideal, and tension sutures "electively" used can avoid later wound dehiscence. Nylon sutures are best avoided in contaminated wounds, and the slowly dissolving sutures of Vicryl and Dexon are reasonable alternatives. Removal of debris and dead tissue helps avoid infection.

Post-Operative Care

Close monitoring with appropriate support systems, frequent reassessments (anticipating possible complications), staged rehabilitation, and continued communication are the major aims. Cancer patients who have undergone surgery can change quickly. Many need a period of intensive care monitoring; all can develop complications.

Complications (Table 3) are best handled by early detection and intervention before they progress to an unmanageable stage. One or two even major complications are usually readily treatable; multiple complications often cause further compromise of organ systems and may not be retrievable. Advance planning for post-operative care allows requirements to be anticipated and avoids the tragedy of a patient's dying from treatable complications simply because monitoring or support facilities, as found in intensive care, were not planned for.

Most patients and families will anxiously await news of what was found and done and will always appreciate frankness with disclosures and judgements. They will expect an opportunity to ask questions will be expected, and may well require patience and understanding for their anxieties to be resolved. The plan for recovery and rehabilitation, including the likely length of stay in hospital, period of rehabilitation, other planned treatments, and follow-up policy, with the need for investigations, should be conveyed not just to patient and family but also to staff involved. When no gain has been made or prognosis is bad, then this must be placed in perspective for the patient. Anxiety is aggravated by

Table 3. Post-operative complications in cancer patients operated upon for visceral obstruction

---

1. Haemorrhage: poor liver function, marrow involvement, prior blood loss, extensive blood replacement
2. Infection: wound, obstructed viscera, septicaemia
3. Acid–base and electrolyte imbalance, liver or renal failure
4. Cardio-respiratory failure: blood loss, poor nutrition, imbalance of other organ function, pulmonary embolus
5. Poor wound healing: hypoxia–anaemia, cardiac failure, infection, poor nutrition
6. Nutritional deficiency: prior deficiency, ileus, infection, surgery to the gastrointestinal tract
7. Psychological reactions: operations, changed prognosis, colostomies and drain tubes, abnormal feeding, intensive support systems

---

uncertainty, and all patients can have a management plan with expectations explained to them, their family and their own family doctor.

Conclusion

There are particular problems in managing cancer patients with visceral obstruction that highlight the requirements for treating cancer patients in general and surgical oncology patients in particular. Careful assessment and planning, patient and honest communication, and particular attention to principles of surgical oncology before, during and after surgery all contribute to optimizing surgical support.

Sexuality: An Unknown Word for Patients with a Stoma?

R.J. Wells

Royal Marsden Hospital, Fulham Road, London SW3 6JJ, United Kingdom

Introduction

Despite enormous developments in cancer treatments and cancer care in particular, and our widely publicised claims in the provision of holistic care for the sick, we still appear to be experiencing great difficulty in addressing the sexuality of our patients, and particularly those who have undergone procedures resulting in altered body image, such as formation of a stoma [1]. In this so-called permissive age, when bare-breasted women and scantily clad males adorn newspapers and magazines, and the human sexual response is capable of, and has been subjected to, measurement in controlled laboratory conditions—when information is available to us in learned texts on what to do and how to do it, and even how much our heart rate increases during orgasm [2]—one would have hoped that human sexuality and the essential part it plays in most of our lives would be given rather more attention in dealing with the sick than it actually is.

When one or more parts of the body function inappropriately, the individual affected is likely to be diagnosed as unhealthy or sick. People thus diagnosed then have recourse to a battery of health care providers who will attempt to make them physically well, or at least restore them to an optimum level of functioning. The responsibility in this for the health care staff is to work as a collegiate members of an interdisciplinary team to deliver, as far as possible, research-based care to help the individual feel better. Rarely, however, if ever, do we investigate the effect that physical ill-health has had on sexual health. The World Health Organisation [3] says that "sexual health is the integration of the somatic, emotional, intellectual and social aspects of sexual being, in ways that are positively enriching and that enhance personality, communication and love. The purpose of sexual health care should be the enhancement of life and personal relationships and not merely counselling and care related to pro-creation or sexually transmitted diseases." Add to this definition the plethora of literature available to us on sexuality and sexual dysfunction, and one really must wonder why we have not yet come to terms with this important and integral part of human functioning.

Why is There a Problem?

It has often been written that health care providers will be unable to come to terms with the sexuality of their patients until they are happy with their own sexuality. But what do we mean by sexuality? All too frequently, I think, we confuse the sex act with sexuality. Sexuality is, I hope, something rather more than erection, penetration and ejaculation. Sexuality is much more comprehensive [4]; of course it includes the sex drive, but it is much more about our human character, our self-image, gender identity, closeness to others, touching, intimacy, expression of maleness and femaleness. Sexuality therefore is not located between the umbilicus and the kneecaps, but is a reflection of our human character [4]. It follows that if we can appreciate this definition of sexuality and apply it to ourselves and be happy with that, then we can use our confidence to help others regain theirs.

However, undoing the welter of complexes about sex and sexuality instilled in us by parents, teachers and religions of all denominations, may not be so easily achieved. If we ourselves have been brain-washed into believing that sexuality is simply to do with sex and that various parts of the anatomy are taboo, then unless the educators and leaders of the professions in health care come to our aid I see very little prospect of holistic care for our patients. What of course I am trying to say is that, delighted though I am to be with you today, it is not enough to have periodic lectures on the subject. If we really believe that the sexual health of our patients is as important as their physical well-being, then we will demand that health care providers are educationally prepared for and professionally supported in this vital aspect of care, and ensure the sexual needs of the individual are fully considered in the planning of a course of treatment.

Altered Body Image

As we mature and are able to recognise self, we become aware of our body image; we pay scant attention to the fact that what we see in the mirror is the wrong way round, and we become accustomed to our reflection. Some will be more happy with what they see than others, and some will make determined efforts to alter their appearance by diverse creative methods. As we grow older our body image changes; this man before you, rapidly approaching fifty, once had masses of black curly hair and an unlined visage! For others the changes may be more troublesome; stretch marks, weight gain, falling breasts, baldness and wrinkles—all affect our perceptions of body image [5]. These changes happen gradually, and many of them can be ameliorated by the use of pills, potions, creams, surgery, wigs and corsets. We can to some extent stem the flow of altered body image, at least for a little while, and maintain our sexuality.

Alterations of body image brought about by disease or the attempts to control disease is not so easily dealt with. Despite our self-criticism of our appearance we would not want it changed—except for the better. For many people with cancer this is often not an option, and even the diagnosis of cancer can have an immediate adverse effect on body image and self-perception. The very mention of the word often brings about nightmare images of virulent cells coursing through the body, with thoughts of contagion, and this sometimes separates people who had previously been close.

Cancer, Altered Body Image and Sexuality

The initial diagnosis of malignant disease is frequently a unifying force in relationships which may previously have been shaky or have fallen into a routine. The threat of imminent death of a partner or family member may help, initially, to cement relationships. How well that bonding continues depends greatly on treatment regimes and how we, health care providers, support people through them. It is at this time, along with all the other things that we need to be cognisant of, that we should begin meeting the sexual needs of people with cancer. Whilst hoping for cure or control of the disease, we need to be mindful of all the problems which will occur before the patient reaches the hoped-for outcome. The responses to the disease and the needs it will provoke, are well documented [6] and frequently ignored. We are extremely adept at distributing patient information literature, and explaining about the sequelae of treatment— *some* of the sequelae of treatment.

Once the immediacy of the potential death of a loved one has receded and treatment has commenced, the closeness brought about by the diagnosis may begin to diminish. The results of treatment will affect not only the patient but those close to him/her, and dealing with pain, hair loss and vomiting can put a tremendous strain on a relationship, as can the thought of making love to someone with a stoma. The strain may become so great that even resolution of the disease fails to restore the previous closeness. Sadly, it is not true for everyone that love conquers all.

I suspect that if you were to visit most cancer patients in most hospitals in most countries of the world, especially those undergoing formation of a stoma, and look at their plan of nursing care, you would be unlikely to see any mention of sexuality, and yet we mouth constant platitudes about the activities of daily living. Our sexuality encompasses many of our human qualities; our spiritual, social, emotional, psychological and physical self is affected by our sexuality. Coughlin [7] suggests that for most of us our quality of life pivots on and around our sexuality. What value, then is, care delivered on the basis of activities of daily living if sexuality is excluded?

I recently reviewed the care of a patient with a nurse and asked her why there was no record of attention to sexuality in his plan of care—he had undergone the formation of a stoma. "He did not mention it", was the response. Jory Graham deals with such situation very succinctly in her book *In the Company of Others* [8]: "Even though the patient does not ask directly 'What will this do to my sex life?' the question still exists and must be answered." At times like this patients do not need nice young ladies, they require professionals who can anticipate their worst fears and help them deal with them." If he'd wanted to know, he'd ask" is not a worthy response from a professional nurse.

Very often, failure of a relationship following a diagnosis of cancer results from the patient rejecting the partner. The patient may be so bereaved by the loss of body image—the missing breast, the bag of faeces hanging on the abdominal wall, the mutilated face—and so fearful of rejection that the partner is held at bay and eventually gives up trying. Perhaps a normal reaction on our part might be, "How could he/she do that?"—'seldom, I suspect, do we stop and muse about our part in this sorry state of affairs. Did we do anything to ameliorate the shame being felt by our patient? Did we do anything to prevent them withdrawing into their own private hell, so bad they couldn't share it with the one they loved? Did we do anything to encourage them to continue to be a sexual person?

People who come to us for care, with hope and trust, do not leave their sexuality at home, any more than they leave their fear behind. Surely it is at this time, before treatment begins, that they need help and support from the whole team to maintain their closeness and physical intimacy and to express their feelings. Excluding the partner increases the sense of aloneness for both, and may eventually result in total exclusion.

What Can We Do?

If we are really serious about addressing sexuality issues arising from cancer and altered body image, then there are ways we can help. But are we serious? Let us assume so.

Pre-treatment counselling of all patients undergoing stoma formation and, where relevant, their partners is essential if they are to emerge at the other end relatively unscathed. Both need to know of the treatment regime and how it will affect both of them in terms of their sexuality. The partner needs to be aware of his/her vital role; being there, understanding, touching, looking, reinforcing feelings with needs, small tokens of love and esteem. Both need equity and truth telling when dealing with potential sexual problems, and help with interventions which might be used as substitutes for sexual intercourse or demonstrations of love: cuddling, visual stimulation, stroking, mutual masturbation, auto-eroticism and fantasies. People frequently need positive reinforcement that cessation of sexual activity will not be permanent though practice may be necessary to achieve success, and this will need constant reinforcement on follow-up visits to the hospital. I remember one unfortunate woman who had carcinoma of the cervix and was told that following caesium insertion she should cease vaginal intercourse; when I was talking to her some 2 years later she asked when I thought she might be able to make love to her husband again.

One system which has been beneficial to diverse health care providers in addressing sexual needs is the P-LI-SS-IT [9] model. The person who devised it is J. S. Annon. PLISSIT stands for:

P   Permission
LI   Limited information
SS   Specific suggestions
IT   Intensive therapy

This model allows four levels of approach, each letter or pair of letters designating a suggested method for handling presenting sexual concerns; the first three levels are viewed as brief therapy and the fourth as intensive therapy. The model has a number of distinct advantages: it can be used in most settings and adapted to whatever length of counselling time is needed. Each level of approach will require increasing amounts of time and professional experience. The model therefore allows health care providers to gear their approach to their level of competence; this also means that it in effect constitutes a plan which aids the determining of referral to other appropriate practitioners. Let us examine it rather more closely [9]:

Level P   The patient has been "given permission" to be sexual and to explore alternative methods of sexual expression. This requires open discussion and communication with the patient.
Level LI   This level covers providing limited information to dispel preconceived and false information which may inhibit recovery. Myths such as that cancer is contagious can be dispelled, and information on sexual impairment which may result from treatment can be offered.
Level SS   Specific suggestion involves the giving of explicit information on alternative sexual techniques or modifying present sexual activities. Although this may be difficult for some practitioners, they can refer patients on to other professionals. It is important, however, that they listen to the patients' concerns and assure them that they will be dealt with by a colleague.
Level IT   Intensive therapy requires interventions by an expert; this may be a clinical nurse specialist, psychologist, psychiatrist, or sex therapist.

The PLISSIT system has been found to work well when care givers recognise the limits and levels of their expertise and ensure appropriate referrals to other practitioners as the need arises.

Conclusion

If the developments taking place in health care at the present time are to be effective—I am thinking specifically of nursing models and primary nursing—then we will have to be seen to be concentrating on the holistic needs of the individual, not just the obvious needs. The sequelae of cancer reach far beyond the individual into his/her extended social network [7], and it is in that milieu that patients will have to function when we have finished with them. How effectively that is achieved depends largely on how effective we have been. If adequate sexual functioning and tolerable sexuality are part of quality of life, then we as professionals can no longer ignore these components of individual care.

I share the view of Seedhouse [10] that there are no limits to nursing. If there are options which are available and will improve autonomy and functioning and we don't take them, then we are not working for health. To put it differently: if you are not part of the solution, then you are part of the problem.

Each individual is a unique human being with needs and wants, whose sexual identity and functioning is threatened by disease and treatment. Our responsibility in attempting sexual rehabilitation is to restore to that individual the capacity to be lovable and loving.

References

1. Ginsberg JJ (1986) Sexual rehabilitation of the cancer patient undergoing ostomy surgery. J Enterostom Ther 13: 148–152
2. Shipes E, Lehr S (1982) Sexuality and the male cancer patient. Cancer Nursing: October
3. World Health Organisation (1975) Technical Report Series, No. 572
4. Webb C (1985) Sexuality, nursing and health. Wiley, London
5. Salter M (ed) (1988) Altered body image: the nurse's role. Wiley, London.
6. MacElveen-Hoehm P, McCorkle R (1985) Understanding sexuality in progressive cancer. Semin Oncol Nurs 1 (1): 56–62
7. Coughlin V (1986) Sexuality and the cancer patient—a deafening silence. Unpublished paper
8. Graham J (1983) In the company of others. Victor Gollancz, London
9. Annon JS (1976) Behavioural treatment of sexual problems. Brief therapy. Harper and Row, New York
10. Seedhouse DF (1988) Ethics: the heart of health care. Wiley, London

Cytokines and Hematopoietins: Physiology, Pathophysiology, and Potential as Therapeutic Agents

R. Mertelsmann, F.M. Rosenthal, A. Lindemann, and F. Herrmann

Abteilung Innere Medizin I–Hämatologie/Onkologie, Medizinische Universitatsklinik, Hugstetter Straße 55, W-7800 Freiburg, FRG

Introduction

Improved understanding of host biology, immunology, and tumor pathophysiology raises the possibility of introducing new treatment modalities for cancer patients: stimulation of host defense mechanisms, including specific and nonspecific immunological approaches, as well as approaches aimed directly at altering tumor growth and differentiation by therapeutically influencing pathophysiological mechanisms. In addition, amelioration of cancer and cancer treatment-associated morbidity offers new possibilities for improving the quality of life for many patients, as well as options for increased dose-intensity regimens, with the potential of achieving higher cure rates in some patient groups. In this chapter we will focus on insights gained into the in vivo physiology of human cytokines and on the experience gained so far with the use of cytokines in cancer therapy.

Cytokines are polypeptide products of activated cells that in most instances provide short range communication between cells by influencing their proliferation, differentiation, and state of activation. These hormone-like agents are produced by multiple cell types and several of them have pleiotropic and overlapping, sometimes synergistic or additive, activities, not being restricted to influencing one cell lineage only. The majority of growth factors appear to have the capacity of inducing other cytokines in activated white blood cells. This complex network of interactions makes the evaluation of clinical studies conducted with these factors very complicated, since multifaceted direct and indirect effects on many organ systems have to be expected. The potential clinical use of human cytokines can arbitrarily be divided into four strategies:

1. Stimulation of the immune response in order to enhance immunosurveillance of neoplasms (e.g., interleukin-2)
2. Mitigation of cancer- and cancer therapy-related immuno- and myelosuppression and augmentation of nonspecific mechanisms of host resistance

Recent Results in Cancer Research, Vol. 121
© Springer-Verlag Berlin · Heidelberg 1991

(e.g., granulocyte-macrophage colony-stimulating factor, granulocyte colony-stimulating factor, erythropoietin)

3. Indirect improvement of antitumor response and survival by reducing toxicity and thus altering the definition of the maximum tolerated doses of conventional chemotherapeutic regimens (colony-stimulating factors, interleukin-1 and -3)

4. Direct influence on tumor cell growth and differentiation via cytotoxic, cytostatic, or regulatory mechanisms (e.g., interferons, tumor necrosis factor).

Apart from this potential use in cancer therapy, there are a number of nonneoplastic disorders associated with cytopenias in which the use of growth factors may prove to be beneficial.

Cytokines involved in immunoregulation or cell proliferation can be divided into several groups (Table 1), such as hematopoietic growth factors, interleukins, interferons, tumor necrosis factors, and others. While many of the names of these factors are based on the original assay system of detection, most more recently identified cytokines have been called interleukins, in view of their pleiotropic activities. Since most cytokines possess multiple biologic properties and target cells, there are overlapping activities between groups, making any classification somewhat arbitrary.

Hematopoietic Growth Factors

The hematopoietic growth factors (HGFs) are a family of glycoprotein hormones which regulate survival, proliferation, and differentiation of hematopoietic progenitor cells as well as the functional activities of mature cells [1]. During the past few years the genes for five of the human factors have been defined, cloned, and recombinant forms of the proteins produced and purified. The different factors have been operationally defined by prefixes based on the predominant type of colony found in vitro in response to these molecules. The factors currently under active clinical investigation include multipotential colony-stimulating factor (multi-CSF or interleukin-3), granulocyte-macrophage CSF (GM-CSF), granulocyte CSF (G-CSF), macrophage CSF (M-CSF), and erythropoietin (EPO).

Granulocyte-Macrophage Colony-Stimulating Factor

The human gene encoding GM-CSF is located on chromosome 5q21-5q32 [2]. Probably due to variable glycosylation, the molecular mass of the mature protein, which comprises 127 amino acids, ranges from 14 to 35 kD [3]. A variety of cells producing GM-CSF have been identified, among them monocytes, fibroblasts, endothelial cells, epithelial cells, and T lymphocytes [4]. GM-CSF

Table 1. Cytokines involved in immunoregulation and hematopoietic blood cell development

Family	Molecules	Synonyms	Chromosomal localization	Molecular weight[a] (kD)
1. Growth factors	Multi-CSF	IL-3	5q23–q31	14–28
	GM-CSF	CSF-α	5q21–q32	14–35
	G-CSF	CSF-β	17q11–q22	18–22
	M-CSF	CSF-1	5q33	47–74
	EPO		7q11–q22	34–39
2. Interleukins	IL-1	Hematopoietin-1	2q14	31; 17
	IL-2	TCGF	4q26–q28	15
	IL-3	Multi-CSF	5q23–q31	14–28
	IL-4	BSF-1	5q	15–20
	IL-5	BCGF-II, TRF	5q	12–18
	IL-6	BSF-2	7q	24
	IL-7			
	IL-8			
	IL-9			
3. Interferons	IFN-α	Leukocyte-IFN	9	18–20
	IFN-β	Fibroblast-IFN	9	23
	IFN-γ	Immune-IFN	12	20–25
4. Tumor necrosis factors	TNF-α	Cachectin	6	17
	TNF-β	Lymphotoxin	6	25
5. Others (examples)	PDGF	Platelet derived growth factor		
	TGF-α	Transforming growth factor α		
	TGF-β	Transforming growth factor β		

[a] Variations in molecular weight are in most cases due to different degrees of glycosylation.
TCGF, T-cell growth factor; BSF, B-cell stimulatory factor; BCGF, B-cell growth factor; TRF, T-cell replacing factor; PDGF, platelet derived growth factor; TGF, transforming growth factor. For other abbreviations see text.

stimulates granulocyte/macrophage and eosinophil colony formation in vitro and acts in combination with erythropoietin as erythroid burst-promoting activity [5]. In addition to its effect on progenitor cell differentiation, GM-CSF also induces a variety of functional changes in mature cells. It increases neutrophil phagocytic activity, inhibits the migration of neutrophil granulocytes [6], and induces the production of other cytokines (e.g., tumor necrosis factor, interleukin-1) by these same cells [7, 8]. It also induces macrophage tumor cytotoxicity [9], activates macrophages to synthesize MHC class II molecules, to augment antigen presentation [10], and to release oxygen radicals [11].

Although these in vitro findings suggested a possible role for inducing indirect and direct antitumor effects, no such effects of GM-CSF have been observed as yet in any of the clinical studies [12–14]. Induction of in vivo tumor cytotoxicity might be achieved by combining GM-CSF with other macrophage activating factors like interferon-γ (IFN-γ), GM-CSF delivering large numbers of effector cells and IFN-γ triggering the response. Apart from its possible role as antitumor agent, which requires further evaluation, GM-CSF shows activity in reducing chemotherapy-associated morbidity.

Severe and prolonged myelosuppression after chemotherapy in neoplastic disease is a fundamental problem. Complications during this myelosuppressive period often limit the practicability of chemotherapeutic regimens. Frequently, patients receiving high-dose chemotherapy develop neutropenia that often results in bacterial and secondary fungal infections. Shortening the period and degree of neutropenia should decrease the incidence and severity of infections, thereby also shortening the hospital stay, and may reduce the mortality associated with chemotherapy.

In our own phase II clinical trial, it was shown that the neutrophil nadir was significantly elevated and the period of relevant neutropenia abbreviated with a single daily subcutaneous dose of GM-CSF (250 μg/m^2 body surface area) given over a period of 10 days [15]. Patients were protected from febrile events and, somewhat surprisingly, the incidence of mucositis was reduced as well. No significant effect was seen in regard to platelet counts, hemoglobin levels, or duration of chemotherapy-related thrombocytopenia and anemia.

At higher doses (several-fold higher than required for amelioration of chemotherapy-induced neutropenia), the dose-limiting toxicities reported were fever and, during continuous infusion into small veins, thrombosis [16–21].

Effects of GM-CSF were also studied in the clinical setting of autologous bone marrow transplantation [17, 22, 23]. It has been shown that this GM-CSF accelerates the rate of neutrophil recovery and increases the circulating pool of peripheral blood hematopoietic progenitors. No difference was seen between GM-CSF treated patients and nontreated patients with respect to the first appearance of neutrophils in the circulation [24].

Administration of GM-CSF to patients with myelodysplastic syndrome has been described to normalize red cell, white cell, and platelet counts in some patients [25]. More recent studies, however, have not been able to confirm this optimistic report, demonstrating rises in neutrophil counts only. At higher GM-

CSF doses an increase in leukemic blast cells in the blood and bone marrow has been seen, indicating that GM-CSF can stimulate the proliferation of human leukemic blast cells as well as of normal hematopoietic cells in vivo [19, 20, 26]. Even a possible progression to frank leukemia has been observed [26]. Some ongoing studies are exploring the use of GM-CSF in acute myeloblastic leukemia, by augmenting the proportion of malignant cells recruited into the S-phase of the cell cycle and thus obtaining enhanced cytotoxic effects with drugs such as Ara-C, that kill cycle-activated cells [27, 28].

The value of GM-CSF in the treatment of aplastic anemia appears to be limited to those patients with residual hematopoiesis as reported by Champlin and Nissen and their colleagues [29, 30]. Combinations of hematopoietic growth factors acting on early progenitors with later-acting factors might have synergistic effects in accelerating repopulation of the bone marrow and warrant further investigation in this disease.

Ultimately, GM-CSF may find a place in the treatment of other nonmalignant conditions characterized by leukopenia (e.g., acquired immune deficiency syndrome) [31] or in the improvement of host defense in infectious disease [32].

Granulocyte Colony-Stimulating Factor

Due to alternative splicing, two cDNAs representing a 177 amino acid protein form and a 174 amino acid protein form of human G-CSF have been isolated [33–35]. The shorter version of the molecules seems to be more active in vivo. The gene which encodes for G-CSF is located on chromosome 17 in region q11–q22 [36].

G-CSF is a rather lineage-specific hematopoietic growth factor, in that it acts on cells capable of forming one differentiated cell type: the neutrophil granulocyte. In combination with other hematopoietic growth factors it acts synergistically to stimulate a broader spectrum of colony-forming cells [33]. In addition, G-CSF increases antibody-dependent cellular cytotoxicity of peripheral blood granulocytes as well as several other aspects of neutrophil activity [37]. Like GM-CSF, G-CSF has been utilized in the prevention of chemotherapy-induced neutropenia [38–42] and in the setting of autologous bone marrow transplantation [22, 43]. A dose-dependent increase in absolute neutrophil counts (at least three-fold) and shortening of the neutropenic period was observed. At higher doses up to ten-fold increase in monocytes was also seen [40]. In one study the incidence of severe infections was reduced following those cycles of chemotherapy combined with G-CSF [39].

Neutropenia caused by marrow infiltration with low grade lymphoma (hairy cell leukemia) also improved after treatment with G-CSF [44].

Toxicities in G-CSF trials in general have been minimal, essentially being limited to bone pain, presumably secondary to bone marrow expansion. This adverse effect was seen in up to 25% of patients treated with an intravenous bolus $\geq$ 30 μg/kg body weight; with subcutaneous administration and lower doses it was less frequently encountered. In some patients reversible elevation of serum alkaline phosphatase and lactic dehydrogenase have been noted, and occasionally evidence of overshooting neutrophil activation such as the acute neutrophilic dermatosis (Sweet's syndrome) has been observed [44]. Some studies have shown a reduction in platelet counts after repeated subcutaneous injections of G-CSF (240 μg/m^2 per day for 14 days of repeated 21-day chemotherapy cycles) or continuous intravenous infusion at higher doses ($\geq$ 30 μg/kg).

Again, like GM-CSF, G-CSF is currently being tested by a number of investigators for its usefulness in the treatment of neutropenic disorders due to malignancies, as well as in congenital (Kostmann's syndrome), cyclic, or idiopathic neutropenia [45–47]. From the promising preliminary data it can be anticipated that in the near future some of these disorders will be at least ameliorated by the use of recombinant G-CSF.

Erythropoietin

EPO is a glycoprotein hormone produced predominantly in the kidney and to a limited extent in the liver. It regulates the proliferation and differentiation of erythroid progenitor cells to mature erythrocytes [48]. Recent work has suggested that the EPO-producing cell in the kidney is a peritubular interstitial cell found mainly in the inner renal cortex [49, 50]. In the adult only 10%–20% of plasma EPO is produced in the liver, but the exact site of synthesis has not been identified as yet [51]. In the fetus the liver is the primary site of EPO formation [52].

The mechanism by which a hypoxic stimulus triggers the production and release of EPO is still unknown. Evidence has been presented that the oxygen sensor is a heme protein [53].

EPO is a heavily glycosylated, 166 amino acid protein with a molecular mass of 34–39 kD. The EPO gene has been localized to chromosome 7q11–q22 by in situ hybridization [54]. Like those of its natural counterpart, the major target cells of recombinant EPO have been identified as colony-forming progenitor cells committed to the erythroid lineage (CFU-E, colony-forming unit–erythroid) and to a minor extent as more immature erythroid progenitor cells, the BFU-E (burst-forming unit–erythroid). Although some in vivo data have been accumulated indicating that EPO induces the proliferation of megakaryocyte (CFU-MK) and granulocyte/macrophage (CFU-GM) progenitor cells [55, 56, and W. Oster, personal communication], in most of the recent clinical trials no significant changes in circulating leukocyte or platelet numbers were seen. This, however, may be related to the dose and time schedule of EPO administration in these studies.

Clinical studies have clearly documented the effectiveness of recombinant EPO in correction of anemia in patients with end-stage renal disease [57, 58] as well as in predialysis patients [59]. In these patients only low levels of EPO can be demonstrated in the serum. Although, pathogenetically, anemia in tumor patients is not characterized by EPO deficiency, we investigated whether EPO levels exceeding normal values could stimulate erythropoiesis in these patients and thus contribute to correcting transfusion-dependent anemia.

The therapeutic effect of EPO in correcting chemotherapy-induced anemia in patients with normal renal function was demonstrated recently [60]. A significant and sustained increase in hemoglobin and hematocrit was demonstrated with EPO given twice weekly as a bolus injection using an escalating dose schedule (150–300 U/kg body weight). EPO response was accompanied by a decrease in serum ferritin. The requirement for red blood cell transfusion was eliminated by EPO therapy. EPO was also shown to be beneficial in the treatment of anemia of malignancy due to neoplastic bone marrow infiltration [61]. One patient with multiple myeloma showed an increase in platelet counts to >75% above baseline level, which was maintained for 3 months after discontinuation of EPO therapy.

This result underlines that the potential role of EPO as a thrombopoietic growth factor needs further evaluation.

No side effects were noted during EPO therapy. This conflicts with results in patients with endstage renal disease, in whom EPO therapy was associated with increases in blood pressure and where even thromboses, strokes, and seizures, induced presumably by increases in peripheral vascular resistance and blood viscosity, were seen. This difference may possibly be explained by a predisposition of patients with renal disease to vascular complications and to their lack of functioning kidneys to regulate the fluid balance.

Interleukin-3 (Multi-CSF)

As for GM- and G-CSF, the gene for interleukin-3 (IL-3) has been located on the long term of chromosome 5 in region q23–q31 [62]. The protein is produced by activated T lymphocytes and has a molecular mass of 14–28 kD. IL-3 is a multilineage hematopoietin which promotes the growth and differentiation of various myeloid progenitor cells including early multipotent progenitors such as blast colony-forming units and mixed colonies. The colonies produced in response to IL-3 contain eosinophils, basophils, neutrophils, mast cells, megakaryocytes, macrophages, and erythroid cells.

In preclinical murine and primate models IL-3 has been shown to significantly elevate numbers of circulating leukocytes [63, 64]. A phase I/II trial in patients with advanced malignancies with or without bone marrow failure has revealed the following dose related hematological responses: increases in platelet counts, absolute leukocyte counts including neutrophils, monocytes, eosinophils, lymphocytes and, to a lesser extent, basophils, reticulocyte counts, and bone marrow cellularity [65]. Side effects included fever, flushing, headache, and local irritation at the site of the subcutaneous injection. More efficacy is to be expected from the use of combinations of hematopoietins acting on early progenitor cells with late-acting myeloid growth factors.

Macrophage Colony-Stimulating Factor

M-CSF is the last of the human hematopoietic growth factors available in recombinant form which has just progressed from the laboratory into clinical use. Definite data with respect to biological activity and toxicity in humans are not available yet.

M-CSF is a glycoprotein of 47–74 kD comprising two identical subunits [66]. The gene is located on chromosome 5 in close proximity to the IL-3 gene (5q33). Monocytes, fibroblasts, and endothelial cells have been shown to be able to produce this factor.

Interleukins

Of all interleukins known to affect the immune response, IL-2 has received the most attention in cancer therapy.

IL-2, previously known as T cell growth factor, is a 15.5-kD glycoprotein secreted predominantly by T helper lymphocytes after exposure to mitogens or antigens. It induces T cell proliferation and the proliferation and differentiation of B cells, resulting in the secondary induction of other lymphokines including IL-4 [67], tumor necrosis factor (TNF) [68], and IFN-γ [69, 70]. IFN-γ in turn is the prototype of a macrophage-activating factor, enhancing, for example, the ability of macrophages to kill intracellular pathogens and tumor cells [71–74].

IL-2 also directly augments the cytotoxicity of human monocytes [75] and stimulates the activation of nonspecific cytolytic effector cells, designated lymphokine-activated killer (LAK) cells. Most of the IL-2-induced cytolytic activity was found to be mediated by activated natural killer (NK) cells [76].

Experiments with sublethally irradiated tumor-bearing animals suggested that recombinant IL-2 does not cause tumor regression by direct action on the tumor but rather by activation of a radiosensitive host component, presumably a cellular component of the immune system [77]. The potential clinical use of IL-2 thus depends on its ability to activate endogenous or exogenous cells able to exert antitumor effects.

Initial clinical studies with IL-2 were performed by Rosenberg and colleagues using adoptive immunotherapy with high dose IL-2 and ex vivo activated LAK cells in patients with metastatic malignant melanoma (MM), renal cell carcinoma (RCC), or colorectal cancer [78, 79]. This protocol consists of an intravenous bolus injection of IL-2 10^4–10^5 U/kg body weight every 8 h for 5 days to stimulate LAK precursor cells, followed by the harvest of peripheral blood lymphocytes by leukapheresis and subsequent in vitro cultivation and stimulation with IL-2. These LAK cells are then reinfused into the patient with additional systemic IL-2 therapy. West and colleagues described a continuous infusion regimen for IL-2 plus LAK cells which produced comparable results with apparently lower toxicity [80].

Antitumor activity was also demonstrated in patients with MM or RCC receiving IL-2 therapy without LAK cells, indicating that exogenous LAK cells are not an absolute requirement for antitumor activity of IL-2.

Overall response rates achieved by IL-2 treatment with or without LAK cells ranged from 0%–50% in RCC and 11%–50% in MM [79, 81–83].

Side effects of IL-2 were significant in patients treated on high-dose protocols. The dose-limiting toxicities included fever and chills, hypotension, and interstitial pulmonary edema, due to the development of a capillary leak syndrome. These effects resolved within 24–48 h after discontinuation of therapy. Other commonly encountered side effects were nausea/vomiting, diarrhea, and bone marrow toxicity (anemia, thrombocytopenia). In the pathogenesis of adverse events IL-2-induced release of prostaglandins and other secondary mediators like TNF-α or IL-1 are thought to play a role [84–86].

An interesting phenomenon that is frequently reported and also observed in our ongoing study with IL-2 plus IFN-α (repeated cycles of a 96-h infusion of IL-2 at a dosage of MU/m^2 per day and subcutaneous injection of IFN-α at a dosage of 6 MU/m^2 per day on day 1 and 4) in patients with MM and RCC is the mixed response, suggesting a different susceptibility of metastases to treatment depending on their anatomical site. Preliminary results of this trial show comparable efficacy (response rate of 21%) to the trial using IL-2 and LAK cells with reduced toxicity (unpublished observations). To investigate the possible synergistic effects of IL-2 with chemotherapeutic agents, clinical studies using IL-2 in conjunction with low-dose cyclophosphamide in patients with MM and RCC have been conducted [87–89]. The rationale for adding this cytotoxic drug was to block induction of counter-acting suppressor T lymphocytes by IL-2. In the clinical trials no objective responses were achieved in patients with RCC and 15%–43% remission rates (complete and partial remissions and mixed responses) were seen in melanoma patients.

Responses to IL-2 alone or in combination with LAK cells or cyclophosphamide have been seen with a variety of doses and schedules, but at the present time no optimum regimen can be defined.

Another immunotherapeutic approach to the treatment of patients with malignant melanoma has been reported by Rosenberg [90]. With the systemic administration of ex vivo expanded tumor-infiltrating lymphocytes (TIL) in conjunction with IL-2 and pretreatment of patients with cyclophosphamide, higher response rates were apparently achieved in a preliminary clinical trial than with the treatment with LAK cells. Duration of response, however, was often short.

Tumor Necrosis Factor-α

TNF-α, a secretory product of activated macrophages [68, 91, 92], NK cells, T lymphocytes, B lymphocytes, and also granulocytes [93, 94], is an endogenous mediator of inflammation and various immunological reactions. The protein has a molecular weight of 17 kD and is encoded by a gene located on the short arm of chromosome 6 [95, 96]. It has been shown that TNF can activate neutrophils [97], augment macrophage [98] and NK cell [99] cytotoxicity, and induce other cytokines such as IL-1 and IL-6 [100]. In vitro experiments have also demonstrated several effects of TNF on vascular endothelium, such as induction of MHC antigens [101], increased adherence for granulocytes [102], inhibition of endothelial growth [103], and also, paradoxically, stimulation of angiogenesis [104].

The cytotoxic activity shown by TNF in many transformed cell lines but not normal cells [105] and its antitumor activity in animal models [106, 107] led to its clinical evaluation in cancer patients. However, in phase I and II studies with single agent TNF the overall response rate was disappointingly low, ranging around 5%, and toxicity was substantial. Slightly higher response rates were seen in gastrointestinal tumors and RCC [108, 109].

At lower doses general weakness, fever, and chills dominated the clinical picture. As reported for IL-2, the dose-limiting toxicity was hypotension and interstitial fluid retention. Other, also mainly dose-dependent adverse effects, were nausea/vomiting, diarrhea, headache, and myalgia [110]. The most frequently observed laboratory abnormality was a temporary decrease in absolute leukocyte counts. This is most likely due to margination of circulating leucokytes by TNF-induced increased endothelial adherence [111, 112].

The effects by which TNF exerts its antitumor activity are pleiotropic and not yet understood. Evidence has been presented that direct and indirect vascular effects via activation of the arachidonic acid cascade are involved in the induction of tumor necrosis and also in TNF-induced side effects. Animal experiments have shown that the administration of oxygen scavengers could prevent lethality without impairment of the antitumor activity [113]. It remains to be seen whether in clinical trials pretreatment with oxygen scavengers or the combination of TNF with other immunoregulatory agents reduces side effects without inhibiting antitumor effects.

Interferons

Interferons (IFNs) are a heterogeneous family of proteins which have been broadly classified into three groups: α, β, and γ. IFN-α and IFN-β ("type I IFNs") have similar biological and physicochemical properties and are produced following viral infections by leukocytes and fibroblasts respectively. IFN-γ or immune IFN ("type II IFN") is secreted by antigen- or mitogen-activated T lymphocytes. The properties attributed to the various IFNs are numerous and include antiviral activity and antiproliferative and immunomo-dulatory effects. The antineoplastic activity would seem to result from both a direct inhibitory effect on cell growth and multiplication [114] and an indirect effect by modification of the immune system. The latter effect includes augment-ation of NK cell activity [115], increased expression of surface antigens [116], and suppression or enhancement of some B and T cell functions [117, 118]. IFN-γ is also a potent activator of macrophage function [74, 119].

Up to now the most impressive clinical results have been achieved with IFN-α in hematologic disorders, especially in hairy cell leukemia [120] and chronic myelogenous leukemia [121]. IFN-α has also been recommended for the treatment of AIDS-related Kaposi's sarcoma [122] and malignant melanoma [123].

Clinical trials with IFN-α in patients with hairy cell leukemia have shown remission rates between 70% and 90%, with 10%–30% complete remissions [124]. After cessation of treatment up to 40% of the patients in complete remission relapsed within 9–12 months. However, remissions could be easily reinduced in these patients by resumption of IFN-α therapy [125].

The mechanism by which TFN-α acts in hairy cell leukemia is uncertain. There is evidence that exogenous IFN-α may interrupt a paracrine loop by which microenvironmental cells produce cytokines (e.g., TNF) which inhibit normal hematopoiesis and stimulate the growth of hairy cells [126, 127].

Chronic myelogenous leukemia is also sensitive to IFN-α. Recently, Talpaz described a 73% complete hematologic remission rate in 96 patients with early benign phase disease [128]; 19% of the patients achieved a cytogenetic remission with complete suppression of the clone carrying the Philadelphia chromosome. Of responding patients, 60% have sustained complete cytogenetic responses for more than 6 months, the median duration being 30 months. Also, patients who relapse with chronic myelogenous leukemia after allogenic bone marrow transplantation might benefit from IFN-α therapy [129].

The results in late chronic phase (more than 1 year after diagnosis) have been less favorable. Here, a possible approach might be a combination treatment of IFN-α and low-dose cytosine arabinoside [130].

Adverse events observed with IFN therapy are predominantly flu-like symptoms such as fever, chills, fatigue, and myalgias. Anorexia, weight loss, nausea/vomiting, and diarrhea have also been frequently reported.

The laboratory abnormalities seen during therapy with IFN indicated mild hematologic (leukopenia, anemia, neutropenia, thrombocytopenia), renal (pro-teinuria, elevated blood urea nitrogen), and hepatic (elevated glutamic oxalo-acetic transaminase and bilirubin) toxicity [131].

Other indications in oncology for which IFN has proved promising, but for which definitive data are still lacking, include multiple myeloma [124], T-cell lymphoma [132], non-Hodgkin's lymphoma [133] and RCC [134].

References

1. Nicola NA (1987) Why do hematopoietic growth factor receptors interact with each other? Immunol Today 8: 134–139
2. Hueber K, Isobe M, Croce CM, Golde DM, Kaufman SE, Gasson JC (1985) The human gene encoding GM-CSF is a 5q29–q32, the chromosome region deleted in the 5q-anomaly. Science 230: 1282–1285
3. Donahue RE, Wang EA, Foutch L, Leary AC, Witek-Giametti JS, Metzger M, Hewick RM, Steinbrink DR, Shaw G (1986) Effects of N-linked carbohydrate on the in vivo properties of human GM-CSF. Cold Spring Harbor Symp Quant Biol 51: 685–692
4. Herrmann F, Oster W, Meuer SC, Klein K, Lindemann A, Mertelsmann R (1988) Interleukin-1 stimulates T lymphocytes to produce GM-CSF. J Clin Invest 81: 1415–1418
5. Donahue RE, Emerson SG, Wang EA, Wong GG, Clark SC, Nathan DG (1985) Demonstration of burst-promoting activity of recombinant human GM-CSF on circulating erythroid progenitors using an assay involving the delayed addition of erythropoietin. Blood 66: 1479–1481
6. Metcalf D, Begley CG, Johnson GR, Nicola NA, Vadas MA, Lopez AF, Williamson DJ, Wong CG, Clark SC, Wang EA (1986) Biologic properties in vitro of recombinant human granulocyte-macrophage colony-stimulating factor. Blood 67: 37–45
7. Lindemann A, Riedel D, Oster W, Meuer SC, Blohm D, Mertelsmann R, Herrmann F (1988) GM-CSF induces secretion of interleukin-1 by polymorpho-nuclear neutrophils. J Immunol 140: 837–839
8. Herrmann F, Riedel D, Bambach T, Mertelsmann R (1987) Recombinant granulocyte/macrophage-colony stimulating factor (RGM-CSF) inhibits growth of clonogenic cells in monoblast line U937 due to induction of tumor necrosis factor-alpha (TNF-ALPHA) and interleukin 1 (IL-1). Proc Am Soc Clin Oncol 6: A71
9. Grabstein KH, Urdal DL, Tushinsi RJ, Mochizuki DY, Price VL, Canterell MA, Gillis S, Conlon PJ (1986) Induction of macrophage tumoricidal activity by GM-CSF. Science 32: 506–508
10. Fischer H-G, Frosch S, Reske K, Reske-Kunz AB (1988) GM-CSF activates macrophages derived from bone marrow cultures to synthesis of MHC class II molecules and to augmented antigen presentation function. J Immunol 141: 3882–3888
11. Reed SG, Nathan CF, Pihl DL, Rodricks P, Shanebeck K, Conlon PJ, Grabstein PJ (1987) Recombinant granulocyte/macrophage colony stimulating factor activates macrophages to inhibit *Trypanosoma cruzi* and release hydrogen peroxide: Comparison with γ-interferon. J Exp Med 166: 1734–1746
12. Herrmann F, Schulz G, Lindemann A, Meyenburg W, Oster W, Krumwieh D, Mertelsmann R (1988) Yeast-expressed granulocyte-macrophage colony-stimulating factor in cancer patients: a phase Ib clinical study. Behring Inst Mitt 83: 107–118
13. Steis RG, Clark J, Longo DL (1989) A phase Ib evaluation of recombinant granulocyte-macrophage colony-stimulating factor. In: Berger HG et al. (eds) Cancer therapy. Springer, Berlin Heidelberg New York, pp 103–111
14. Herrmann F, Schulz G, Lindemann A, Meyenburg W, Oster W, Krumwieh D, Mertelsmann R (1989) Hematopoetic responses in patients with advanced malig-

nancy treated with recombinant human granulocyte-macrophage colony-stimulating factor. J Clin Oncol 7: 159–167

15. Herrmann F, Wieser M, Schulz G, Lindemann A, Oster W, Mertelsmann R (1988) Single daily subcutaneous administration of rhGM-CSF ameliorates hematopoietic toxicity of chemotherapy in outpatients (abstract). Blood 72: 390

16. Link H, Freund M, Kirchner H, Stoll M, Schmid H, Bucsky P, Seidel J, Schulz G, Schmidt RE, Riehm H, Poliwoda H, Welte K (1989) Enhancement of autologous bone marrow transplantation with recombinant granulocyte-macrophage colony-stimulating factor (rhGM-CSF). In: Berger HG et al. (eds) Cancer therapy. Springer, Berlin Heidelberg New York, pp 96–102

17. Brandt SJ, Peters WP, Atwater SK, Kurtzberg J, Borowitz MJ, Jones RB, Shpall EJ, Bast RC, Gilbert CJ, Oette DH (1988) Effect of recombinant human granulocyte-macrophage colony-stimulating factor on hematopoietic reconstitution after high-dose chemotherapy and autologous bone marrow transplantation. N Engl J Med 318: 869–876

18. Antman KS, Griffin JD, Elias A, Socinski MA, Ryan L, Cannistra SA, Oette D, Whitley M, Frei E, Schnipper LE (1988) Effect of recombinant human granulocyte-macrophage colony-stimulating factor on chemotherapy-induced myelosuppression. N Engl J Med 319: 593–598

19. Ganser A, Völkers B, Greher J, Ottmann OG, Walther F, Becker R, Bergmann L, Schulz G, Hoelzer D (1989) Recombinant human granulocyte-macrophage colony-stimulating factor in patients with myelodysplastic syndromes – a phase I/II trial. Blood 73: 31–37

20. Ganser A, Völkers B, Greher J, Walther F, Hoelzer D (1989) Application of granulocyte-macrophage colony-stimulating factor in patients with malignant hematological diseases. In: Berger HG et al. (eds) Cancer therapy. Springer, Berlin Heidelberg New York, pp 90–95

21. Herrmann F, Ganser A, Lindemann A, Wieser M, Schulz G, Hoelzer D, Mertelsmann R (1989) Stimulation of granulopoiesis in patients with malignancy by rhGM-CSF: assessment of two routes of administration. J Biol Response Mod (in press)

22. Peters WP (1989) The effect of recombinant human colony-stimulating factors on hematopoietic reconstitution following autologous bone marrow transplantation. Semin Hematol 26: 18–23

23. Peters WP, Atwater S, Kurtzberg J (1989) The use of recombinant human granulocyte macrophage colony-stimulating factor in autologous bone marrow transplantation. In: Gale R, Champlin R (eds) Bone marrow transplantation: current controversies. Liss, New York, pp 595–606

24. Socinski MA, Cannistra SA, Elias A, Antman KH, Schnipper L, Griffin JD (1988) Granulocyte-macrophage colony stimulating factor expands the circulating hematopoietic progenitor cell compartment in man. Lancet I: 1194–1198

25. Vadhan-Raj S, Keating M, LeMaistre A, Hittelman WN, McCredie K, Trujillo JM, Broxmeyer HE, Henney C, Gutterman JU (1987) Effects of recombinant human granulocyte-macrophage colony-stimulating factor in patients with myelodysplastic syndrome. N Engl J Med 317: 1545–1552

26. Herrmann F, Lindemann A, Klein H, Luebbert M, Schulz G, Mertelsmann R (1989) Effect of recombinant human granulocyte-macrophage colony-stimulating factor in patients with myelodysplastic syndrome with excess blasts. Leukemia 3: 335–338

27. Cannistra SA, Groshek P, Griffin JD (1989) Granulocyte-macrophage colony-stimulating factor enhances the cytotoxic effects of cytosine-arabinoside in acute myeloblastic leukemia and in the myeloid blast crisis phase of chronic myeloid leukemia. Leukemia 3: 328–334

28. Andreeff M, Hegewisch-Becker S, Tafuri A, Bressler J, Redner A, Haimi J, Souza L, Welte K (1989) Recruitment of leukemic cells in vitro by colony-stimulating factors (G-CSF, GM-CSF, interleukin-3): evidence of increased cell kill and of differentiation by high- and low-dose cytosine arabinoside. Blut (in press)

29. Champlin RE, Nimer SD, Ireland P, Oette DH, Golde DW (1989) Treatment of refractory aplastic anemia with recombinant human granulocyte-macrophage colony-stimulating factor. Blood 73: 694–699

30. Nissen C, Tichelli A, Gratwohl A, Speck B, Milne A, Gordon-Smith EC, Schaedelin J (1988) Failure of recombinant human granulocyte-macrophage colony-stimulating factor therapy in aplastic anemia patients with severe neutropenia. Blood 72: 2045–2047

31. Groopman J, Mitsuyasu RT, DeLero M, Oette DH, Golde DW (1987) Effect of recombinant human granulocyte-macrophage colony-stimulating factor on myelopoiesis in the acquired immuno-deficiency syndrome. N Engl J Med 317: 593–598

32. Mooney DP, Ganelli RL, O'Reeilly M, Herbert JC (1988) Recombinant human granulocyte colony-stimulating factor and pseudomonas burn wound sepsis. Arch Surg 123: 1353–1357

33. Welte K, Platzer E, Lu L, Gabrilove JL, Levi E, Mertelsmann R, Moore MAS (1985) Purification and biological characterization of human pluripotent hematopoietic colony-stimulating factor. Proc Natl Acad Sci USA 82: 1526–1530

34. Nagata S, Tsuchiya M, Asano S, Kaziro Y, Yamazaki T, Yamamozo O, Hirata N, Kubota N, Oheda H, Nomura H, Ono M (1986) Molecular cloning and expression of cDNA for human granulocyte colony-stimulating factor. Nature 319: 415–418

35. Souza LM, Boone TC, Gabrilove JL, Lai PH, Zsebok M, Murdock DC, Chazin VR, Bruszewski J, Lu H, Chen KK, Barendt J, Platzer E, Moore MAS, Mertelsmann R, Welte K (1986) Recombinant human granulocyte colony-stimulating factor: effects on normal and leukemic myeloid cells. Science 232: 61–65

36. Simmers RN, Webber LM, Shannon MF, Garson OM, Wong MA, Sutherland GR (1987) Localization of the G-CSF gene on chromosome 17 proximal to the breakpoint in the t(15; 17) in acute promyelocytic leukemia. Blood 70: 330–332

37. Platzer E, Oez K, Welte, K, Sandler A, Gabrilove JL, Mertelsman R, Moore MA, Kalden JR (1987) Human pluripotent hematopoietic colony stimulating factor; activities on human and murine cells. Immunobiology 172: 185–193

38. Asano S, Shirafuji N, Watari K, Matsuda S, Uemura N, Jeki R, Kodo H, Takaku F (1988) Phase I clinical study for recombinant human granulocyte colony-stimulating factor. Behring Inst Mitt 83: 222–228

39. Bronchud M, Scarfte JH, Thatcher N, Crowther D, Souza LM, Alton NK, Testa NG, Dexter TM (1987) Phase I/II study of recombinant human granulocyte colony-stimulating factor in patients receiving intensive chemotherapy for small cell lung cancer. Br J Cancer 56: 809–813

40. Gabrilove JL, Jakubowski A, Scher H, Sternberg C, Wong G, Gron J, Yagoda A, Fain K, Moore MAS, Clarkson B, Oettgen HF, Alton K, Welte K, Souza L (1988) Effect of granulocyte colony-stimulating factor on neutropenia and associated morbidity due to chemotherapy or transitional cell carcinoma of the urothelium. N Engl J Med 318: 1414–1422

41. Lindemann A, Herrmann F, Oster W, Meyenburg W, Haffneer P, Souza L, Mertelsmann R (1989) Hematologic effects of recombinant human granulocyte colony-stimulating factor in patients with malignancy. Blood (in press)

42. Morstyn G, Campbell L, Souza LM, Alton NK, Keech J, Green M, Sheridan W, Metcalf D, Fox R (1988) Effect of granulocyte colony-stimulating factor on neutropenia induced by cytotoxic chemotherapy. Lancet I: 667–672

43. Sheridan W, Morstyn G, Green M et al. Phase II study of granulocyte colony-stimulating factor (G-CSF) in autologous one marrow transplantation (ABMT) (abstract) Proc Am Soc Clin Oncol (in press)

44. Glapsy JA, Baldwin GC, Robertson PA, Souza L, Vincent M, Ambersley J, Golde DW (1988) Therapy for neutropenia in hairy cell leukemia with recombinant human granulocyte colony-stimulating factor. Ann Intern Med 109: 789–795

45. Jakubowski AA, Souza L, Kelly F, Fain K, Budman D, Clarkson B, Bonilla MA, Moore MAS, Gabrilove J (1989) Effects of granulocyte colony-stimulating factor in a patient with idiopathic neutropenia. N Engl J Med 320: 38–42

46. Hammond WP, Price TH, Souza LM, Dale DC (1989) Treatment of cyclic neutropenia with granulocyte colony-stimulating factor. N Engl J Med 320: 1306–1311

47. Bonilla MA, Gillio AP, Ruggiero M, Kernan NA, Brochstein JA, Abboud MA, Fumagalli L, Vincent M, Welte K, Souza LM, O'Reilly RI (1988) In vivo recombinant human granulocyte colony-stimulating factor (rhG-CSF) corrects neutropenia in patients with congenital agranulocytosis. (abstract) Blood 72: 349

48. Spivac JL (1986) The mechanism of action of erythropoietin. Int J Cell Cloning 4: 139–166

49. Koury ST, Bondurant MC, Koury MJ (1988) Localization of erythropoietin synthesizing cells in murine kidneys by in situ hybridization. Blood 71: 524–527

50. Lacombe C, DaSilva JL, Bruneval P, Fournier JG, Wendling F, Casadevall N, Camilleri JP, Bariety J, Varet B, Tambourin P (1988) Peritubular cells are the site of erythropoietin synthesis in the murine hypoxic kidney. J Clin Invest 81: 620–623

51. Fried W (1972) The liver as a source of extrarenal erythropoietin production. Blood 40: 671–677

52. Zanjani ED, Poster J, Burlington H, Mann LI, Wasserman LR (1977) Liver as the primary site of erythropoietin formation in the fetus. J Lab Clin Med 89: 640–644

53. Goldberg MA, Dunning SP, Bunn HF (1988) Regulation of the erythropoietin gene: evidence that the oxygen sensor is a heme protein. Science 242: 1412–1415

54. Law ML, Cai C-H, Lin F-K, Wei A, Huang S-Z, Hartz J-H, Morse H, Lin C-H, Jones C, Kao F-T (1986) Chromosomal assignment of the human erythropoietin gene and its DNA polymorphism. Proc Natl Acad Sci USA 83: 6920–6924

55. Ganser A, Bergmann M, Voelkers B, Gruetzmacher P, Scigalla P, Hoelzer D (1989) In vivo effects of recombinant human erythropoietin on circulating human haematopoietic progenitor cells. Exp Hematol 17: 433–435

56. Geissler K, Stockenhuber F, Kabrna E, Hinterberger W, Balcke P, Lecher K (1989) Recombinant human erythropoietin and haematopoietic progenitor cells in vivo. Blood 73: 2229

57. Adamson JW (1989) The promise of recombinant human erythropoietin. Semin Hematol 26: 5–8

58. Eschbach JW, Egrie JC, Downing MR, Browne JK, Adamson JW (1987) Correction of the anemia of end-stage renal disease with recombinant human erythropietin. N Engl J Med 316: 73–80

59. Lim VS, DeGowin RL, Zavala D, Kirchner PT, Abels R, Perry P, Fangman J (1989) Recombinant human erythropoietin treatment in pre-dialysis patients. Ann Intern Med 110: 108–114

60. Oster W, Herrmann F, Cicco A, Gamm H, Zeile G, Brune T, Lindemann A, Schulz G Mertelsmann R (1989) Erythropoietin prevents chemotherapy-induced anemia. Blut 59: 1–5

61. Oster W, Herrmann F, Gamm H, Zeile G, Lindemann A, Müller G, Brune T; Kraemer H-P, Mertelsmann R, Erythropoietin (EPO) for the treatment of anemia of malignancy due to neoplastic bone marrow infiltration. J Clin Oncol (in press)

62. Yang Y-C, Ciarletta AB, Temple PA, Chung MP, Kovacic S, Witek-Giannotti JS, Leary AC, Kirz R, Donahue RE, Wong GG, Clark SC (1986) Human IL-3 (multi-CSF): identification by expression cloning of a novel hematopoietic growth factor related to murine IL-3. Cell 47: 3–10

63. Donahue RE, Wang EA, Stone DK, Kamen R, Wong GG, Sehgal PK, Nathan DG, Clark SC (1986) Stimulation of hematopoiesis in primates by continuous infusion of recombinant human GM-CSF. Nature 321: 872–875

64. Welte K, Bonilla MA, Gillio AP, Boone TC, Potter GK, Gabrilove JL, Moore MAS, O'Reilley, Souza LM (1987) Recombinant human G-CSF: effects on hematopoiesis in normal and cyclophosphamide treated primates. J Exp Med 165: 941–948

65. Ganser A, Lindemann A, Seipelt G, Ottmann OG, Herrmann F, Schulz G, Mertelsmann R, Hoelzer D (1989) Effect of recombinant human interleukin-3 (rhIL-3) in patients with bone marrow failure – a phase I/II trial (abstract). Blood (74): 177

66. Stanley ER, Hansen G, Woodcock J, Metcalf D (1975) Colony stimulating factor and the regulation of granulopoiesis and macrophage production. Fed Proc 34: 2272–2278

67. Howard M, Matis L, Malek TR, Shevach E, Kehl W, Cohen D, Nakanishi K, Paul WE (1983) Interleukin-2 induces antigen reactive T cell lines to secrete BCGF-1. J Exp Med 158: 2024–2039

68. Nedwin GE, Svedersky LP, Bringman TS, Palladino MA, Goeddel DV (1985) Effect of interleukin-2, γ-interferon, and mitogens on the production of tumor necrosis factor alpha and beta. J Immunol 135: 2492–2497

69. Farrar WL, John HM, Farrar J (1981) Regulation of the production of immune interferon and cytotoxic T-lymphocytes by IL-2. J Immunol 126: 1120–1125

70. Kawase I, Brooks CG, Kuribayashi K, Olabunenaga S, Newman W, Gillis S, Henney CS (1983) Interleukin-2 induces γ-interferon production: participation of macrophages and NK-like cells. J Immunol 131: 288–292

71. Black CM, Catterall JR, Remington, JS (1987) In vivo and in vitro activation of alveolar macrophages by recombinant γ-interferon. J Immunol 138: 491–495

72. Murray HW, Spitalney GL, Nathan CF (1985) Activation of mouse peritoneal macrophages in vitro and in vivo by γ-interferon. J Immunol 134: 1619–1622

73. Nathan CF, Murray HW, Wiebe ME, Rubin BY (1983) Identification of γ-interferon as the lymphokine that activates human macrophage oxidative metabolism and antimicrobial activity. J Exp Med 158: 670–689

74. Schreiber RD, Celada A (1985) Molecular characterisation of γ-interferon as a macrophage activating factor. In: Pick E (ed) Lymphokines, Academic, New York, pp 87–118

75. Malkovsky M, Loveland B, North M, Asherson GL, Gao L, Ward P, Fiers W (1987) Recombinant interleukin-2 directly augments the toxicity of human monocytes. Nature 325: 262–265

76. Phillips JH, Lanier LL (1986) Dissection of the lymphokine-activated killer phenomenon. Relative contribution of peripheral blood natural killer cells and T lymphocytes to cytolysis. J Exp Med 164: 814–825

77. Rosenberg SA, Mule JJ, Spiess PJ, Reichert CM, Schwarz SL (1985) Regression of established pulmonary metastases and subcutaneous tumor mediated by the systemic administration of high-dose recombinant interleukin-2. J Exp Med 61: 1169–1188

78. Rosenberg SA, Lotze MT, Muul LM, Leitman S, Chang AE, Ettinghausen SE, Matory YL, Skibber JM, Shilari E, Vetto JT, Seipp CA, Simpson C, Reichert CM (1985) Observations on the systemic administration of autologous lymphokine-activated killer cells and recombinant interleukin-2 to patients with metastatic cancer. N Engl J Med 313: 1485–1492

79. Rosenberg SA, Lotze MT, Muul LM, Chang AE, Avis FP, Leitman S, Linehan WM, Robertson CN, Lee RE, Rubin JT, Seipp CA, Simpson CG, White DE (1987) A progress report on the treatment of 157 patients with advancd cancer using lymphokine-activated killer cells and interleukin-2 or high-dose interleukin-2 alone. N Engl J Med 316: 889–879

80. West WH, Tauer KW, Yanelli JR, Marshall GD, Orr DW, Thurman GB, Oldham RK (1987) Constant-infusion recombinant interleukin-2 in adoptive immune therapy of cancer. N Engl J Med 316: 898–905

81. Dutcher JP, Creekmore S, Weiss GR, Margolin K, Markowitz AB, Roper MA, Parkinson D (1989) A phase II study of interleukin-2 and lymphokine activated killer cells in patients with metastatic malignant melanoma. J Clin Oncol 7: 477–485

82. Fischer RI, Coltman CA, Doroshow JH, Rayner AA, Hawkins MJ, Mier JW, Wiernik P, McMannis JD, Weiss GR, Margolin KA, Gemlo BT, Hoth DF, Parkinson DR, Paietta E (1988) Metastatic renal cell cancer treated with interleukin-2 and lymphokine-activated killer cells. A phase II clinical trial. Ann Inten Med 108: 518–523

83. Lotze MT, Matory YL, Rayner AA, Ettinghausen SE, Vetto JT, Seipp CA, Rosenberg SA (1986) Clinical effects and toxicity of interleukin-2 in patients with cancer. Cancer 58: 2764–2772

84. Gemlo BT, Palladino MA, Jaffe HS, Espevik TP, Rayner AA (1988) Circulating cytokines in patients with metastatic cancer treated with recombinant interleukin 2 and lymphokine-activated killer cells. Cancer Res 48: 5864–5867

85. Fraser-Scott K, Hatzakis H, Seong D, Jones CM, Wu KK (1988) Influence of natural and recombinant interleukin 2 on endothelial cell arachidonate metabolism. Induction of de novo synthesis of prostaglandin H synthase. J Clin Invest 82: 1877–1883

86. Mier JW, Vachino G, Van der Meer J, Numerof RP, Adams S, Cannon JG, Bernheim HA, Atkins MB, Parkinson DR, Dinarello CA (1988) Induction of circulating tumor necrosis factor as the mechanism for the febrile response to interleukin-2 in cancer patients. J Clin Immunol 8: 426–436

87. Lindemann A, Hoeffken K, Schmidt RE, Diehl V, Kloke O, Gamm H, Hayungs J, Oster W, Böhm M, Kolitz JE, Franks CR, Herrmann F, Mertelsmann R (1989) A phase II study of low-dose cyclophosphamide and recombinant human interleukin-2 in metastatic renal cell carcinoma and malignant melanoma. Cancer Immunol Immunother 28: 275–281

88. Mitchell MS (1989) Low-dose cyclophosphamide and IL-2 in the treatment of advanced melanoma. In: Berger HG et al. (eds) Cancer therapy. Springer, Berlin Heidelberg New York, pp 85–89

89. Mitchell MS, Kempf RA, Harel W, Shau H, Boswell WD, Lind S, Bradley EC (1988) Effectiveness and tolerability of low-dose cyclophosphamide and low-dose intravenous interleukin-2 in disseminated melanoma. J Clin Oncol 6: 409–424

90. Rosenberg SA, Packard BS, Aebersold PM, Solomon D, Topalian SL, Toy ST, Simon P, Lotze MT, Yang JC, Seipp CA, Simpson C, Carter C, Bock S, Schwartzenhuber D, Wei JP, White DE (1988) Use of tumor-infiltrating lymphocytes and interleukin-2 in the immunotherapy of patients with metastatic melanoma. N Engl J Med 319: 1676–1680

91. Bate CAW, Taverne J, Playfair JHL (1988) Malarial parasites induce TNF production by macrophages. Immunology 64: 227–231

92. Sayers TJ, Macker I, Chung J, Kugler E (1987) The production of tumor necrosis factor by mouse bone marrow-derived macrophages in response to bacterial LPS and chemically synthesised monosaccharide precursors. J Immunol 138: 2935–2940

93. Cuturi MC, Murphy M, Costa-Giomi MP, Weinmann R, Perussia B, Trinchieri G (1987) Independent regulation of tumor necrosis factor and lymphotoxin production by human peripheral blood lymphocytes. J Exp Med 165: 1581–1594

94. Degliantoni G, Murphy M, Kobayashi M, Francins MK, Perussia B, Trindieri G (1985) Natural killer (NK) cell-derived hematopoietic colony inhibiting activity and NK cytotoxic factor: relationship with tumor necrosis factor and synergisms with immune interferon. J Exp Med 162: 1512–1530

95. Nedwin GE, Naylor SL, Sakaguchi AY, Smith D, Nedwin JJ, Pennica D, Goeddel DV, Gray PW (1985) Human lymphotoxin and tumor necrosis factor genes. Structure, homology and chromosomal location. Nucleic Acids Res 13: 6361–6373

96. Pennica D, Nedwin GE, Hayflick JS, Seeburg PH, Derynek R, Palladino MA, Kohr WJ, Aggarwal BB, Goeddel DV (1984) Human tumor necrosis factor. Precursor, structure, expression and homology to lymphotoxin. Nature 312: 724–729

97. Shalaby MR, Aggarwal BB, Rinderknecht E, Svedersky LP, Finkle BS, Palladino MA (1985) Activation of human polymorpho-nuclear neutrophil functions by interferon-gamma and tumor necrosis factor. J Immunol 135: 2069–2073

98. Hori K, Ehrke MH, Mace K, Mihich E (1987) Effect of recombinant tumor necrosis factor on tumoricidal activation of murine macrophages. synergism between tumor necrosis factor and γ-interferon. Cancer Res 47: 5868–5874

99. Ostensen ME, Thiele DL, Lipsky PE (1987) Tumor necrosis factor alpha enhances cytolytic activity of human natural killer cells. J Immunol 138: 4185–4191

100. Old LJ (1985) Tumor necrosis factor (TNF). Science 230: 630–632

101. Collins T, Lapierre LA, Fiers W, Strominger JL, Prober JS (1986) Recombinant human tumor necrosis factor increases mRNA levels and surface expression of HLA-A,B antigens in vascular endothelial cells and dermal fibroblasts in vitro. Proc Nat Acad Sci USA 83: 446–450

102. Pohlman TH, Stanness KA, Beatty PG, Ochs HD, Harlan JM (1986) An endothelial cell surface factor(s) induced in vitro by lipopolysaccharide, interleukin-1 and tumor necrosis factor-alpha increases neutophil adherence by a CDw 18-independent mechanism. J Immunol 135: 4548–4533

103. Van De Wiel PA, Pieters RHH, Bloksma N (1987) Synergistic action of recombinant TNF and endotoxin on cultured endothelial cells. Immunobiology 175: 75

104. Leibovich SJ, Polverini PJ, Shephard MJ, Wiseman MJ, Shively DM, Nuseir V (1987) Macrophage-induced angiogenesis is mediated by tumor necrosis factor alpha. Nature 329: 630–632

105. Sugarman BJ, Aggarwal BB, Hass PE, Figari IS, Palladino MA, Shepard HM (1985) Recombinant human tumor necrosis factor-alpha: effects on proliferation of normal and transformed cells. Science 230: 943–945

106. Carswell EA, Old LJ, Kassel RL, Green S, Fiore D, Williamson B (1975) An endotoxin induced serum factor that causes necrosis of tumors. Proc Natl Acad Sci USA 72: 3666–3670

107. Haranaki K, Carswell EA, Williamson B, Pentergast JS, Satomi N, Old LJ (1986) Purification, characterisation and antitumor activity of nonrecombinant mouse tumor necrosis factor. Proc Natl Acad Sci USA 83: 3949–3953

108. Blick M, Sherwin SA, Rosenblum M, Gutterman J (1987) Phase I study of recombinant tumor necrosis factor in cancer patients. Cancer Res 47: 2986–2989

109. Gamm H, Herrmann F, Mull R, Flener R, Mertelsmann R, Recombinant human tumor necrosis factor-alpha in advanced cancer: a phase I clinical trial. (AACR Abstract)

110. Mertelsmann R, Gamm H, Flener R, Herrmann F (1987) Recombinant human tumor necrosis factor alpha (rhTNF-α) in advanced cancer: a phase I clinical trial (abstract) Proc AACR 28: 1583

111. Bevilacqua MP, Pober JS, Mendrick DL, Cotram RS, Gimbrone MA (1988) Identification of an inducible endothelial leukocyte adhesion molecule, E-LAM 1. Proc Nat Acad Sci USA (in press)
    Pober JS, Gimbrone MA, Lapierre LA, Mendrick DL, Fiers W, Rothlein R, Springer TA (1986) Overlapping patterns of activation of human endothelial cells by interleukin-1, tumor necrosis factor and immune interferon. J Immunol 137: 1893–1896

113. Haranaka K, Satomi N, Sakurai A, Haranaka R (1986) Necrotizing activity of tumor necrosis factor and its mechanism. Ann Inst Pasteur Immunol 139: 288–294

114. Strander H (1977) Anti-tumor effects of interferon and its possible use as an anti-neoplastic agent in man. Tex Med 35: 429

115. Herberman RB, Ortaldo JR, Mantovani A, Hobbs DS, Kung HF, Pestka S (1982) Effect of human recombinant interferon on cytotoxic activity of natural killer (NK) cells and monocytes. Cell Immunol 67: 160–167

116. Lindahl P, Gresser I, Leary P et al. (1976) Enhanced expression of histocompatibility antigens of lymphoid cells treated with interferon. J Infect Dis 133 [suppl]: A66

117. Brodeur BR, Merigan TC (1975) Mechanism of the suppressive effect of interferon on antibody synthesis in vivo. J Immunol 114: 1323–1328

118. Schnaper HW, Aune TM, Pierce CW (1983) Suppressor T cell activation by human leucocyte interferon. J Immunol 131: 2301–2306

119. Vilcek J, Gray PW, Rinderknecht E, Sevastopoulos CG (1985) Interferon-γ: a lymphokine for all seasons. In: Pick E (ed) Lymphokines. Academic, New York, pp 1–32

120. Quesada JR, Keuben J, Manning JJ, Hersh EM, Gutterman JU (1984) Alpha interferon for induction of remission in hairy cell leukemia. N Engl J Med 310: 15–18

121. Talpaz M, Kantarjian HM, McCredie K, Trujillo JM, Keating MJ, Gutterman JU (1986) Hematologic remission and cytogenetic improvement induced by recombinant human interferon alpha in chronic myelogenous leukemia. N Engl J Med 314: 1065–1069

122. Groopman JE, Gottlieb MS, Godman J, Hisugasu RT, Conant MA, Prince H, Faney JU, Derezin M, Weinstein WM, Casavante C, Rothman J, Rudnik SA, Volberding PA (1984) Recombinant alpha-2-interferon therapy for Kaposi's sarcoma associated with acquired immunodeficiency syndrome. Ann Intern Med 100: 671–676
123. Creagan ET, Ahmann DL, Green SJ, Long HJ, Frytak S, O'Fallon JR, Itri LM (1984) Phase II study of recombinant leukocyte A interferon in disseminated malignant melanoma. J Clin Oncol 1984 2: 1002–1005
124. Niederle N, Kummer G (1989) The role of interferon in the management of patients with hairy cell leukemia and multiple myeloma. In: Berger HG et al. (eds) Cancer therapy. Springer, Berlin Heidelberg New York, pp 112–123
125. Aulitzky W, Gastl G, Tilg H, von Lüttichau I, Flener R, Huber C (1986) Recurrence of hairy cell leukemia upon discontinuation of IFN treatment. Blut 53: 215
126. Porzsolt F, Digel W, Buck C, Raghavachar A, Stefanic M, Schöniger W (1989) Possible mechanism of interferon action in hairy cell leukemia. In: Berger HG et al. (eds) Cancer therapy. Springer, Berlin Heidelberg New York, pp 126–131
127. Lindemann A, Ludwig WD, Oster W, Mertelsmann R, Herrmann F (1989) High level secretion of TNF-alpha contributes to hematopoietic failure in hairy cell leukemia. Blood 73: 880–884
128. Talpaz M, Kantarjian H, Kurzrock R, Trujillo JM, Gutterman JU (1989) Sustained complete cytogenetic response among Philadelphia positive chronic myelogenous leukemia (CML PH¹) patients treated with alpha interferon (abstract). Blood 74: 289
129. Higano CS, Raskind W, Durnam D, Singer JW (1989) Alpha interferon (IF) induces cytogenetic remissions in patients who relapse with chronic myelogenous leukemia (CML) after allogenic bone marrow transplantation (BMT) (abstract). Blood 74: 307
130. Kantarjian H, Keating M, McCredie K, Gutterman J, Freireich E, Deisseroth A, Talpaz M (1989) Treatment of advanced stages of Philadelphia-chromosome (Ph)-positive chronic myelogenous leukemia (CL) with alpha interferon (IFN-α) and low-dose cytosine arabinoside (Ara-C) (abstract). Blood 4: 878
131. Jones GJ, Itri LM (1986) Safety and tolerance of recombinant interferon alpha-2a (Roferon-A) in cancer patients. Cancer 57: 1709–1715
132. Bunn PA, Foon KA, Ihde DC, Longo DL, Eddy, J, Winkler CF, Weach SR, Zeffren J, Sherwins S, Oldham R (1984) Recombinant leukocyte A interferon: an active agent in advanced cutaneous T-cell lymphomas. Ann Intern Med 101: 484–487
133. Foon KA, Sherwin SA, Abrams PG, Kongo DU, Fer MF, Stevenson HC, Ochs JJ, Bottino GC, Schoenberger CS, Zeffren J, Jaffe ES, Oldhorn RK (1984) Treatment of advanced non-Hodgkin's lymphoma with recombinant leucocyte A interferon. N Engl J Med 311: 1148–1152
134. Einzig AI, Krown SE, Oettgen HF (1984) Recombinant leukocyte A interferon (rIFNa-A) in renal cell cancer (RCC) (abstract). Proc Am Soc Clin Oncol 3: C-209

Hemopoietic Growth Factors in the Treatment of Acute Leukemias and Myelodysplastic Syndromes

G. Seipelt, A. Ganser, and D. Hoelzer

Abteilung für Hämatologie, Zentrum der Inneren Medizin, Klinikum der
Johann Wolfgang Goethe-Universität, Theodor-Stern-Kai 7, W-6000 Frankfurt 70, FRG

Introduction

The potential useful effects of hemopoietic growth factors (HPGF) alone or in combination with cytotoxic drugs in acute myeloblastic leukemias (AML) and myelodysplastic syndromes (MDS) include: (a) enhancement of marrow recovery after chemotherapy, which would decrease the risk of infection and possibly reduce the requirement for transfusion of red blood cells and platelets; (b) synchronization of malignant cells prior to treatment with cycle-specific drugs; and (c) a possible induction of maturation in leukemic blast cells. In this report the in vitro effects of HPGF on AML blast cells and the results of initial clinical trials of HPGF in patients with AML as well as in patients with MDS will be discussed.

In Vitro Effect of HPGF on AML Cells

Receptor Studies. The action of HPGF on hemopoietic cells may depend on the presence or absence of receptors for these molecules. Cell surface receptors for HPGF have been detected by binding studies with biologically active radioiodinated granulocyte colony-stimulating factor (G-CSF) on leukemia cell lines (Souza et al. 1986; Nicola et al. 1985), with marked heterogeneity being found in the number of receptors on individual cells (Begley et al. 1988). No correlation was found between the level of receptor expression in cells from AML patients and the frequency of AML cells that are able to form colonies of leukemic blasts in semisolid media (termed the AML colony-forming unit, or AML-CFU) when stimulated with G-CSF. Several groups have published data aimed at characterizing the human receptor granulocyte-macrophage CSF for (GM-CSF). Both normal human neutrophils and human leukemia cell lines such as HL-60 and KG-1 possess an extremely low number of high-affinity GM-CSF receptors, estimated at between 50 and 260 receptors per cell (Gasson et al. 1986; Park et al. 1986). Examination of GM-CSF binding to fresh blast cells from AML patients has revealed significantly lower binding than to normal human neutrophils (Di Persio et al. 1988; Kelleher et al. 1988). Whether normal myeloblasts also have low numbers of GM-CSF receptors compared with more mature myeloid cells has to be assessed. It is possible that in AML blast cells the cell surface receptors may be continually occupied or downmodulated by autonomously produced GM-CSF, as might be predicted by an autocrine model of AML.

Differentiation and Proliferation Induction by HPGF. Many investigators have demonstrated that leukemic cell lines such as the murine myelomonocyte leukemia cell line WEHI-3B can be induced to differentiate into mature granulocytes with G-CSF (Platzer et al. 1985; Souza et al. 1986; Nicola et al. 1985; Begley et al. 1987), whereas GM-CSF showed little or no differentiation-inducing activity in murine myeloblastic cell lines (Nicola et al. 1985). The effect of HPGF on human leukemic blast cells is very heterogeneous. In most but not all patients GM-CSF stimulates the in vitro proliferation of AML blast cells (Platzer et al. 1985; Griffin et al. 1986; Griffin and Löwenberg 1986; Souza et al. 1986; Kelleher et al. 1987; Vellenga et al. 1987), including the clonogenic stem cell. Studies on human HL-60 cells have indicated that both G-CSF and GM-CSF have some ability to induce morphological differentiation and suppress stem cell self-regeneration in HL-60 cells (Begley et al. 1987). However, no in vitro effect of HPGF on differentiation of blast cells in 20 patients with AML was observed by Vellenga et al. (1987), and Jinnai (1990) could show differentiation induction in only 2 out of 14 AML patients. The import of these findings remains unresolved, since the percentage of mature neutrophils also increased without addition of HPGF in these two patients. Carlo-Stella and coworkers (1990) showed that only G-CSF and interleukin-6 (IL-6) had a marked differentiation-inducing activity in CD34-positive AML cells in eight AML patients, but not interleukin-3 (IL-3) and GM-CSF. In conclusion, the in vitro data indicate that IL-3 and GM-CSF promote selfrenewal of clonogenic cells, while G-CSF and IL-6 preferentially promote differentiation. Whether this is relevant in vivo is unclear since there is evidence for leukemic clone maturation in vivo (Hittelman et al. 1988).

Rationale for Combined Treatment with GM-CSF and Cytotoxic Drugs

Since cells in S-phase are more susceptible to chemotherapy, combined treatment with HPGF and cytotoxic drugs could improve the killing of leukemic cells. Inducing leukemic clonogenic cells to proliferate appears to enhance the cytotoxicity of the cell cycle-specific drug cytosine arabinoside (ara-C) (De Witte et al. 1988; Cannistra et al. 1989). In five of six patients demonstrating clonogenic cell growth in response to GM-CSF, Cannistra et al. (1989) found a significant increase in leukemic clonogenic cell kill compared to treatment with ara-C alone. Enhancement of cytotoxicity appears to be related to recruitment from G_0 but not to an increase in S-phase (Tafuri et al. 1989). An increase in the percentage of cells in S-phase did not result in increased cell kill. These findings are supported by another study showing that the kill of myeloid blast cells by ara-C is not related to the GM-CSF-induced rise in the percentage of cells in S-phase, but rather to a change in ara-C metabolism (Hiddeman et al. 1989). After exposure to GM-CSF, a significantly higher incorporation of ^{3}H-labeled ara-C into the myeloid blast cells was found in 14 out of 16 patients. As shown by Muhm and coworkers (1989), GM-CSF in vivo effectively recruits leukemic blast cells into S-phase too.

Clinical Trials Using GM-CSF in AML

Different approaches have been used to combine GM-CSF and chemotherapy in patients with AML, with the rationale of recruiting leukemic blast cells into S-phase prior to chemotherapy and possibly shortening neutropenia after chemo-therapy in these patients (Table 1) Muhm and coworkers (1989) treated 12 patients with de novo AML with GM-CSF (250 μg/m^2 per day, continuous i.v.) in combination with a standard cytotoxic chemotherapy regimen. GM-CSF was started 48 or 24 h prior to chemotherapy in nine patients. In three patients with initially high leukocyte counts, GM-CSF was started after chemotherapy-induced reduction in the white blood cell count to below 30 000/μl. GM-CSF infusion was discontinued when neutrophil counts had returned to above 500 cells/μl after chemotherapy-induced aplasia. During the pretreatment phase with GM-CSF, neutrophils increased in all patients and blast cells in six of nine patients. Recruitment of leukemic blast cells into S-phase in vivo and a subsequent cell killing by cytotoxic drugs were demonstrated. Ten patients achieved complete remission, seven within the first cycle. Duration of aplasia was significantly shortened in these patients when compared with historical controls (absolute neutrophil count > 500/μl: 21.6 vs 25.2 days).

In a study by Büchner and coworkers (1989) undertaken to evaluate possible shortening of chemotherapy-induced neutropenia by GM-CSF in patients with acute leukemia and at high risk of early death, 29 elderly or relapsed patients (23 with AML, 6 with acute lymphoblastic leukemia, ALL) were entered into the study. On day 4 after chemotherapy, continuous i.v. infusion of GM-CSF (250 μg/m^2 per day) was started. Median recovery of neutrophil counts in 16 patients receiving the TAD9 protocol (thioguanine, ara-C, daunorubicin) was shortened to 10 days, compared to 15 days in historical controls. Corresponding data after the S-HAM protocol with high-dose ara-C (and mitoxantrone) were 14 days vs 23 days. The chemotherapy-induced nadir in the white blood cell count was followed by regrowth of blasts in three AML patients; this disap-peared, however, in two patients after discontinuation of GM-CSF. DNA aneuploidy, as detected by bone marrow flow cytometry, persisted after chemotherapy in one AML patient but disappeared following GM-CSF treat-ment. Of the three patients with regrowth of blasts, two had residual leukemic colony growth in vitro prior to GM-CSF. Pretherapeutic growth stimulation by GM-CSF mostly failed to predict later progression of the leukemia.

In a study by Teshima et al. (1989), G-CSF was administered to 24 leukemia patients. In nine patients who underwent allogeneic bone marrow transplan-

Table 1. GM-CSF therapy in AML

Authors	Patients	Induction	GM-CSF		Dose	n	CR(%)	ED	Increase in	
			Time						Neutrophils	Blast cells
Muhm et al. 1989	de novo	ara-C,-D	prior 48 h+ during CT		250 µg/day CI until NC > 500/µl	12	58	2	9/9	6/9 prior to CT
Büchner et al. 1989	age > 65, relapse	TAD, HD ara-C/ Mitox	post CT		250 µg/day CI until NC > 500/µl	23	55			2 transient 1 persistent
Estey, personal communi- cation.	Poor risk	HD ara-C	during CT		120 µg/day CI until NC > 1000/µl	5	4	1	3/4	0

CI, continuous infusion; CT, chemotherapy; ED, early death; HD, high-dose; NC, neutrophic count.

tation a shortening of neutropenia was observed, with recovery of neutrophil counts $> 500/\mu l$ on day 11.3 compared with 26.8 days in historical controls. In seven of eight patients who received G-CSF after the first remission-induction therapy, neutrophil counts increased from $< 300/\mu l$ to $> 4000/\mu l$ within 10 days. Blast cells did not increase in any patient, including four with acute non-lymphocytic leukemia.

Clinical side effects in the patients treated with GM-CSF or G-CSF were mild and tolerable. As in the phase I studies with HPGF, fever, weight gain, pleural effusions, bone pain, and diarrhea were the most common side effects observed.

Growth Factors in MDS

Before the efficacy of HPGF in AML was studied, these agents had been used in the treatment of MDS patients. Seven clinical trials with GM-CSF alone have been published to date (Table 2). An increase in circulating neutrophils was found in 88% of the patients. The effect on other cell lineages was less uniform: in reticulocytes an increase occurred in 27% of patients and a decrease in 5%, and in platelets an increase was observed in 13% and a decrease in 16% (Antin et al. 1988; Ganser et al. 1989; Herrmann et al. 1989; Vadhan-Raj et al. 1988; Thompson et al. 1989; Estey 1990; Hoelzer et al. 1989). In 15 patients (19%) an increase in the marrow and/or peripheral blood blast cells was noted. Ten patients progressed to AML, particularly patients with $> 15\%$ bone marrow blasts. Five out of 11 patients 2 refractory anemia with excess blasts, RAEB; 1 refractory anemia with excess blasts in transformation, RAEB-T; 2 chronic myelomonocytic leukemia, CMML) treated with GM-CSF in a phase I/II trial at our institution had an increase in blast cells; four received treatment with low-dose ara-C and one, conventional polychemotherapy (Ganser et al. 1989b). In nine patients with RA receiving GM-CSF alone for three 14-day cycles, no appearance of blasts was noted (Hoelzer et al. 1989). The final answer as to whether the progression is due to the administration of HPGF or to the natural course of the underlying disease can only be provided by a randomized trial comparing GM-CSF with a placebo control group.

To date, two studies have been reported using G-CSF in MDS patients. Twenty-three patients have been treated, of whom twenty-one had an increase in neutrophil counts. Three had an increase in reticulocytes, and no substantial changes in platelet counts were noted. A decrease of infectious episodes was noted at times of neutrophil improvements in patients on long-term mainten-ance therapy (Greenberg et al. 1990; Kobayashi et al. 1989).

Erythropoietin and IL-3 in MDS

Additional growth factors that have been studied in MDS are erythropoietin and Il-3. These HPGF were used to study whether the defective proliferation of the hemopoietic precursors in MDS could be overcome by pharmacological

Table 2. Treatment of MDS with GM-CSF

Authors	Dose ($\mu g/m^2$)	Schedule Route	Days	n	Neutrophils +	Neutrophils −	Reticulocytes +	Reticulocytes −	Platelets +	Platelets −
Vadhan-Raj et al. 1988	60–500	i.v. (24 h)	14	8	8		7		3	
Antin et al. 1988	15–240	i.v. (1–12 h)	14	7	6	1	7			
Thompson et al. 1989	0.3–10	s.c.	10	16	12		3	1	2	
Ganser et al. 1989	15–150	i.v. (8 h)	7–14	11	9		2		1	1
Herrmann et al. 1989	5–750	i.v. (0.5 h)	5	4	4					
Hoelzer et al. 1989	250	s.c.	3×14	9	7	1	2	3	2	2
Estey et al. 1989	120	i.v. (24 h)	84	22	22				2	9
Total				77	68(88%)	2(3%)	21(27%)	4(5%)	10(13%)	12(16%)

doses of erythropoietin and IL-3, thereby stimulating erythropoiesis, granu-lopoiesis, and megakaryopoiesis.

Erythropoietin. The effect on transfusion requirements were evaluated during long-term treatment with erythropoietin (Table 3). Six patients with MDS were treated with recombinant human erythropoietin (patients 1–5, 450 U/kg twice weekly, i.v.; patient 6 10 kU 5 days/week, s.c.). One patient showed a marked response with a rise in hemoglobin and hematocrit and a decrease in serum ferritin. The serum level of erythropoietin was lower in this responding patient than in three other patients in whom pretreatment erythropoietin levels had been determined. Although a study by Bowen et al. (1990) showed only a weak correlation between endogenous erythropoietin level and hemoglobin level in MDS patients, indicating that not only decreased responsiveness to erythro-poietin plays a role in MDS, a low serum erythropoietin level could be of predictive value for the response to erythropoietin therapy.

Interleukin-3. Preclinical studies have demonstrated that IL-3 effectively stimu-lates myelopoiesis, erythropoiesis, and thrombopoiesis in several murine and non-human primate models (Kindler et al. 1986; Metcalf et al. 1986; Broxmeyer et al. 1987; Donahue et al. 1988; Krumwieh and Seiler 1989; Mayer et al. 1989). On the basis of these data, nine patients (6 refractory anemia, RA; 3 RAEB) were treated with IL-3 as part of a phase I/II trial (Table 4). IL-3 was administered for 15 days s.c. at doses between 250 and 500 µg/day. Most patients showed a rise in neutrophils, eosinophils, basophils, monocytes, and lymphocytes. Platelet counts increased in six of the patients and reticulocyte counts in three. In one patient with secondary RAEB the proliferative effect of IL-3 resulted in an increase in blast cells in the bone marrow and peripheral blood. In the remaining patients, there was no increase in blast numbers in the bone marrow or in the peripheral blood, indicating that the malignant cell populations remained under differentiative control. Dysplastic features in the bone marrow persisted with IL-3 treatment (Ganser et al. 1990).

Combined Treatment Schedules in Patients with MDS

In a European multicenter phase II trial[1] we are at present evaluating the efficacy of a combination of low-dose ara-C and GM-CSF on poor-prognosis MDS

---

[1] MDS study group: Hoelzer D., Ganser A., Dept. of Hematology, University of Frankfurt; Höffken K., Becher R., Dept. of Internal Medicine, University of Essen; Lutz D., Krieger O., Dept. of Internal Medicine, Hanusch Hospital, Vienna; Diehl V., Lathan B., Dept. of Internal Medicine, University of Cologne; Boogaerts M.A., Verhaef G., University Hospital, University of Leuven; Ferrant A., Martiat P., Hospital Erasme, University of Brussels; De Witte T., van der Lelly N., Div. of Hematology, University of Nijmegen; Klausmann M., Dept. of Internal Medicine, University of Marburg; Herrmann F., Mertelsmann R., Dept. of Internal Medicine, University of Freiburg; Schulz G., Clinical Research Oncology, Behring-Werke AG, Marburg.

Table 3. Recombinant human erythropoietin in patients with MDS

Patient no.	Diagnosis	Sex	Age (years)	Erythropoietin (mU/ml)	Hemoglobin (g/dl)		Hematocrit (%)		Reticulocytes (‰)	
					pre	post	pre	post	pre	post
1	RA	f	79	204	7.2	8.4	24.2	24.8	0.16	0.2
2	RA	m	68		8.4	7.4[a]	25.6	21.8[a]	0.0	0.1
3	RA	f	67	71	9.1	11.8	28.9	36.7	1.2	1.1
4	RA	m	76	286	5.7	7.9[a]	17.3	23.0[a]	0.1	0.4
5	RAEB	f	50	244	7.2	8.3[a]	21.7	25.9[a]	0.07	0.29
6	RAEB	m	30		5.9	7.5[a]	16.0	21.5[a]	0.31	0.05
Mean					7.3	8.6	22.3	25.6	0.31	0.37

[a] Unchanged transfusion dependency.

Table 4. Treatment of MDS with IL-3

Patient no.	Diagnosis	Dosage ($\mu g/m^2$)	Leukocytes ($\times 10^3/\mu l$)		Neutrophils ($\times 10^3/\mu l$)		Platelets ($\times 10^3/\mu l$)		Reticulocytes (%)[a]		Blast cells ($\times 10^3/\mu l$)	
			pre	post	pre	post	pre	post	pre	post	pre	post
1	RA	250	3.3	13.2	2.04	10.82	188	260	0.04	0.21	0	0
2	RA	250	3.0	5.0	1.59	1.75	137	134	0	0.56	0	0
3	RA	500	3.6	10.0	2.10	4.50	364	426	0.27	0.29	0	0
4	RA	500	3.7	5.8	1.89	3.81	50	86	0	0.07	0.12	0.17
5	RA	500	4.4	15.9	2.42	9.86	156	226	0.56	0.32	0	0.14
6	RA	250	2.0	5.9	0.36	1.53	8	NC	0.74	0.81	0	0.04
7	RAEB	250	3.8	7.1	1.18	2.56	8	NC	1.21	1.21	0	0.36
8	RAEB	500	1.4	4.5	0.30	0.39	7	22	0.06	0.14	0.02	0.05
9	RAEB	500	1.5	2.5	0.20	0.62	5	31	1.07	1.07	0.05	0.10
Mean			2.97	7.77	1.34	3.95	102	133	0.44	0.52	0.02	0.09

The maximum response during the study is given.

NC, no change.

[a] Corrected reticulocyte count (%).

patients (Fig. 1). Patients with RAEB, RAEB-T, or CMML were treated with three 14-day courses of recombinant human GM-CSF (250 μg/m^2 per day, s.c., at 8 a.m.) and low-dose ara-C (20 mg/m^2 per day, s.c., at 8 p.m.). Patients with RA received GM-CSF only.

Between April 1988 and October 1989, 58 patients with MDS (median age 59 years, range 31–85) entered this trial. Sixteen patients had RA, 20 RAEB, and 19 RAEB-T. In four patients with CMML the myelomonocytic cells increased and the protocol was discontinued thereafter. Fifteen patients with RAEB or RAEB-T received three cycles of the combined treatment; platelet counts increased in eight of these patients, remained unchanged in three, and decreased in four. The neutrophil counts increased from $1.11 \pm 0.41/\mu$l to $11.61 \pm 3.24/\mu$l. Blast cells in the bone marrow decreased substantially in 7 out of 11 patients (from 21% to 4%), but two patients with RAEB-T progressed to AML.

A different treatment schedule involving GM-CSF and low-dose ara-C has been used in a randomized phase II trial by the EORTC leukemia group in patients with RAEB/RAEB-T (Gerhartz et al. 1989). Low-dose ara-C (2×10 mg/m^2 per day, s.c.) was given for 2 weeks and recombinant human GM-CSF (2×150 μg/day, s.c. was given either during the 3rd week (arm 1) or during the 2nd week (arm 2). After completion of three cycles, 27 patients were eligible

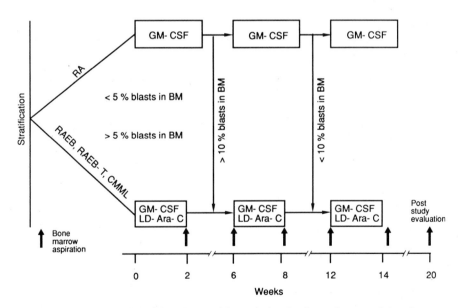

Fig. 1. Treatment schedule for patients with myelodysplastic syndromes. *RA*, refractory anemia; *RAEB*, refractory anemia with excess blasts; *RAEB-T*, refractory anemia with excess blasts in transformation; *CMML*, chronic myelomonocytic leukemia; *BM*, bone marrow; *GM-CSF*, granulocyte-macrophage colony stimulating factor; *LD-Ara-C*, low-dose cytosine arabinoside. From Hoelzer et al. (1990)

and evaluable for outcome. Fifteen out of 23 patients had a favorable response (complete remission 8, partial remission 7).

Discussion

As initial clinical trials have shown, HPGF can be used safely in patients with AML. There are several arguments which may justify the combination of stimulation and cytotoxic treatment in patients with AML. In vitro studies have shown that GM-CSF recruits leukemic blast cells into the cell cycle or has an influence on the metabolism of the blast cells, thereby rendering them more susceptible to cytotoxic drugs, as could be demonstrated by combining GM-CSF and ara-C in vitro. Muhm and coworkers (1989) showed that GM-CSF can effectively recruit leukemic blast cells into S-phase in vivo too, making treatment with cycle-specific drugs more potent. In addition, it has been demonstrated (Büchner et al. 1989; Teshima et al. 1989) that the neutropenic phase after chemotherapy is significantly shortened by GM-CSF. Since the vast majority of deaths in AML are due to infections during the aplasia following chemotherapy, shortening of the neutropenic period may improve the overall treatment results.

In the trial by Büchner et al. (1989) three of 23 AML patients had a regrowth of leukemic blast cells. Two of the three patients had a residual leukemic colony growth in vitro prior to GM-CSF. After discontinuation of GM-CSF, the blast cells disappeared, and there was no evidence of a continuing GM-CSF-induced progression of AML or reduction of remission duration. Thus, GM-CSF seems to reduce treatment toxicity in AML patients and may allow more effective antileukemic treatment strategies in future.

The treatment of refractory anemia MDS patients with GM-CSF or G-CSF showed that the neutrophil count increased in all patients without stimulation of blast cells. These HPGF given as long-term maintenance therapy to patients with severe neutropenia could play a role in lowering the frequency of infectious episodes. Treatment with IL-3 showed that megakaryopoiesis can be stimulated in the majority of patients, whereas the elevation in reticulocyte counts in 33% of the patients did not result in a response in hemoglobin or hematocrit. Long-term IL-3 treatment could possibly lead to more promising results in stimulating erythropoiesis. The lack of stimulation of erythropoiesis by erythropoietin in the majority of patients might be overcome by combining erythropoietin with IL-3, which could more effectively lower transfusion requirements and stimulate megakaryopoiesis.

Combined treatment with GM-CSF and low-dose ara-C resulted in a prolonged increase in platelet counts in 8 out of 15 RAEB/RAEB-T patients. Blast cells decreased in 7 out of 11 patients, but whether the progression to AML in two patients was due to the administration of GM-CSF or due to the natural course of the underlying disease is not clear. The definitive answer to this can only be provided by randomized trials comparing patients treated with HPGF with a placebo control group.

While initial results seem very promising, more studies, both in vitro and in vivo, are required to evaluate the role of hemopoietic growth factors in the treatment of both MDS and AML.

References

Antin JH, Smith BR, Holmes W, et al. (1988) Phase I/II study of recombinant human granulocyte-macrophage colony stimulating factor in aplastic anemia and myelodysplastic syndrome. Blood 72: 705–713

Begley CG, Metcalf D, Nicola NA (1987) Purified colony stimulating factors (G-CSF and GM-CSF) induce differentiation in human HL60 leukemic cells with suppress of clonogenicity. Int J Cancer 39: 99–105

Begley CG, Metcalf D, Nicola NA (1988) Binding characteristics and proliferative action of purified granulocyte colony-stimulating factor (G-CSF) on normal and leukemic human promyelocytes. Exp Hematol 16: 71–79

Bowen DT, Jacobs A, Mary P, et al. (1990) Serum erythropoietin and erythropoiesis in patients with myelodysplastic syndromes. Eur J Haematol 44: 30–32

Broxmeyer HE, Williams D, Hangoc G, et al (1987) Synergistic myelopoietic actions in vivo after administration to mice of combinations of purified natural murine colony-stimulating factor 1, recombinant murine interleukin-3 and recombinant murine granulocyte/macrophage colony-stimulating factor. Proc Natl Acad Sci USA 84: 3871–3875

Büchner T, Hiddemann W, Königsmann M, et al. (1989) Hematologic and therapeutic effects of recombinant human GM-CSF following chemotherapy in patients with acute leukemias at higher age or after relapse. Blood 74 (Suppl 1): 271a

Cannistra SA, Groshek P, Griffin JD (1989) Granulocyte-macrophage colony-stimulating factor enhances the cytotoxic effects of cytosine arabinoside in acute myeloblastic leukemia and in the myeloid blast crisis phase of chronic myeloid leukemia. Leukemia 3: 328–334

Carlo-Stella C, Mangoni L, Almici A, et al. (1990) Effect of recombinant growth factors on the in vitro growth of CD34-positive acute myeloid leukemia cells. Third symposium on minimal residual disease in acute leukemia, Rotterdam 1990, p 107

De Witte T, Muus P, Haanen C, et al. (1988) GM-CSF enhances sensitivity of leukemic clonogenic cells to long-term low dose cytosine arabinoside with sparing of the normal clonogenic cells. Behring Inst Mitt 83: 301–307

DiPersio J, Billing P, Kaufman S, et al. (1988) Characterization of human granulocyte-macrophage colony-stimulating factor receptor. J Biol Chem 263: 1834–1841

Donahue RE, Seehra J, Metzger M, et al. (1988) Human IL-3 and GM-CSF act synergistically in stimulating hematopoiesis in primates. Science 241: 1820–1823

Estey E et al. (1990) In: Acute myelogenous leukemia. UCLA symposia on molecular and cellular biology, New series (in press)

Ganser A, Völkers B, Greher J, et al. (1989) Recombinant human granulocyte-macrophage colony-stimulating factor in patients with myelodysplastic syndromes – a phase I/II trial. Blood 73: 31–37

Ganser A, Seipelt G, Lindemann A, et al. (1990) Effects of recombinant human interleukin-3 in patients with myelodysplastic syndromes. Blood 1990 (in press)

Gasson JC, Kaufman SE, Weisbart RH, et al. (1986) High-affinity binding of granulocyte-macrophage colony-stimulating factor to normal and leukemic human myeloid cells. Proc Natl Acad Sci USA 83: 669–673

Gerhartz HH, Visani G, Delmer A, et al. (1989) Randomized phase II trial with GM-CSF and low-dose Ara-C in patients with "high risk" myelodysplastic syndromes. Blood 74 (Suppl 1): 119a

Griffin JD, Löwenberg B (1986) Clonogenic cells in acute myeloblastic leukemia. Blood 68: 1185–1195

Griffin JD, Young D, Herrmann F, et al. (1986) Effects of recombinant human GM-CSF on proliferation of clonogenic cells in acute myeloblastic leukemia. Blood 67: 1448–1453

Herrmann F, Lindemann A, Klein H, et al. (1989) Effect of recombinant human granulocyte-macrophage colony-stimulating factor in patients with myelodysplastic syndrome with excess blasts. Leukemia 3: 335–338

Hiddemann W, Kiehl M, Schleyer E, et al. (1989) Stimulatory effect of GM-CSF and IL-3 on the metabolism and cytotoxic activity of cytosine-arabinoside in leukemic blasts from patients with acute myeloid leukemia. Blood 74 (Suppl 1): 230a

Hittelman WN, Agbor P, Petkovic I, et al. (1988) Detection of leukemic clone maturation in vivo by premature chromosome condensation. Blood 72: 1950–1960

Hoelzer D, Ganser A, Völkers B, et al. (1988) In vitro and in vivo action of recombinant human GM-CSF in patients with myelodysplastic syndromes. Blood Cells 14: 551–559

Hoelzer D, Ganser A, Seipelt G, et al. (1989) Simultaneous treatment with recombinant human granulocyte-macrophage colony-stimulating factor and low-dose cytosine arabinoside in patients with myelodysplastic syndromes. Blood 74 (Suppl 1): 118a

Hoelzer D, Ganser A, Ottmann OG, et al. (1990) Effect of treatment with rhGM-CSF and low-dose cytosine arabinoside on leukemic blast cells in patients with myelodysplastic syndromes. Haematol Blood Transfusion 33: 763–769

Jinnai I (1990) In vitro growth response to G-CSF and GM-CSF by bone marrow cells of patients with acute myeloid leukemia. Leukemia Res 14: 227–240

Kelleher CA, Miyauchi J, Wong G, et al. (1987) Synergism between recombinant growth factors, GM-CSF and G-CSF, acting on the blast cells of acute myeloblastic leukemia. Blood 69: 1498–1503

Kelleher CA, Wong GG, Clark SC, et al. (1988) Binding of iodinated recombinant human GM-CSF to the blast cells of acute myeloblastic leukemia. Leukemia 2: 211–215

Kindler V, Thorens B, de Kossodo S, et al. (1986) Stimulation of hematopoiesis in vivo by recombinant bacterial murine interleukin-3. Proc Natl Acad Sci USA 83: 1001–1005

Kobayashi Y, Okabe T, Ozawa K, et al. (1989) Treatment of myelodysplastic syndromes with human granulocyte colony-stimulating factor: a preliminary report. Am J Med 86: 178–182

Krumwieh D, Seiler FR (1989) In vivo effects of recombinant colony stimulating factors on hematopoiesis in cynamolgus monkeys. Transplant Proc 21: 379–383

Mayer P, Valent P, Schmidt G, et al. (1989) The in vivo effect of recombinant human interleukin-3: demonstration of basophil differentiation factor, histamine-producing activity and priming of GM-CSF-responsive progenitors in nonhuman primates. Blood 74: 613–621

Metcalf D, Begley CG, Johnson GR, et al. (1986) Effects of purified bacterially synthesized murine multi-CSF (IL-3) on hematopoiesis in normal adult mice. Blood 68: 46–57

Muhm M, Andreeff M, Geissler K, et al. (1989) RhGM-CSF in combination with chemotherapy—a new strategy in the therapy of acute myeloid leukemia. Blood 74 (Suppl 1): 117a

Negrin RS, Haeuber DH, Nagler A, et al. (1989) Treatment of myelodysplastic syndromes with recombinant human granulocyte colony-stimulating factor. A phase I–II trial. Ann Intern Med 110: 976–984

Nicola NA, Begley CG, Metcalf D (1985) Identification of the human analogue of a regulator that induces differentiation in murine leukaemic cells. Nature 314: 625–628

Park LS, Friend D, Gillis S, et al. (1986) Characterization of the cell surface receptor for human granulocyte/macrophage colony-stimulating factor. J Exp Med 164: 251–262

Platzer E, Welte K, Gabrilove JL, et al. (1985) Biological activities of a human pluripotent hemopoietic colony stimulating factor on normal and leukemic cells. J Exp Med 162: 1788–1801

Souza LM, Boone TC, Gabrilove J, et al. (1986) Recombinant pluripotent human granulocyte colony-stimulating factor: effects on normal and leukemic myeloid cells. Science 232: 61–65

Tafuri A, Lemoli RM, Gulati S, et al. (1989) Rationale and limitations of combined cytokine chemotherapy treatment of acute myeloblastic leukemia. Blood 74 (Suppl 1): 231a

Teshima H, Ishikawa J, Kitayama H, et al. (1989) Clinical effects of recombinant human granulocyte colony-stimulating factor in leukemia patients: a phase I/II study. Exp Hematol 17: 853–858

Thompson JA, Douglas JL, Kidd P, et al. (1989) Subcutaneous granulocyte macrophage colony-stimulating factor in patients with myelodysplastic syndrome: toxicity, pharmacokinetics, and hematological effects. J Clin Oncol 7: 629–637

Vadhan-Raj S, Kellagher MJ, Keating M, et al. (1988) Phase I study of recombinant human granulocyte-macrophage colony stimulating factor in patients with myelodysplastic syndrome. N Engl J Med 317: 1545–1552

Vadhan-Raj S, Broxmeyer HE, Spitzer G, et al. (1989) Stimulation of nonclonal hematopoiesis and suppression of the neoplastic clone after treatment with recombinant human granulocyte-macrophage colony-stimulating factor in a patient with therapy-related myelodysplastic syndrome. Blood 74: 1491–1498

Vellenga E, Ostapovicz D, Griffin JD (1987) Effects of recombinant IL-3, GM-CSF, and G-CSF on proliferation of leukemic clonogenic cells in short-term and long term cultures. Leukemia 1: 584–589

Recombinant Human GM-CSF in Small Cell Lung Cancer: A Phase I/II Study

H. Anderson[1], H. Gurney[1], N. Thatcher[1], R. Swindell[2], J.H. Scarffe[1], and J. Weiner[3]

[1]CRC Department of Medical Oncology, Christie Hospital, Manchester, M20 9BX, United Kingdom
[2]Department of Medical Statistics, Christie Hospital, Manchester M20 9BX, United Kingdom
[3]Glaxo Institute for Molecular Biology SA, Geneva, Switzerland

Introduction

Patients with cancer are at risk of developing infections whilst neutropenic (Bodey 1986). Several studies have shown that haematological growth factors, granulocyte colony-stimulating factor (G-CSF) and granulocyte-macrophage colony-stimulating factor (GM-CSF) may lessen the duration and severity of chemotherapy-induced neutropenia (Antman et al. 1988; Bronchud et al. 1987; Morstyn et al. 1988; Gabrilove et al. 1988). The study by Bronchud et al. (1987) showed that the number of febrile episodes during neutropenia was lower after courses of chemotherapy followed by administration of G-CSF than after chemotherapy not followed by G-CSF.

GM-CSF is a glycoprotein that stimulates the proliferation and differentiation of neutrophil, eosinophil and monocyte precursors in vitro (Metcalf 1985). Recombinant human GM-CSF (Glaxo) is an *Escherichia coli*-derived single-chain polypeptide of 128 amino acid residues with a purity of approximately 97% and a specific activity of $>1.5 \, MU/mg$ protein in the AML-193 cell proliferation assay.

The aim of this study was to assess the safety of GM-CSF given in daily subcutaneous injections to patients with small cell lung cancer, to observe its effect on the blood count and bone marrow before chemotherapy, and to assess its efficacy in preventing chemotherapy-associated neutropenia.

Patients and Methods

Patients were eligible for the study if they had histologically proven small cell lung cancer, were aged <75 years, had an ECOG performance status ≤ 2 and had received no previous therapy. The pre-treatment leucocyte count had to be $>3.0 \times 10^9/l$, the platelet count $>100 \times 10^9/l$, and the transaminases less than 1.5 times their normal level unless due to metastatic disease. Patients with a creatinine clearance of <50 ml/min, tetracycline allergy, serious concurrent medical illness, or a life expectancy of <4 months were excluded from entry into the study.

In the phase I study patients were given subcutaneous GM-CSF at a dosage of 50, 150, 300 or 500 μg/m^2 per day for 10 days. There was no within-patient dose escalation. Subgroup patients were entered into the next dose level after safety and tolerance had been assessed at the previous dose level.

After completion of the phase I study, patients had 4 days off therapy and for phase II were then randomised to receive GM-CSF with either odd or even number courses of chemotherapy. The chemotherapy given was etoposide 120 mg/m^2 i.v. daily for 3 days, doxorubicin 50 mg/m^2 i.v. bolus on day 1 and ifosfamide 5 g/m^2 with equidose mesna as a 24-h infusion on day 1, followed by mesna 3 g/m^2. The mean nadir leucocyte count following this regimen is 0.5×10^9/l. The aim was to give each patient six courses of chemotherapy at 3-weekly intervals. Chemotherapy was given if the leucocyte count was $>3.0 \times 10^9$/l and the platelet count $>100 \times 10^9$/l. GM-CSF was given at the same dose as in phase I, starting 24 h after the last dose of chemotherapy, and continued for 14 days. Blood counts were checked thrice weekly following the first two courses of chemotherapy. The number of febrile episodes and antibiotic courses were documented throughout the study.

Results

Seventeen patients were entered into the study, 14 males and 3 females, with a median age of 58 years (range 43–73 years). In the phase I study GM-CSF was shown to cause a leucocytosis which showed some dose response (Table 1). Following the first injection of GM-CSF there was a rapid fall in the leucocyte count 30–60 min from administration that lasted up to 4 h. The maximum

Table 1. Phase I: dose of GM-CSF and rise in leucocyte count

Dose (μg/m^2)	No. of patients	Mean WCC day 1 (range)	Maximum WCC (range)
50	3	8.7 (8.4–9.1)	21.6 (18.3–26.0)
150	4	6.7 (5.3–8.1)	25.0 (20.2–29.4)
300	6	9.1 (5.7–14.7)	34.3 (18.4–54.6)
500	4	10.1 (6.4–12.2)	39.4 (29.6–54.6)

WCC, white blood cell count.

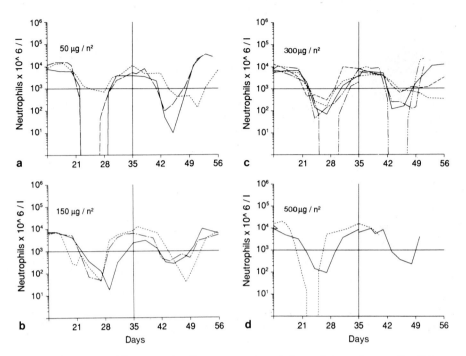

Fig. 1a–d. Neutrophil count after first two cycles of chemotherapy for small cell lung cancer followed by GM-CSF therapy. Chemotherapy given on days 15 and 35. GM-CSF given after odd (*short dashes*) or even (*long dashes*) cycles of chemotherapy, i.e. days 18–32 or days 38–52.

a GM-CSF 50 $\mu g/m^2$:   1 patient with odd cycles
                             2 patients with even cycles
b GM-CSF 150 $\mu g/m^2$:   1 patient with odd cycles
                             2 patients with even cycles
c GM-CSF 300$\mu g/m^2$ 2 patients odd cycles
                             3 patients with even cycles
d GM-CSF 500 $\mu g/m^2$:   1 patient odd cycles
                             1 patient with even cycles

leucocyte count occurred 8–12 h after GM-CSF administration. Platelet and haemoglobin levels were unaffected by GM-CSF.

Neutropenia was significantly reduced following the chemotherapy courses with GM-CSF ($p = 0.04$; Fig. 1).

Toxicity

In the phase I study the most common toxic effect was bone pain, which occurred in 11 (65%) patients at GM-CSF doses of 150–500 $\mu g/m^2$. Two patients (nos. 9 and 15) withdrew because of WHO grade 3 bone pain, (GM-CSF doses 300 and 500 $\mu g/m^2$ respectively). Patient 9 had negative initial bone marrow findings but had malignant infiltration on analysis of the bone marrow sample taken after phase I. A rash occurred in 8 (47%) patients. This commonly was an erythematous rash with induration at the injection sites, occasionally also occurring at distant sites. It settled quickly on cessation of GM-CSF administration and tended not to recur in the phase II study. Transient fever occurred in 4 (24%) patients, lethargy in 2 (12%) and diarrhoea in 2 (12%) patients. One patient (no. 16) receiving a 500 $\mu g/m^2$ dosage withdrew from the study because of anxiety.

Of the patients who received 50 $\mu g/m^2$ GM-CSF in the phase II study, patient 1, who had no rash during the phase I study, developed a transient rash during GM-CSF administration after the first course of chemotherapy. Patient 3 was withdrawn from the study after two courses of chemotherapy because of multiple pulmonary emboli. Of the four who received 150 $\mu g/m^2$, one (no. 4) died of infection, having developed pneumococcal pneumonia and septicaemia with progression of the lung cancer after completion of the phase I study. Her condition improved at first, but she died after the first course of chemotherapy. Patient 7 died of progressive cancer. In his case chemotherapy was stopped after five courses. He had pain and lethargy that could have been due to tumour progression. All five of the six patients going onto the phase II study at the 300 $\mu g/m^2$ dose level reported some toxicity. One reported pain, two had a transient rash and pain (one also had lethargy), one had lethargy alone and one patient left the study after three cycles of chemotherapy because of a left brachial artery embolus. Of the two patients in the phase II study receiving 500 $\mu g/m^2$ GM-CSF, one (no. 14) died unexpectedly at home after two courses of therapy. No autopsy was obtained.

Infections

A total of 56 courses of chemotherapy were given.

Chemotherapy with GM-CSF

Following 26 cycles of chemotherapy with GM-CSF, patients were given antibiotics on seven (27%) occasions. In one case (patient 3) the fever may have been due to multiple pulmonary emboli. In all cases the antibiotics were given intravenously: netilmicin and piperacillin (six occasions) and erythromycin (once, patient 3). One patient (no. 4) suffered a bacteraemia with *Streptococcus pneumoniae* and subsequently died of pneumonia and progressive pulmonary cancer.

Chemotherapy Without GM-CSF

Thirty cycles of chemotherapy were given without subsequent administration of GM-CSF. On 10 (30%) occasions infection developed. Patient 5 received oral antibiotics for a discharging ear infection and patient 14 died at home of presumed infection. On eight occasions netilmicin and piperacillin were given intravenously. Two patients had bacteraemias. Haemolytic streptococci were cultured on two occasions (group B, patient 6; group A, patient 12).

Neutrophil chemiluminescence and chemotaxis were measured before the phase I study and at its completion using methods previously described (Bronchud et al. 1988). The median value of chemiluminescence was 1224 mV (range 955–1679) before and 1148 mV (range 327–2184) after 10 days of GM-CSF treatment. Six patients had a fall and five a rise in chemiluminescence.

The median value for chemotaxis was 152×10^2 mm (range 117–178 mm $\times 10^2$) before therapy and 100 mm $\times 10^2$ range 40–144 mm $\times 10^2$) at the end of the phase I study. Eight Patients had a fall, one no change and one a rise in the value.

Discussion

Despite a significant reduction in neutropenia following chemotherapy, the incidence of infection and use of intravenous antibiotics was not reduced by the administration of GM-CSF after chemotherapy courses. This result contrasts with a previous study from this institute which showed that intravenously administered G-CSF reduced the duration of neutropenia and number of infections in small cell lung cancer patients who received the same chemotherapy (Bronchud et al. 1987).

The neutrophil function tests showed that chemotaxis was reduced following GM-CSF therapy. Peters et al. (1988) have also reported reduced chemotaxis after GM-CSF therapy. Bronchud et al. (1988) reported on neutrophil migration in the patients from their 1987 study in a subsequent paper. They too found that chemotaxis was reduced after G-CSF therapy.

Daily subcutaneous GM-CSF was associated with more toxicity than G-CSF. Our study showed that highest leucocyte counts occurred 8–12 h after GM-CSF. We propose to evaluate the effect of twice daily subcutaneous injections and daily intravenous injection of GM-CSF in this patient group.

Summary

Seventeen patients with small cell lung cancer were entered into a dose ranging phase I–II study using rhGM-CSF (Glaxo). In the phase I study patients received 50, 150, 300 or 500 $\mu g/m^2$ GM-CSF for 10 days by daily subcutaneous injection. Full blood counts were performed thrice weekly. After 4 days off all therapy patients then received chemotherapy with doxorubicin 50 mg/m^2 i.v. bolus, day 1, ifosfamide 5 g/m^2 with mesna 5 g/m^2 over 24 h by continuous infusion followed by mesna 3 g/m^2, and etoposide 120 mg/m^2 i.v. on days 1–3. A total of six courses of chemotherapy were given.

In the phase II study patients received the same dose of GM-CSF as in the phase I. GM-CSF was given 24 h after the last dose of chemotherapy for 14 days. Full blood counts were checked thrice weekly and the incidence of infections noted. Patients were randomised to receive GM-CSF with either odd or even courses of chemotherapy.

The leucocyte count rose from a mean of 8.7 to $21.6 \times 10^9/l$ at the 50 $\mu g/m^2$ GM-CSF dosage and from 11.4 to $39.4 \times 10^9/l$ at the 500 $\mu g/m^2$ dosage during the phase I study. Phase I toxicity was: bone pain in 65% of patients, rash in 47%, fever in 24%, lethargy in 12% and diarrhoea in 12%. In the phase II study the duration of neutropenia was less during the chemotherapy courses with GM-CSF ($p = 0.04$) but the number of infections was similar. Analysis of the 56 courses of chemotherapy showed infection followed 7 (27%) that of the 26 courses with GM-CSF and 10 (33%) of the 30 courses without GM-CSF.

Acknowledgement. We thank Glaxo, Switzerland, for the supply of GM-CSF.

References

Antman KS, Griffin JD, Elias A, Socinski MA, Ryan L, Cannistra SA, Oette D, Whitley M, Frei E, Schnipper LE (1988) Effect of recombinant human granulocyte-macrophage colony-stimulating factor on chemotherapy-induced myelosuppression. N Engl J Med 319: 593–598

Bodey GP (1986) Infection in cancer patients; a continuing association. Am J Med 81 (1A): 11–26

Bronchud MH, Scarffe JH, Thatcher N, Crowther D, Souza LM, Alton NK, Testa NG, Dexter TM (1987) Phase I/II study of recombinant human granulocyte colony-stimulating factor in patients receiving intensive chemotherapy for small cell lung cancer. Br J Cancer 56: 809–813

Bronchud MH, Potter MR, Morgenstern G, Blasco MJ, Scarffe JH, Thatcher N, Crowther D, Souza LM, Alton NK, Testa NG, Dexter TM (1988) In vitro and in vivo analysis of the effects of recombinant human granulocyte colony-stimulating factor in patients (1988). Br J Cancer 58: 64–69

Gabrilove JL, Jakubowski A, Scher H, Sternberg C, Wong G, Grous J, Yagoda A, Fain K, Moore MAS, Clarkson B, Oettgen HF, Alton K, Welte K, Souza L (1988) Effect of granulocyte colony-stimulating factor on neutropenia and associated morbidity due to chemotherapy for transitional-cell carcinoma of the urothelium. N Engl J Med 318: 1414–1422

Metcalf D (1985) The granulocyte-macrophage colony-stimulating factors. Science 229: 16–22

Morstyn G, Campbell L, Souza LM, Alton MK, Keech J, Green M, Sheridan W, Metcalf D, Fox R (1988) Effect of granulocyte colony-stimulating factor in neutropenia induced by cytotoxic chemotherapy. Lancet i: 667–671

Peters WP, Stuart A, Affronti ML, Kim CS, Coleman RE (1988) Neutrophil migration is defective during recombinant human granulocyte-macrophage colony-stimulating factor infusion after autologous bone marrow transplantation in humans. Blood 72: 1310–1315

Recombinant Human Interleukin-3 in Patients with Hematopoietic Failure

A. Ganser[1], A. Lindemann[2], G. Seipelt[1], O.G. Ottmann[1], M. Eder[1], F. Herrmann[2], J. Frisch[3], G. Schulz[3], R. Mertelsmann[2], and D. Hoelzer[1]

[1]Abteilung für Hämatologie, Zentrum der Inneren Medizin, Klinikum der Johann Wolfgang Goethe-Universität, Theodor-Stern-Kai 7, W-6000 Frankfurt 70, FRG
[2]Abteilung Hematologie-Onkologie, Medizinische Universitätsklinik, Hugstetter Straße 55, W-7800 Freiburg, FRG
[3]Behringwerke AG, Klinische Forschung, W-3550 Marburg, FRG

Infections and bleeding are the most frequent causes of death in patients with bone marrow failure secondary to chemotherapy and/or radiotherapy for malignant disease. Treatment of anemia and severe thrombocytopenia has hitherto depended solely on red blood cell and platelet transfusion. With the recent availability of recombinant hematopoietic colony-stimulating factors (CSFs), stimulation of hematopoiesis in vivo has evolved as a new, potentially efficacious treatment modality. The feasibility of this approach is supported by several clinical studies showing that two distinct CSFs, granulocyte-macrophage CSF (GM-CSF) and granulocyte CSF (G-CSF), can indeed elevate total leukocyte counts in patients with bone marrow failure [1–14]. However, improvements in erythropoiesis and thrombopoiesis were observed only sporadically [2, 6, 7, 8].

Interleukin-3 (IL-3) belongs to a family of glycoprotein hormones responsible for regulating hematopoietic and immune functions, although not necessarily under steady-state conditions [15]. IL-3 promotes the survival, proliferation, and development of multipotential hematopoietic stem cells and of committed progenitor cells of the granulocyte/macrophage, erythroid, eosinophil, megakaryocyte, mast cell and basophilic lineages [16–18]. In addition, IL-3 enhances myeloid end cell functions such as phagocytosis, antibody-dependent cellular cytotoxicity, and metabolism of eosinophils [19] but not neutrophils [20], as well as monocyte cytotoxicity [21]. Its range of activities is broader than that of the other CSFs [16, 22, 23], and, in particular, it appears to be a more potent stimulator of megakaryocytopoiesis [24–26] and of ontogenetically very early hematopoietic progenitor cells [17].

Preclinical studies have demonstrated that IL-3 effectively stimulates myelopoiesis, erythropoiesis, and thrombopoiesis in several murine and nonhuman primate models [27–32]. On the basis of these data and the availability of sufficient quantities of human IL-3 (rhIL-3) produced by recombinant DNA techniques [33–36], we have treated nine patients with secondary bone marrow failure in a phase I/II study to evaluate the safety and hematological effects of subcutaneous injections of rhIL-3. Our data demonstrate that rhIL-3 has the capacity to stimulate myelopoiesis, thrombopoiesis, and, to a lesser degree, erythropoiesis at dose levels well tolerated by these patients.

Methods

Patient Selection

In a phase I/II study, nine patients with secondary bone marrow failure and severe cytopenia were treated with rhIL-3: six men and three women, ranging in age from 18 to 74 years (median: 65 years). The underlying diseases and previous therapies are listed in Table 1. Bone marrow hypoplasia due to prolonged chemotherapy for cancer and/or tumor infiltration of the bone marrow was confirmed by bone marrow cytology and histology. These patients had received their last previous dose of chemotherapy between 3 weeks and 14 months (median: 2.5 months) prior to initiation of rhIL-3 treatment. Three of these patients had received additional radiotherapy. Three patients had been treated with recombinant GM-CSF at 6 weeks, 4 months and 8 months respectively prior to entering the present trial, without persisting improvements of peripheral blood counts. In no patient was there any evidence of spontaneous hematopoietic recovery. None of the patients had clinical evidence of bacterial, fungal, or

Table 1. Baseline characteristics of the nine study patients

Male/female ratio	6/3
Age (years):	
median	65
range	18–74
Diagnoses:	
multiple myeloma	2
non-Hodgkin's lymphoma:	
low-grade	3
high-grade	2
germ cell tumor	1
testicular teratoma	1
Chemotherapy	6
Chemo- and radiotherapy	3
Interval to IL-3 therapy (weeks):	
median	11
range	3–62
Transfusion dependency:	6
red blood cells	6
platelets	4

viral infections when entering this study. One patient treated at 500 $\mu g/m^2$ was only evaluable for toxicity but not for hematologic response because rhIL-3 had to be discontinued after 2 days of treatment.

Eligibility criteria included a performance status of more than 50% (Karnofsky Scale), a life expectancy of more than 3 months, preserved hepatic, renal, cardiac, and hemostatic function, and absence of clinically apparent allergies or bronchoalveolar disorders. The study was approved by the local ethics committee. Informed written consent was obtained from the patients before rhIL-3 therapy started.

Recombinant Human IL-3

The cDNA of rhIL-3 was isolated from human peripheral blood lymphocytes and the gene product expressed in yeast [35]. The molecular weight was in the range of 14–16 kD. The rhIL-3 used in this study was produced and provided by Immunex/Behringwerke AG (Seattle/Marburg). The specific activity of this substance was $> 1 \times 10^7$ units/mg protein in a bone marrow proliferation assay. Sterility, pyrogenicity, general safety, and purity studies met the Office of Biologics standard. No endotoxin was measurable with the limulus amebocyte lysate assay (< 10 pg/mg protein).

Study Design

rhIL-3 was administered by subcutaneous bolus injection daily for 15 days. Patients were monitored daily and all constitutional symptoms (fever, bone pain, malaise) were recorded. Before and during the study, patients were regularly monitored by means of complete history and physical examination and laboratory tests including a complete blood count, differential and reticulocyte counts, a chemistry profile, coagulation profile, and urinalysis. An electrocardiogram and chest X-ray were performed before the study and after the final dose. Bone marrow aspirates and biopsy specimens were processed according to conventional methods and evaluated before and after the treatment cycle.

Student's t-test was used to calculate the mean $\pm$ SEM. The Wilcoxon signed rank test for paired data was used to test for significant differences between data before and after administration of rhIL-3.

Toxicity was graded according to the World Health Organization (WHO) criteria [37]. Dose-limiting toxicity was generally defined as WHO grade 3 toxicity or higher. Red cell concentrates were administered if the hemoglobin level dropped below 8 g/dl or if there were symptoms related to anemia. Platelet transfusions were only administered in cases of bleeding. Antipyretics were not given unless the body temperature rose above 39° C.

Results

Both total leukocyte counts and circulating neutrophil counts rose in all evaluable eight patients in response to rhIL 3 (Table 2; Fig. 1). The rise in circulating leukocytes was delayed, but eventually seven out of eight patients reached neutrophil counts above $2000/\mu$l, and no patient had a count below $500/\mu$l after treatment. The median time to peak neutrophil counts was 19 days (range: 6–50). Eosinophils, basophils, and monocytes all peaked at a median time of 13–16 days (range: 14–46 days for eosinophils, 8–50 days for basophils, and 11–46 days for monocytes).

A stimulation of thrombopoiesis with a subsequent 1.3- to 14.3-fold (mean: 6-fold) increase in circulating platelet numbers occurred in five of eight evaluable patients. This increase resulted in discontinuation of platelet transfusions in two out of three patients who had been dependent on repeated substitution. Reticulocyte counts responded to administration of rhIL-3 in three out of eight patients. The reticulocyte counts reached the maximum at a median of 8 days (range: 2–65) and rose 1.1- to 3.7-fold (mean: 2.3-fold). The necessity of red blood cell transfusions was, however, not reduced during the observation period. Serum IgM levels increased dose-independently in all eight evaluable patients from 0.73 ± 0.12 g/l to 2.50 ± 0.99 g/l ($p < 0.01$). Mean serum IgG and IgA levels did not change.

Bone marrow samples obtained before and after the treatment cycles demonstrated increases in cellularity in six out of eight patients, along with increases in megakaryocytes and eosinophils, but not in basophils (Table 3). In one patient (no. 7) the shift to the left in granulopoiesis resulted in an increase of myeloblasts from 1% to 9% and an increase in mostly abnormal promyelocytes. There were no increases in bone marrow-infiltrating tumor or lymphoma cells.

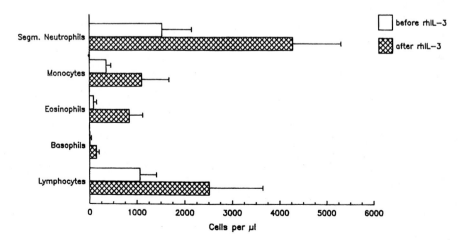

Fig. 1. Effect of treatment with rhIL-3 on leukocyte counts

Table 2. Changes in peripheral blood count during treatment with rhIL-3

Pat. no.	Dosage (µg/m²)	Leukocytes[a]		Neutrophils[a]		Platelets[a]		Hb (g/dl)		Reticulocytes (%)	
		Pre	Post	Pre	Post	Pre	Post	Pre	Post	Pre	Post
1	30	3.4	6.1	0.81	2.86	13	67	10.4	11.7	0.7	2.5
2	60	0.8	1.9	0.16	0.63	7	100	8.9	7.7	0.1	0.3
3	60	1.7	3.6	0	2.38	57	74	10.5	10.3	0.1	0.3
4	60	4.4	13.4	1.19	2.28	18	185	9.4	9.5	0.7	0.8
5	125	1.9	5.6	1.10	4.48	58	122	8.7	8.6	1.0	1.4
6	125	4.5	10.9	3.92	6.21	112	n.c.	10.5	9.8	0.4	1.7
7	250	8.1	15.5	4.62	10.10	17	n.c.	10.4	11.5	4.2	4.5
8	250	1.2	9.3	0.48	5.39	228	392	7.0	10.6	1.0	1.3
9	500[b]	1.8	n.e.	0.11	n.e.	43	n.e.	10.2	n.e.	0.7	n.e.

The maximum response during the study is given. n.c., no change; n.e., not evaluable.

[a] $\times 10^3/\mu l$.

[b] rhIL-3 only given for 2 days.

Table 3. Marrow findings of patients with bone marrow failure before and after administration of rhIL-3

Pat. no.	Cellularity[a]		Megakaryocytes[b]		Blasts & Promyelocytes (%)		Eosinophils (%)		Basophils (%)		M/E ratio	
	Before	After	Before	After	Before	After	Before	After	Before	After	Before	After
1	+	+	+	+	0	1	2	6	1	1	0.10	0.93
2	+	++	−	+	n.e.	n.e.	n.e.	n.e.	n.e.	n.e.	n.e.	n.e.
3	+	+	+	+	n.e.	n.e.	n.e.	n.e.	n.e.	n.e.	n.e.	n.e.
4	+	+	+	+	1	0	2	1	0	0	0.82	0.64
5	+	+++	+	++	3.5	14	4	8.5	0	0	0.18	3.45
6	+	+++	+	++	8.5	6.5	3	11	0.5	0	2.26	3.22
7	++	+++	+	++	17	48	1	31	0	0	25.3	20.0
8	+	+++	++	++	12	8.5	3.5	14.5	0	0.5	0.80	2.10
9	+	n.d.	+	n.d.	2.5	n.d.	3.5	n.d.	0	n.d.	4.40	n.d.

n.e., not evaluable because of fibrosis; n.d., not done; M/E, mycloid/erythroid.
a +, hypocellular (10%–30%); ++, normocellular (30%–60%); +++, hypercellular (>60%).
b −, absent; +, reduced; ++, normal; +++, increased.

The toxicity of the treatment schedule was mild. Fever, with a body temperature not exceeding 40° C, was seen in the majority of patients and was usually more pronounced during the first few days of therapy. Headache accompanied by stiffness of the neck also occurred. In the patient receiving 500 μg/m^2, the rhIL-3 therapy had to be discontinued after 2 days because of development of pneumonia. Mild local erythema at the site of subcutaneous injection of rhIL-3 was observed in several patients.

Effects possibly attributable to rhIL-3 on neoplastic cells included a transient rise in circulating atypical B-lymphocytes in one patient with centrocytic lymphoma receiving 60 μg rhIL-3/m^2 and in one patient with immunocytoma receiving 250 μg/m^2. The latter patient also developed palpable lymph nodes and an increase in spleen size, which were all reversible within 2 weeks after the discontinuation of rhIL-3 treatment. No increase in paraprotein levels was observed in the two patients with multiple myeloma.

Discussion

Treatment with rhIL-3 clearly induced a multilineage hematopoietic response, with an increase in leukocytes, platelets, and reticulocytes. Although the increase in leukocytes did not start as soon as after treatment with GM-CSF [1–9] or G-CSF [10–14], it was nevertheless so pronounced that the risk of infection due to neutropenia could be reduced.

The equally, if not more, important response to rhIL-3 was the increase in platelet and reticulocyte counts, which is only rarely observed after treatment with GM-CSF [1–9] or G-CSF [10–14]. The basis of this response again seems to be stimulation at the level of the multipotential and lineage-committed progenitor cells, resulting in a delayed response of platelets and reticulocytes [16–18, 25, 38, 39]. The hematopoietic response in these patients thus repeats the observations in vivo in mice [28] and nonhuman primates [30–32] which have shown IL-3 to stimulate thrombopoiesis and erythropoiesis.

Stimulation of lymphopoiesis was evinced by both a rise in lymphocyte counts and increases in the concentration of IgM in the serum. The increase in T lymphocytes was unselective, affecting both T helper and T suppressor subsets. Why only the IgM and not the IgG, IgA and IgE gradients increased after rhIL-3 remains unresolved, since IL-3 has been shown to induce production of IgG by human B lymphocytes in vitro [40].

Recombinant rhIL-3 was well tolerated, apart from headache and neck stiffness at the higher doses of subcutaneous bolus administration, which máy be indirectly due to release of other cytokines. Although no anticancer effects were seen in these patients, the duration of the treatment periods was too short for possible effects to occur. However, patients with nonhematopoietic tumors did not exhibit any obvious acceleration of tumor growth either, as could have occurred according to in vitro studies [41, 42]. By contrast, stimulation of malignant B cells was seen in two patients with lymphoma. The transient increase in circulating lymphoma cells and in the size of the lymph nodes, with regression after discontinuation of rhIL-3 treatment, indicates that the lymphoma cells apparently were receptive to rhIL-3 stimulation. In one patient, treatment with rhIL-3 resulted in development of the morphological characteristics of a myelodysplastic syndrome. Presumably, the anemia and thrombocytopenia in this patient resulted from a pre-existing myelodysplastic syndrome which became overt after stimulation of the immature blast cells by the IL-3 [43]. It should further be noted that this particular patient was the only one in whom the low platelet counts did not increase after treatment with rhIL-3.

In conclusion, rhIL-3 appears to be a potent and well-tolerated multilineage stimulant of thrombopoiesis, leukocytopoiesis, and erythropoiesis in man. It therefore appears to be of considerable value in the treatment of either chemo- or radiotherapy-induced or disease-related pancytopenic disorders.

Summary

Nine patients with bone marrow failure and prolonged severe cytopenias were treated with recombinant human interleukin-3 (rhIL-3) at doses ranging from 30 μg/m^2 to 500 μg/m^2. rhIL-3 was administered in a subcutaneous bolus injection daily for 15 days. Platelet counts increased by a mean of 6-fold (range: 1.3- to 14.3-fold) in five out of eight evaluable patients. Reticulocyte counts increased 2.9-fold in three patients, and neutrophil counts increased by a mean of 3.1-fold in all eight patients. Platelet transfusions could be discontinued after treatment with rhIL-3 in two out of three evaluable transfusion-dependent patients. Only mild side effects, mainly fever and headache, were observed. These results indicate that rhIL-3 functions as a multilineage hematopoietic growth factor in vivo in patients with secondary bone marrow failure.

Acknowledgment. We are indebted to Karin Leibold-Meid for coordinating data collection and evaluation, and to Dr. U. Essers, Aachen, for patient referral.

References

1. Groopman JE, Mitsuyasu RT, DeLeo MJ, Oette DH, Golde DW (1987) Effect of recombinant human granulocyte-macrophage colony-stimulating factor on myelopoiesis in the acquired immunodeficiency syndrome. N Engl J Med 317: 593–598
2. Vadhan-Raj S, Keating M, LeMaistre A, Hittelmann WN, McCredie K, Trujillo JM, Broxmeyer HE, Henney C, Gutterman JU (1987) Effects of recombinant human granulocyte-macrophage colony-stimulating factor in patients with myelodysplastic syndromes. N Engl J Med 317: 1545–1552
3. Antin JH, Smith BR, Holmes W, Rosenthal DS (1988) Phase I/II study of recombinant human granulocyte-macrophage colony-stimulating factor in aplastic anemia and myelodysplastic syndrome. Blood 72: 705–713

4. Vadhan-Raj S, Buescher S, Broxmeyer HE, LeMaistre A, Lepe-Zuniga JL, Ventura G, Jeha S, Horwitz L, Trujillo JM, Gillis S, Hittelman WN, Gutterman JU (1988) Stimulation of myelopoiesis in patients with aplastic anemia by recombinant human granulocyte-macrophage colony-stimulating factor. N Engl J Med 319: 1628–1634

5. Vadhan-Raj S, Buescher S, LeMaistre A, Keating M, Walters R, Ventura C, Hittelman W, Broxmeyer HE, Gutterman JU (1988) Stimulation of hematopoiesis in patients with malignancy by recombinant human granulocyte-macrophage colony-stimulating factor. Blood 72: 134–141

6. Ganser A, Voelkers B, Greher J, Ottman OG, Walther F, Becher R, Bergmann L, Schulz G, Hoelzer D (1989) Recombinant human granulocyte-macrophage colony-stimulating factor in patients with myelodysplastic syndromes — a phase I/II study. Blood 73: 31–37

7. Thompson JA, Lee DJ, Kidd P, Rubin E, Kaufmann J, Bonnem EM, Fefer A (1989) Subcutaneous granulocyte-macrophage colony-stimulating factor in patients with myelodysplastic syndrome: toxicity, pharmacokinetics and hematological effects. J Clin Oncol 7: 629–637

8. Ganser A, Ottmann OG, Erdmann H, Schulz G, Hoelzer D (1989) The effect of recombinant human granulocyte-macrophage colony-stimulating factor on neutropenia and related morbidity in chronic severe neutropenia. Ann Intern Med 111: 887–892

9. Herrmann F, Lindemann A, Klein H, Lubbert M, Schulz G, Mertelsmann R (1988) Effect of recombinant human granulocyte-macrophage colony-stimulating factor in patients with myelodysplastic syndrome with excess blasts. Leukemia 3: 355–338

10. Negrin RS, Haeuber DH, Nagler A, Olds LC, Donlon T, Souza LM, Greenberg PL (1989) Treatment of myelodysplastic syndromes with recombinant. human granulocyte colony-stimulating factor. A phase I–II trial. Ann Intern Med 110: 976–984

11. Glaspy JA, Baldwin GC, Robertson PA, Souza L, Vincent M, Ambersley J, Golde DW (1988) Therapy for neutropenia in hairy cell leukemia with recombinant human granulocyte colony-stimulating factor. Ann Intern Med 109: 789–795

12. Kobayashi Y, Okabe T, Ozawa K, Chiba S, Hino M, Miyazono K, Urabe A, Takaku F (1989) Treatment of myelodysplastic syndromes with recombinant human granulocyte colony-stimulating factor: a preliminary report. Am J Med 86: 178–182

13. Jakubowski AA, Souza L, Kelly F et al. (1989) Effects of human granulocyte colony-stimulating factor in a patient with idiopathic neutropenia. N Engl J Med 320: 38–42

14. Bonilla MA, Gillio AP, Ruggeiro M, Kernan NA, Brochstein JA, Abboud M, Fumagalli L, Vincent M, Gabrilove JL, Welte K, Souza LM, O'Reilly RJ (1989) Effects of recombinant human granulocyte colony-stimulating factor in patients with congenital agranulocytosis. N Engl J Med 320: 1574–1580

15. Ihle J, Keller J, Oroszlan S, Henderson LE, Copeland TD, Fitch F, Prystowsky MB, Goldwasser E, Schrader JW, Palazynski E, Dy M, Lebel B (1983) Biologic properties of homogenous interleukin 3. J Immunol 131: 282–287

16. Leary AG, Yang YC, Clark SC, Gasson JC, Golde DW, Ogawa M (1987) Recombinant gibbon interleukin 3 supports formation of human multilineage colonies and blast cell colonies in culture: comparison with recombinant human granulocyte-macrophage colony-stimulating factor. Blood 70: 1343–1348

17. Saeland S, Caux C, Favre C, Aubry LP, Mannoni P, Pebusque MJ, Gentilhomme O, Otsuka T, Ykotay T, Arai N, Banchereau J, de Vries JE (1988) Effects of recombinant human interleukin 3 on CD34-enriched normal hematopoietic progenitors and on myeloblastic leukemia cells. Blood 72: 1580–1588

18. Sonoda Y, Yang YC, Wong GG, Clark SC, Ogawa M (1988) Analysis in serum-free culture of the targets of recombinant human hemopoietic growth factors: interleukin 3 and granulocyte-macrophage colony-stimulating factor are specific for early development stages. Proc Natl Acad Sci USA 85: 4360–4363

19. Rothenberg ME, Owen WF Jr, Silberstein DS, Woods J, Sobermann RJ, Austen KF, Stevens RL (1988) Human eosinophils have prolonged survival, enhanced functional properties, and become hypodense when exposed to human interleukin 3. J Clin Invest 81: 1986–1992

20. Lopez AF, Dyson PG, To LB, Elliott J, Milton SE, Russell JA, Juttner CA, Yang YC, Clark SC, Vadas MA (1988) Recombinant human interleukin-3 stimulation of hematopoiesis in humans: loss of responsiveness in differentiation in the neutrophilic myeloid series. Blood 72: 1797–1804

21. Cannistra SA, Vellenga E, Groshek P, Rambaldi A, Griffin JD (1988) Human granulocyte-monocyte colony-stimulating factor and interleukin 3 stimulate monocyte cytotoxicity through a tumor necrosis factor-dependent mechanism. Blood 71: 672–676

22. Lopez AF, To LB, Yang Y-C, Gamble JR, Shannon MF, Burns GF, Dyson PG, Juttner CA, Clark S, Vadas MA (1987) Stimulation of proliferation, differentiation and function of human cells by primate interleukin 3. Proc Natl Acad Sci USA 84: 2761–2765

23. Emerson SG, Yang YC, Clark SC, Long MW (1988) Human recombinant granulocyte-macrophage colony-stimulating factors and interleukin 3 have overlapping but distinct hematopoietic activities. J Clin Invest 82: 1282–1287

24. Bruno R, Briddell R, Hoffman R (1988) Effect of recombinant and purified hematopoietic growth factors on human megakaryocyte colony formation. Exp Hematol 16: 371–377

25. Lu L, Briddell RA, Graham CD, Brandt JE, Bruno E, Hoffman R (1988) Effect of recombinant and purified human haematopoietic growth factors on in vitro colony formation by enriched populations of human megakaryocyte progenitor cells. Br J Haematol 70: 149–156

26. Teramura M, Katahira J, Hoshino S, Motoji T, Oshimi K, Mizoguchi H (1988) Clonal growth of human megakaryocyte progenitors in serum-free cultures: effect of recombinant human interleukin-3. Exp Hematol 16: 843–848

27. Kindler V, Thorens B, de Kossodo S, Allet B, Eliason JF, Thatcher D, Farber N, Vassalli P (1986) Stimulation of hematopoiesis in vivo by recombinant bacterial murine interleukin 3. Proc Natl Acad Sci USA 83: 1001–1005

28. Metcalf D, Begley CG, Johnson GR, Nicola NA, Lopez AF, Williamsen DJ (1986) Effects of purified bacterially synthezised murine multi-CSF (IL-3) on hematopoiesis in normal adult mice. Blood 68: 46–57

29. Broxmeyer HE, Williams D, Hangoc G, Cooper S, Gillis S, Shadduck RK, Bicknell DC (1987) Synergistic myelopoietic actions in vivo after administration to mice of combinations of purified natural murine colony-stimulating factor 1, recombinant murine interleukin-3, and recombinant murine granulocyte/macrophage colony-stimulating factor. Proc Natl Acad Sci USA 84: 3871–3875

30. Donahue RE, Seehra J, Metzger M, Lefebvre D, Rock B, Carbone S, Nathan DG, Garnick M, Sehgal PK, Laston D, la Vallie E, McCoy J, Schendel PF, Norton C, Turner K, Yang YC, Clark SC (1988) Human IL-3 and GM-CSF act synergistically in stimulating hematopoiesis in primates. Science 241: 1820–1823

31. Krumwieh D, Seiler FR (1989) In vivo effects of recombinant colony stimulating factors on hematopoiesis in cynamolgus monkeys. Transplant Proc 21: 379–383

32. Mayer P, Valent P, Schmidt G, Liehl E, Bettelheim P (1989) The in vivo effect of recombinant human interleukin-3: demonstration of basophil differentiation factor, histamine-producing activity and priming of GM-CSF-responsive progenitors in nonhuman primates. Blood 74: 613–621

33. Yang Y-C, Charletta AB, Temple PA, Chung MP, Kovacic S, Witek-Giannotti JS, Leary AC, Kriz R, Donahue RE, Wong GG, Clark SC (1986) Human IL-3 (multi-CSF): identification by expression cloning of a novel hematopoietic growth factor related to murine IL-3. Cell 47: 3–10

34. Dorssers L, Burger H, Bot F, Delwel R, van Kessel HMG, Löwenberg B, Wagemaker G (1987) Characterization of a human multilineage colony-stimulating factor cDNA clone identified by a conserved noncoding sequence in mouse inter-leukin-3. Gene 55: 115–124

35. Gillis G, Urdal DL, Clergenger W, Kluske R, Sassenfeld H, Price V, Cosman D (1988) Production of recombinant human colony stimulating factors in yeast. Behring Inst Mitt 83: 1–7

36. Otsuka T, Miyajima A, Brown N, Otsu K, Abrams J, Saeland S, Caux C, Malefijt RDW, De Vries R, Meyerson P, Yokota K, Gemmel L, Rennick D, Lee F, Arai N, Arai KI, Yokota T (1988) Isolation and characterization of an expressible cDNA encoding human IL-3. Induction of IL-3 mRNA in human T cell clones. J Immunol 140: 2288–2295

37. Miller AB, Hoogstraaten B, Staquet M, Winkler A (1981) Reporting results of cancer treatment. Cancer 47: 201–206

38. Migliaccio AR, Migliaccio G, Adamson JW (1988) Effect of recombinant hemopoie-tic growth factors on proliferation of human marrow progenitor cells in serum-deprived liquid culture. Blood 72: 1387–1392

39. Messner HA, Yamasadi K, Jamal N, Minden MM, Yang YC, Wong GG, Clark SC (1987) Growth of human hemopoietic colonies in response to recombinant gibbon interleukin-3: comparison with human granulocyte and granulocyte-macrophage colony-stimulating factor: Proc Natl Acad Sci USA 84: 6765–6769

40. Tadmori W, Feingersh D, Clark SC, Choi YS (1989) Human recombinant IL-3 stimulates B cell differentiation. J Immunol 142: 1950–1955

41. Berdel WE, Danhauser-Riedl S, Steinhauser G, Winton EF (1989) Various human hematopoietic growth factors (interleukin-3, GM-CSF, G-CSF) stimulate clonal growth of nonhematopoietic tumor cells. Blood 73: 80–83

42. Anderson KC, Jones RM, Morimoto C, Leavitt P, Barut BA (1989) Response patterns of purified myeloma cells to hematopoietic growth factors. Blood 73: 1915–1924

43. Delwel R, Dorssers I, Touw I, Wagemaker G, Löwenberg B (1987) Human recombinant multilineage colony stimulating factor: stimulation of acute myelocytic leukemia progenitor cells in vitro. Blood 70: 333–336

Recombinant Human Granulocyte–Macrophage Colony-Stimulating Factor for the Intensification of Cytostatic Treatment in Advanced Cancer

L. Schmid, B. Thürlimann, M. Müller, and H.-J. Senn

Abteilung für Onkologie und Hämatologie, Medizinische Klinik C, Kantonsspital, 9007 St. Gallen, Switzerland

Introduction

Recombinant human granulocyte–macrophage colony-stimulating factor (GM-CSF) is a glycoprotein that stimulates granulocyte and macrophage progenitor cells to form mature colonies of granulocytes and/or macrophages [1–3]. Clinically, GM-CSF may have a role in stimulating myelopoietic regeneration after irradiation, treatment with cytostatic drugs, bone marrow transplantation and other treatments.

In combining GM-CSF with cytostatic drugs, two goals may be achieved: intensification of cytostatic treatment and/or reduction of the toxicity associated with agranulocytosis.

To study the toxicity and feasibility of dose intensification we started a series of phase I/II studies with 1–3 cycles of intensive chemotherapy plus GM-CSF. This paper gives a short overview of the preliminary results obtained up to January 1990, mainly concerning toxicity, focusing especially on haematotoxicity.

Patients and Method

Patients

Thirteen patients – seven men and six women – were entered in a phase I/II study. The mean age was 38 years, with a range from 18 to 66 years. All patients were suffering from advanced tumours without bone marrow involvement, and all of them had a performance index of 0 or 1 according to SAKK criteria. There were four cases of breast cancer, three of soft tissue sarcoma, and two each of testicular carcinoma, osteogenic sarcoma and Hodgkin's lymphoma.

Cytostatic Treatment

All patients were treated with a first cycle of cytostatics, followed by treatment with GM-CSF for 10–12 days. If possible (i.e. if toxicity allowed), a second cycle of the same cytostatic regimen was given after 14 days, and again GM-CSF was administered for 10–12 days. If a response was observed, a third cycle of the cytostatic drugs was given as early as possible, followed by a final course of GM-CSF treatment.

Up to 32 cycles of therapy were completed. Fifteen cycles consisted of ifosfamide + epirubicin, six of thio-tepa + epirubicin, four of ifosfamide + etoposide + cisplatin, three of bleomycin + etoposide + cisplatin, and two each of ifosfamide + etoposide + VLB and thio-tepa + carboplatin.

The median dosage of ifosfamide per cycle was 7.5 g/m^2 body surface area in cycle 1, 9.5 g/m^2 in cycle 2 and 12.5 g/m^2 in cycle 3. The median dosages of thio-tepa were about 40 mg/m^2 in cycle 1, 42.5 mg/m^2 in cycle 2 and 52 mg/m^2 in cycle 3. The median dosage of epirubicin reached 120 mg/m^2 in cycle 1, 122 mg/m^2 in cycle 2 and 125 mg/m^2 in cycle 3.

Recombinant Human GM-CSF Treatment

Recombinant human GM-CSF (Schering) was given immediately after the chemotherapy for 10–12 days. The first ten treatments with GM-CSF were given as a continuous intravenous infusion. During the next 22 cycles GM-CSF was given twice daily as a subcutaneous injection. The median dosage was about 10 μg/kg body weight during cycles 1 and 2 and about 7.5 μg/kg during cycle 3.

Results

The toxicity of the treatment proved to be mainly haematological. The data base consists of 350 blood samples, taken about very 2nd day during therapy.

Toxicity

Haemoglobin

The mean haemoglobin levels of all patients show a slight but constant drop from 120 g/l at the beginning to about 80 g/l (Fig. 1). Red blood cell transfusions were given at levels of 80 g/l. Analysis of nadir values shows that all patients developed anaemia of less than 100 g/l during cycles 2 and 3. Trend analysis also indicates a significant decrease of nadir values from cycle 1 to cycle 3.

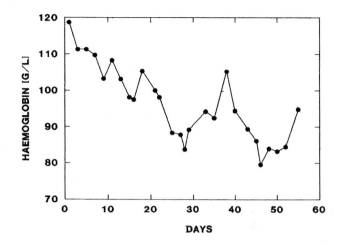

Fig. 1. Mean haemoglobin levels of all patients during chemotherapy cycles 1–3

Granulocytes

Figure 2 shows the course of the mean leucocyte and mean absolute granulocyte counts. Two points are important: (a) the course of the leucocyte counts is essentially mirrored by the circulating cells of granulopoiesis, and (b) during each cycle there is a decrease in the mean granulocyte count to very low values, but the recovery is very rapid.

This is also illustrated by Fig. 3: the median nadir of granulocytes is about 0 during all the cycles. However, only a few patients had WHO grade 4 granulocytopenia for more than 5 days. There is a significant trend toward more prolonged granulocytopenia from cycle 1 to cycle 3.

Another indicator of granulocyte toxicity is the frequency of bacterial infection. Treatment with antibiotics was given in 14 of 31 chemotherapy cycles; 17 (55%) of all cycles could be completed without use of antibiotics. The incidence of use of this type of drugs was higher in cycles 2 and 3 than during cycle 1. At the start of the study we used to administer antibiotics to every patient with a temperature above 38°C and a granulocyte count below 0.5 $\times 10^9$/l. Since GM-CSF can induce fever in most patients, a certain number of these antibiotic treatments may have been redundant.

Platelets

Figure 4 shows the course of the platelet counts during the treatment. Taking all patients together, there is no evidence of alarming platelet toxicity. Analysing the data cycle by cycle, it can be seen that the median platelet nadir drops from about 80×10^9/l during cycle 1 to about 25×10^9/l during cycle 3 (Fig. 5).

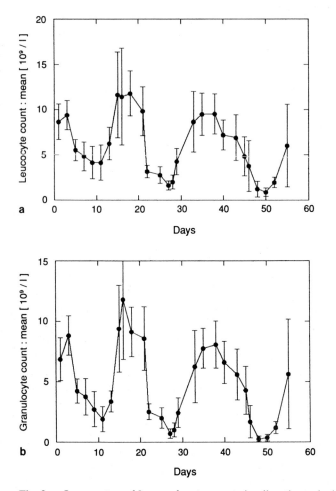

Fig. 2. a Leucocyte and **b** granulocyte counts in all patients during chemotherapy cycles 1–3. Mean ±1 SE

Five patients showed prolonged WHO grade 4 platelet toxicity (defined as a platelet count below $25 \times 10^9/l$), for more than 5 days. Two patients had significant platelet toxicity during cycle 1. In these two cases the planned chemotherapy with thio-tepa plus epirubicin could not be carried out because of cardiotoxicity resulting from previous therapy with anthracyclines, so a combination of thio-tepa plus carboplatin was given. One patient developed grade 4 platelet toxicity for 18 days and the other one for 26 days. In addition, for reasons not clearly understood, efficient substitution of the platelets in these patients was impossible. Only in 5 out of 31 evaluable cycles did platelet transfusions have to be given.

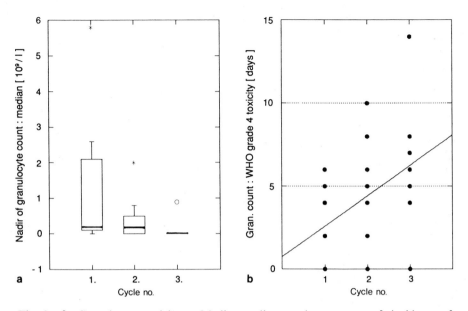

Fig. 3a, b. Granulocyte toxicity. **a** Median nadir granulocyte counts; **b** incidence of WHO grade 4 granulocytopenia. Each dot represents one patient

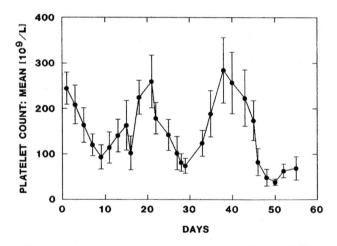

Fig. 4. Platelet counts in all patients during chemotherapy cycles 1–3. Mean ±1 SE

Non-haematological Toxicity

Table 1 summarizes the non-haematological toxicity. Two patients had slight to moderate pleural pain during treatment with GM-CSF. There was no evidence of pulmonary embolism. The only WHO grade 4 non-haematological toxicity

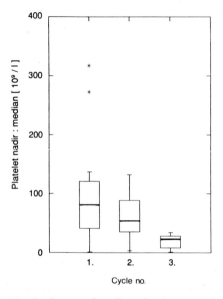

Fig. 5. Course of median platelet count nadir in all patients in chemotherapy cycles 1–3

Table 1. Non-haematological toxicity[a]

Symptom	N	Intensity [WHO grade]	Regimen	Remarks
Pleural pain	1	2	Ifo + epi	GM-CSF?
Respiratory distress	1	4	T-tepa + epi	GM-CSF?
Phlebothrombosis	1	?	BEP	
Lethargy	1	1	Ifo + epi	
Somnolence	1	3	Ifo + epi	
Erythema [face]	1	1	BEP	GM-CSF?
Skin infiltrate	2	2	BEP	GM-CSF
			T-tepa + epi	
Fever	8	2	All	GM-CSF

[a] Hair loss and gastrointestinal toxicity as expected.
Ifo, ifosfamide; epi, epirubicin; t-tepa, thio-tepa; BEP, bleomycin + etoposide + cisplatin.

was observed after the third cycle of thio-tepa plus epirubicin in a patient with breast cancer: a respiratory distress syndrome developed after the end of GM-CSF treatment. The patient recovered after symptomatic therapy without artificial respiration and is now a fully active housewife.

One patient with testicular cancer developed thrombosis of the left subclavian vein during the first treatment cycle with GM-CSF. Two other patients suffered from central nervous symptoms during chemotherapy with ifosfamide and epirubicin. Some metabolites of ifosfamide may be responsible for this type of toxicity.

One patient had a red face during infusion of GM-CSF; two developed mild to moderate skin infiltration locally at the site of subcutaneous administration of GM-CSF.

The majority of patients (eight) developed fever above 38° C during GM-CSF therapy. Two of these eight patients had slight other flu-like symptoms.

Response

Although this phase I/II study was mainly conducted to analyse toxicity and feasibility, a short comment on the overall response rate is given (Fig. 6). In five (38%) of the patients a complete response was obtained; three (23%) had a good partial response. The remission rate of the 13 patients treated is 62%. Up to now one patient has died, 12 are still alive and in good to fair condition. It is too early to draw any further conclusion concerning the efficacy of this type of high-dose chemotherapy.

Discussion

In patients with solid tumours, GM-CSF and G-CSF have up to now been used mainly to intensify cytostatic treatment and/or to reduce the toxicity associated with agranulocytosis [4–7]. Dose intensification may be achieved by raising the dosage of drugs with low non-haematological toxicity and/or by reduction of the intervals between cycles of cytostatic treatment. It is presumed, but largely still

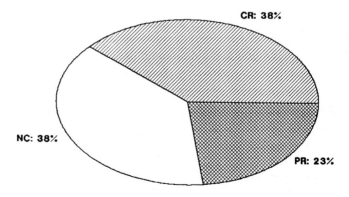

Fig. 6. Overall response rate. *CR*, complete response; *PR*, partial response; *NC*, no change

unproven, that dose intensification will result in a better response of longer duration than conventional treatment.

Reduction of toxicity ought to consist of a shorter duration of granulocytopenia. This may result in decreased incidence of bacterial infection, reduction of the use of antibiotics, and shorter hospital stays. There is convincing clinical evidence that the duration of agranulocytosis induced by cytostatic treatment can be reduced by the use of GM-CSF or G-CSF [4–8].

Although in vitro data with haematopoietic precursors showed some stimulation of megakaryopoiesis by GM-CSF, there are, at least in patients with solid tumours, no clinical data to support this hypothesis. GM-CSF will most probably not influence cytostatically induced thrombocytopenia [9–11].

The ideal dosage and sequence of cytostatic drugs in combination with the use of GM-CSF needs to be investigated in prospective randomized trials. Our preliminary data show that dose intensification by dose elevation and reduction of time intervals between the cycles seems to be a reasonable way.

Both the interference by GM-CSF in the growth of tumour cells and the influence of the intensified cytostatic treatment on the stimulated haematological precursor cells remain to be examined in more detail.

Conclusions

From the results presented we draw the following preliminary conclusions:

1. The combination of up to three cycles of high-dose chemotherapy with GM-CSF seems to be safe and feasible.
2. Recombinant human GM-CSF gives adequate protection from chemotherapy-induced granulocytopenia.
3. Protection against anaemia and thrombocytopenia seems to be relatively poor.

References

1. Metcalf D, Burgess AW (1982) Clonal analysis of progenitor cell commitment to granulocyte or macrophage production. J Cell Physiol 111: 275
2. Metcalf D, Merchav S (1982) Effects on GM-CSF deprivation on precursors of granulocytes and macrophages. J Cell Physiol 112: 411
3. Gasson JC, Weisbart RH, Kaufmann SE (1986) Purified human granulocyte-macrophage colony-stimulating factor: direct action on neutrophils. Science 226: 1339–1342
4. Gabrilove JL, Jakubowski A, Scher H, Sternberg C, Wong G, Grous J, Yagoda A, Fain K, Moore MAS, Clarkson B, Oettgen HF, Alton K, Welte K, Souza L (1988) Effect of granulocyte-colony-stimulating factor on neutropenia and associated morbidity due to chemotherapy for transitional-cell carcinoma of the urothelium. N Engl J Med 318: 1414–1422

5. Vadhan-Ray S, Buescher S, LeMaistre A, Keating M, Walters R, Ventura C, Hittelmann W, Broxmeyer HE, Gutterman JU (1988) Stimulation of hematopoiesis in patients with bone marrow failure and in patients with malignancy by recombinant human granulocyte-macrophage colony-stimulating factor. Blood 72: 134–141
6. Morstyn G, Campbell L, Souza LM, Alton NK, Keech J, Green M, Sheridan W, Metcalf D, Fox R (1988) Effect of granulocyte colony stimulating factor on neutropenia induced by cytotoxic chemotherapy. Lancet I: 667–672
7. Brandt SJ, Peters WP, Atwater SK, Kurtzberg J, Borowitz MJ, Jones RB, Shpall EJ, Bast RC, Gilbert CJ, Oette DH (1988) Effect of recombinant human granulocyte-macrophage colony-stimulating factor on hematopoietic reconstitution after high-dose chemotherapy and autologous bone marrow transplantation. N Engl J Med 318: 869–976
8. Weisbart RH, Gasson JC, Golde DW (1989) Colony-stimulating factors and host defense. Ann Intern Med 110: 297–303
9. Migliaccio G, Migliaccio AR, Adamson JW (1988) In vitro differentiation of human granulocyte/macrophage and erythroid progenitors: comparative analysis of the influence of recombinant human erythropoietin, G-CSF, GM-CSF, and IL-3 in serum-supplemented and serum-deprived cultures. Blood 72: 248–256
10. Broxmeyer HE, Cooper S, Williams DE, Hangoc G, Gutterman JU (1988) Growth characteristics of marrow hematopoietic progenitor/precursor cells from patients on a phase I clinical trial with purified recombinant human granulocyte-macrophage colony-stimulating factor. Exp Hematol 16: 594–602
11. Herrmann F, Schulz G, Lindemann A, Meyenburg W, Oster W, Krumwieh D, Mertelsmann R (1989) Hematopoietic responses in patients with advanced malignancy treated with recombinant human granulocyte-macrophage colony-stimulating factor. J Clin Oncol 7: 159–167

The Potential for the Use of Colony-Stimulating Factors in Autologous Bone Marrow Transplantation

W.P. Peters

Duke University Medical Center, Durham, NC 27710, USA

Introduction

Experimental and clinical evidence suggests that there is a steep dose–response effect for chemotherapy in the treatment of a variety of human malignancies [1]. In the leukemias and lymphomas, the use of dose intensification, including, if necessary, the use of bone marrow transplantation, has resulted in the development of curative approaches in even advanced malignancies [2]. In solid tumors, as well, increasing evidence exists for a dose–response effect in treatment results. Hyruniuk and his colleagues have demonstrated using retrospective analyses in both metastatic and primary disease that the average dose intensity planned or administered correlates with the objective response rate and with the disease-free survival [3, 4]. Similar results have been obtained for various treatment programs of ovarian cancer and Hodgkins' disease. Prospective randomized trials evaluating the effect of dose intensification are currently underway in several cooperative groups. Simultaneously with these efforts, other groups, including our own, have explored the use of high-dose combination chemotherapy in the treatment of resistant solid tumors, particularly breast cancer [5–8]. The use of autologous bone marrow support permits a 2- to 200-fold intensification of dose for individual agents over that attained with conventional doses. The limitation is that the high-dose treatment is associated with significant morbidity and mortality, and efforts to try to ameliorate this toxicity are required.

We have reported that in the autologous bone marrow transplant setting, the dominant cause of treatment-related morbidity and mortality is infection, with nearly 40% of patients dying of bacterial or fungal-related causes. Hemorrhage and organ system toxicity are secondary causes. In his classic work, Bodey demonstrated that both the severity and the duration of myelosuppression was critical in the development of infectious complications [9] and, thus, if one could either shorten the period of myelosuppression or reduce its severity, it should be possible to reduce the toxicity associated with bone marrow transplantation or other forms of intensive chemotherapy.

With the recent isolation, molecular cloning, *in vitro* expression and formulation of the colony-stimulation factors, the opportunity has arisen to determine whether these factors can reduce the period of myelosuppression associated with intensive chemotherapy and thereby reduce the toxicity of transplantation. The colony-stimulating factors are a series of glycoproteins which interact with specific receptors on hematopoietic progenitors and other cells. The factors will affect the survival, proliferation, and differentiation in the target cells. Factors have been named for the lineages which they predominantly, though not exclusively, affect. Hence, granulocyte colony-stimulating factor (G-CSF) produces primarily proliferation of granulocytic precursors from the promyelocyte onward. Macrophage colony-stimulating factor (M-CSF) affects predominantly monocytes and macrophages, activating their function, increasing their proliferation, and promoting their survival. Granulocyte–macrophage colony-stimulating factor (GM-CSF) affects both neutrophils and monocyte precursors, but has more diverse activities such as stimulation of burst-forming units and effects on megakaryocytes. Thus, there is no true lineage fidelity to the use of the colony-stimulating factors. Indeed, even the most specific CSFs, *in vitro*, can affect other lineages, depending on the dose at which they are administered. Hence, the overall effect of these compounds may be related not only to the specific agent that is employed, but also the relative dose which is utilized. GM-CSF, for instance, predominantly affects monocytes at low doses, whereas its effects at high doses are predominantly for the stimulation of myeloid progenitors.

The colony-stimulating factors do not in general act by themselves but, rather, work in concert with or in opposition to other CSFs that are present in circulation. GM-CSF, for instance, is a potent inducer of intracellular tumor necrosis factor (TNF) and interleukin 1 (IL-1) in monocytes, and, in the setting of a secondary event, pretreatment with GM-CSF can lead to an increase in the TNF released into circulation and associated subsequently with enhancement of toxicity (W.P. Peters and C. Dinarello, unpublished observations). The interactions between the multiplicity of colony-stimulating factors and the cascade effects induced by their utilization in patients are only beginning to be discovered, let alone understood.

GM-CSF and G-CSF: Effects in Bone Marrow Transplantation

Intensive chemoradiation therapy used in both autologous and allogeneic bone marrow transplantation procedures is associated with an extended period of panmyelosuppression. Generally between 14 and 21 days of severe panmyelosuppression is present following the high-dose chemotherapy and the infusion of autologous or allogeneic marrow. The period of myelosuppression is dependent upon the preparative regimen employed and the type of underlying disease being treated. Nonetheless, in all of these settings, it is during the period of panmyelosuppression that the greatest risk to the patient occurs. Infectious complications, both bacterial and fungal, are directly related to the duration and severity of the myelosuppression. Organ system toxicity manifested as renal, hepatic, or pulmonary dysfunction also appears related to the duration of severe myelosuppression. We have reported that the average organ system toxicity in the transplantation setting is related in a linear fashion to the length of myelosuppression following intensive chemotherapy. Hence, if the period of severe panmyelosuppression could be reduced, the toxicity of intensive from both therapy, infectious and other causes, may well be reduced. Several groups have now utilized the colony-stimulating factors as adjuncts in the bone marrow transplant setting [10–12]. It is not the intent of this review to detail these experiences but, rather, to summarize the concepts that have evolved from these early experiences.

Effects of GM-CSF

The first factor to be tested in the marrow transplant setting was GM-CSF, in which an acceleration of hematopoietic recovery was demonstrated in autografts for breast cancer and melanoma [13]. Hematopoietic reconstitution studied with GM-CSF has demonstrated that the period of *absolute leukopenia* following marrow infusion is not shortened by the use of GM-CSF compared to historical controls. Once cells begin to appear, there is an acceleration of the rate of hematopoietic recovery during the infusion of colony-stimulating factor. When administration of the CSF is discontinued, leukocyte and neutrophil counts fall to levels achieved without colony-stimulating factor, and hematopoiesis proceeds as in the historical controls. Consequently, with the use of the colony-stimulating factors, there has been a reduction in the frequency of documented bacterial infections and in the organ system toxicity associated with the use of chemotherapy. This pattern of hematologic recovery has been seen in several studies in which GM-CSF has been evaluated.

The use of GM-CSF has been evaluated in patients where marrow has been treated *ex vivo* with 4-hydroperoxycyclophosphamide. This marrow processing results in reduction of the number of CFU-GMs present in the marrow. In this setting, GM-CSF was not effective in enhancing hematopoietic recovery [14]. This is consistent with the premise that GM-CSF can only work on a committed progenitor and that the generation of this progenitor from the earlier precursors is required before the greatest efficacy of this compound is likely to be seen in settings where the number of infused progenitors is high, particularly in settings where mature myeloid progenitors can be utilized.

It is worthwhile to note that in the settings in which GM-CSF has been employed, the period of absolute leukopenia has not been shortened. This is consistent with the model that GM- and G-CSF work on mature, committed progenitors and that these progenitors are required before the full effect of this compound can be seen.

The effect on platelets has been variable from study to study. Several studies have reported improvement of platelets following the use of GM-CSF, and others reported no effect. Myalgias, fever, flu-like syndromes and fluid retention, often more severe at higher doses, have been reported with GM-CSF use.

Effects of G-CSF

Three groups have utilized G-CSF in the autologous bone marrow transplant setting [15–17]. Each group has reported acceleration of hematopoietic recovery. Again, a period of absolute myelósuppression which is not limited by the use of the compound. Infectious complications and organ system injury has been reduced. G-CSF has been well tolerated in the transplant setting, with few toxicities attributed to its use.

Progenitor Cells

Neither GM- nor G-CSF affects the period of absolute leukopenia following high-dose chemotherapy and autologous bone marrow transplants. Hence, alternatives attempting to modify this setting have been considered. The observation of a defined period of absolute leukopenia is consistent with a model in which hematopoietic stem cells must mature to a given point in differentiation before the mature acting CSFs can be efficacious. Hence, there is a minimal time period required for the "stem cells" to differentiate to the point of becoming committed progenitors; during this time, GM- or G-CSF is unlikely to have a major effect on hematopoietic reconstitution. Thus, to eliminate the period of absolute myelosuppression would require either supplying these progenitors, or altering the quality of the marrow harvested in such a way that committed progenitors were present in the marrow in sufficient numbers to be acted upon with these "early acting" CSFs.

One strategy for approaching this situation is to utilize collections of peripheral blood progenitor cells stimulated by colony-stimulating factor or after chemotherapy to enhance hematopoietic recovery when administered with additional CSF. These approaches have been prompted by four considerations: First, the recognition that GM- or G-CSF will enhance the number of peripheral blood progenitors in circulation; secondly, that there is a dose-dependent effect upon marrow progenitors in terms of a proliferative response to colony-stimulating factor; thirdly, that the mature progenitor is the cell most responsive to the effects of the colony-stimulating factor; and fourth, that progenitor cells, by themselves, would only modestly reduce the period of time of absolute myelosuppression, given that the survival of the progenitors is dependent upon the presence of exogenous CSF.

Gianni and his colleagues have demonstrated that the use of peripheral blood progenitors as collected after treatment with high-dose cyclophosphamide, if administered with GM-CSF, shortens the period of absolute myelosuppression and further was associated with a reduction in the number of platelet transfusions required by the patient [18].

Our group, utilizing both GM- and G-CSF, has demonstrated that using either GM- or G-CSF as the priming agent for collecting progenitor cells produces a marked increase in the number of progenitors circulating that can be collected by leukopheresis procedures [19]. Collection of these cells permits large numbers of progenitors to be readministered after high-dose chemotherapy. This has resulted in a reduction in the period of absolute leukopenia and an associated reduction in infectious complications and other organ system toxicity. Hepatic and renal toxicity have been reduced, and overall patient tolerance of intensive chemotherapy programs appear to be improved. Requirements for critical care are reduced. These types of observations have major implications for the application of intensive chemotherapy approaches to the treatment of solid tumors, in that the major limitation to date has been the development of infectious and organ system toxicities. The use of colony-stimulating factors to collect and utilize progenitor cells with bone marrow has been associated with a marked reduction of hematopoietic and nonhematopoietic toxicity.

Myelohematopoiesis Following Bone Marrow Transplantation

The observations with a variety of colony-stimulating factors that have been employed so far suggest that hematopoietic development occurs in a systematic manner following marrow transplantation, and that the understanding of these developmental pathways can provide certain heuristics which can be useful in the further application of the colony-stimulating factors. It appears from abundant clinical data at this point that GM- and G-CSF will act only on a relative mature, committed progenitor, and that unless this progenitor is present in sufficient numbers, GM- or G-CSF is unlikely to have a potent effect upon hematopoietic reconstitution. Consequently, it is unreasonable to expect in marrow ablative procedures that a period of absolute leukopenia will not be present when bone marrow is utilized alone, even with a maximal dose of a mature-acting CSF. The committed progenitor must be present in order for the mature-acting CSF to have effect.

Collection of these progenitors and their readministration with colony-stimulating factor has shortened the period of myelosuppression and offered a tool for further studying the role of the hematopoietic progenitor cells in hematopoietic reconstitution. The characteristics of the progenitor cells suggest that there is an augmentation, not only of the more mature committed progenitors, but perhaps also of an earlier progenitor type that is more closely related to a stem cell.

The use of IL-3 (multi-CSF) has the potential of further reducing the period of hematopoietic recovery. IL-3, from experimental data, appears to increase the number of progenitors capable of responding to GM- or G-CSF. It is probable that responses directly to administered IL-3 will take too long to be of much use if the IL-3 is applied in the post-transplant setting. Hence, if applied in the post-transplant setting, the sequential use of IL-3 followed by GM-CSF would unlikely be better than the use of GM-CSF alone. However, the ability of IL-3, particularly by itself, to prime the marrow offers the opportunity to enhance the quality of marrow prior to collection for use in this type of procedure. A marrow primed with IL-3 should have increased numbers of progenitor cells present that will be responsive to GM- or G-CSF.

This effect may be even more profound with IL-1. The stimulation and preparation of the marrow for subsequent responsiveness to mature-acting CSFs may be most appropriate. In addition, these compounds would be expected to increase the number of peripheral blood progenitors so that a strategy utilizing both progenitor cells and bone marrow could be envisioned with these compounds, as well. Colony-stimulating factors are completely altering the concept of how we approach myelosuppression associated with marrow transplantation, but it is unlikely that one can use these without the presence of either marrow or progenitor cells collected from the periphery. The successful application of these techniques should permit the further reduction of the toxicity associated with intensive chemotherapy programs and, as importantly, opened the door to future therapeutic efforts to improve the therapy of cancer by dose intensification.

References

1. Frei E, Canellos GC (1980) Dose: a critical factor in cancer therapy. Am J Med 69: 585–594
2. Thomas ED (1983) Marrow transplantation for malignant diseases (Karnofsky Memorial Lecture). J Clin Oncol 1: 517–531
3. Hryniuk W, Bush H (1984) The importance of dose intensity in chemotherapy of metastatic breast cancer. J Clin Oncol 2: 1281–1288
4. Hryniuk W, Levine MN (1986) Analysis of dose intensity for adjuvant chemotherapy trials in stage II breast cancer. J Clin Oncol 4: 1162–1170
5. Peters WP, Eder JP, Henner WD, Schryber S, Wilmore D, Finberg R, Schoenfeld D, Bast R, Antman K, Kruskall MS, Gargone B, Schnipper L, Frei E III (1986) High dose combination alkylating agents with autologous bone marrow support: a phase I trial J Clin Oncol 4: 646–654
6. Jones RB, Shpall EJ, Shogan J, Moore J, Gockerman J, Peters WP (1988) AFM induction chemotherapy followed by intensive consolidation with autologous bone marrow (ABM) support for advanced breast cancer. Proc Am Soc Clin Oncol 7: 8
7. Antman K, Eder JP, Schryber S, Andersen J, Peters WP, Henner WD, Finberg R, Elias AD, Shea T, Wilmore D, Kaplan W, Lew M et al. (1986) Fifty-eight solid tumor patients treated with a high dose combination alkylating agent preparative regimen with autologous bone marrow support: the DFCI/HIH experience. Proc Am Soc Clin Oncol 5: 154
8. Mulder NH, Sleijfer D, deVries EGE, Willemse PHB (1988) Intensive induction chemotherapy and intensification with autologous bone marrow reinfusion in patients with stage IIIB and IV breast bancer. Proc Am Soc Clin Oncol 7: 8
9. Williams S, Bitran J, Desser R, Golick J, Beschorner J, Fullem L, Golomb H (1988) A phase II study of induction chemotherapy followed by intensification with high

dose chemotherapy with autologous stem cell rescue (ASCR) in stage IV breast cancer. Proc Am Soc Clin Oncol 7: 9

10. Link H, Freund M, Kirchner H, Stoll M, Schmid H, Bucsky P, Seidel J, Schulz G, Schmidt RE, Riehm H et al. (1988) Recombinant human granulocyte-macrophage colony-stimulating factor (rh GM-CSF) after bone marrow transplantation. Behring Inst Mitt 83: 313–319

11. Applebaum FR, Nemunaitis J (1988) Recombinant human granulocyte macrophage colony stimulating factor (rhGM-CSF) following autologous marrow transplantation in man. Behring Inst Mitt 83: 145–148

12. Devereaux S, Linch DC, Gribben JG, McMillan A, Patterson K, Goldstone AH (1989) GM-CSF accelerates neutrophil recovery after autologous bone marrow transplantation for Hodgkin's disease. Bone Marrow Transplant, 4: 49–54

13. Brandt SJ, Peters WP, Atwater SK, Kurtzberg J, Borowitz MJ, Jones RB, Shpall EJ, Gilbert CJ, Bast RC Jr, Oette DH (1988) Effect of recombinant human granulocyte-macrophage colony-stimulating factor on hematopoietic reconstitution following high-dose chemotherapy and autologous bone marrow transplantation. N Engl J Med 318: 869–876

14. Blazar BR, Widmer MB, Kersey JH, Ramsay NK, McGlave PB, Urdal DL, Gillis S, Henney C, Vallera DA (1988) Recombinant granulocyte/macrophage-colony stimulating factor in human and murine bone marrow transplantation. Behring Inst Mitt 83: 170–180, 1988.

15. Peters WP, Kurtzberg J, Atwater S, Borowitz M, Gilbert C, Rao M, Currie M, Shogan J, Jones RB, Shpall EJ, Souza L (1988) Comparative effects of rHuG-CSF and rHuGM-CSF on hematopoietic reconstitution and granulocyte function following high dose chemotherapy and autologous bone marrow transplantation (ABMT). Blood 72: 130a

16. Sheridan WP, Morstyn G, Wolf M, Dodds A, Lusk J, Maher D, Layton JE, Green MD, Souza L, Fox RM (1989) Granulocyte colony-stimulating factor and neutrophil recovery after high-dose chemotherapy and autologous bone marrow transplantation. Lancet ii: 891–895

17. Taylor KM, Jagannath S, Spitzer G, Spinolo JA, Tucker SL, Fogel B, Cabanillas FF, Hagemeister FB, Souza LM (1989) Recombinant human granulocyte colony-stimulating factor hastens granulocyte recovery after high-dose chemotherapy and autologous bone marrow transplantation in Hodgkins' disease. J Clin Oncol 7: 1791–1799

18. Gianni AM, Siena S, Bregni M, Tarella C, Stern AC, Pileri A, Bonadonna G (1989) Granulocyte-macrophage colony-stimulating factor to harvest circulating haemopoietic stem cells for autotransplantation. Lancet ii: 580–585

19. Peters, WP, Kurtzberg J, Kirkpatrick G, Atwater S, Gilbert C, Borowitz M, Shpall E, Jones R, Ross M, Affronti M, Coniglio D, Mathias B, Oette D (1989) GM-CSF primed peripheral blood progenitor cells (PBPC) coupled with autologous bone marrow transplantation (ABMT) will eliminate absolute leukopenia following high dose chemotherapy (HDC). Blood 74: 50a

Surgical Experiences with 191 Implanted Venous Port-a-Cath Systems

U. Laffer, M. Dürig, H.R. Bloch, and J. Landmann

Department für Chirurgie, Kantonsspital, Spitalgasse 21,
4031 Basel, Switzerland

Introduction

Central venous access remains a problem in patients needing long-term intravenous therapy. Parenteral treatment with the common catheter systems proved to be possible for a short time only, being usually limited by catheter-induced sepsis, thrombosis, or perivascular problems.

At the beginning of the last decade the introduction of completely implantable catheter systems enabled safe and permanent access to the venous system in various medical specialities, but especially in the cytostatic treatment of tumors and in the management of tumor pain and of chronic infections. The use of these systems has increased steadily over the past few years, but unfortunately this increase has also been accompanied by a simultaneous increase of complications, mainly infections (Fuchs et al. 1987; Bothe et al. 1984; Smith and Flanigan 1987; Meurette et al. 1985; Kondi et al. 1988). Although the implantation of a catheter into the venous system does not appear highly demanding from the technical point of view, it should not be considered as one of the procedures which can be carried out quickly by the inexperienced surgeon. The complications caused by the catheter systems and described in the literature can be avoided if a carefully standardized implantation technique is followed and interdisciplinary aftercare of the system is started immediately after implantation.

Standard Implantation Technique

At the University Hospital of Basel we prefer a closed implantation technique employing puncture of the subclavian vein. All implantations are performed in the operating room under the usual antiseptic conditions. Except in already hospitalized patients, the operation is done as an outpatient procedure. The patient is placed on the operating table in a supine, head-down position

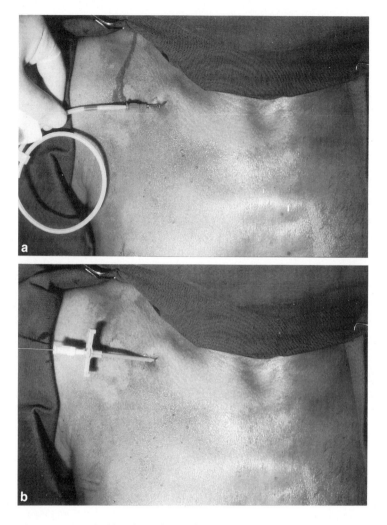

Fig. 1a–d. Surgical implantation technique. **a** Passing the straightened guidewire through the needle into the subclavian vein. **b** Introducing the 9 French sheath-introducer assembly into the vein. **c, d** see p. 191

with a towel placed along the thoracic spine. The supinated arm on the puncture side should be stretched parallel to the body, the head being turned to the opposite side. Under local anesthesia, starting with a small skin incision, the vein is percutaneously punctured. The puncture should be carried out along the medial third of the clavicle and the needle should be directed as near as possible to the bone; this in most cases avoids an accidental pneumothorax. However, placing the needle too near to the clavicle can lead to a compression of the introducer sheath later on, causing an obstruction which makes it difficult to pass the catheter.

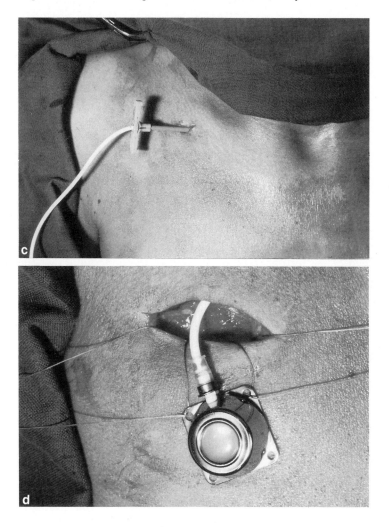

Fig. 1. c Advancing the catheter through the sheath. **d** Connecting the catheter with the portal and suturing two of the four portal corners

When the subclavian vein has been entered, the straightened guidewire is passed through the needle into the vein (Fig. 1a). Leaving the guidewire in place, the needle is withdrawn and a 9 French sheath-introducer assembly is twisted onto the guidewire. The subcutaneous tissue and vein opening are dilated. The assembly is advanced approximately halfway into the vein (Fig. 1b). Introducer and guidewire are then removed, leaving the sheath in place. Now the catheter is advanced through the sheath to the desired central position (Fig. 1c), the correct position being confirmed by the image intensifier. Holding this position, the sheath can be withdrawn. To avoid dislocation we suture the catheter at the vein entry side.

Next, the skin over the proposed portal pocket (the side depends upon the surgeon's and patient's preference) is infiltrated with local anesthetic. After suitable skin incision, the subcutaneous tissue is prepared by sharp or blunt dissection. The portal should lie approximately 0.5–1 cm below the skin surface; a portal placed too deeply may be difficult both to palpate and access, while a portal placed too superficially may cause undue skin irritation.

Using a surgical clamp, a subcutaneous tunnel is prepared from the portal pocket to the vein entry side and the catheter is drawn through this tunnel. The catheter is cut to the required length and then attached to the portal (Fig. 1d). The system is flushed with an antibiotic solution using Cefotiam 1 g in 10 ml NaCl; at the same time the system is tested to see whether blood sampling can be done easily. After this procedure the system is filled up with 5 ml heparinized saline at 50 units ml. The portal is positioned in the subcutaneous pocket and two of the four corners are sutured to the underlying tissue using permanent sutures.

After skin closure the system is ready for immediate use. Following implantation, an X-ray of the thorax is performed as a reference to ensure the catheter tip does not change position and to rule out the occurrence of a pneumothorax. In general, the patients have to stay less than 4 h in the hospital.

Patients and Procedure

From 1983 to 1990 a total of 286 fully implantable catheter systems were implanted (Fig. 2). A small number of intraperitoneal and arterial systems were implanted in the years from 1985 to 1988, both of them less frequently in the last couple of years. In the same period 191 patients received a venous catheter system. The age was 50.2 years on average, ranging from 9.7 years to almost 90 years. There were 126 female patients and 65 male patients.

The indication for permanent venous access was in 141 cases the administration of systemic chemotherapy. There were 36 patients who needed long-term parenteral antibiotic therapy; in 11 cases the system was used for blood sampling and long-term analgesic therapy, and in 3 cases it was used for parenteral nutrition when peripheral venous access was used up.

Among the cancer patients, who represent the main population for the introduction of a Port-a-Cath (Pharmacia Deltec, USA) breast cancer (Fig. 3) was the most common diagnosis, followed by gastrointestinal and ovarian cancer. A second large patient group was made up of those with sepsis and osteitis (Fig. 4) needing long-term parenteral antibiotic chemotherapy. They were followed by patients with malignant lymphoma. The requirements of a fourth heterogeneous group ranged from therapy with cytostatic agents for a carcinoid tumor to blood transfusion for aplastic anemia.

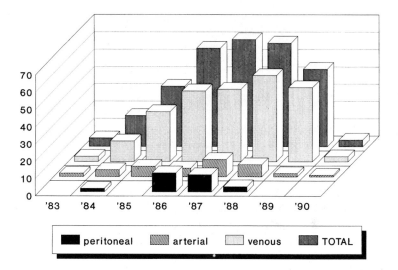

Fig. 2. Overview of the different types of catheter device implanted from 1983 to 1990 at the Department of Surgery, University Hospital, Basel

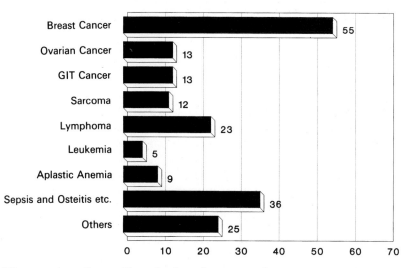

Fig. 3. Diagnoses in patients with an implanted venous catheter system

With few exceptions the venous catheters were implanted using the Seldinger technique. In most cases ($n = 181$) the subclavian vein (129 right and 62 left) was punctured. In 3 cases when puncture of the subclavian vein failed the external jugular vein was used. One hundred and seventy-eight patients were operated on under local anaesthesia and 13 patients under general anesthesia. The indication in one of these cases was an allergy to lidocaine; in the rest, the implantation of

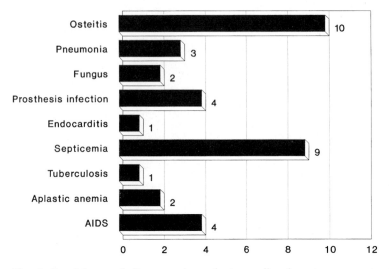

Fig. 4. Breakdown of diagnoses in patients needing long-term parenteral antibiotic chemotherapy

the catheter system was performed in the course of another operation demanding general anesthesia.

Results

In 182 patients the standard venous Port-a-Cath, and in 9 patients the newly developed peripheral access system (P.A.S. Port; Pharmacia Deltec, USA) was implanted.

The total indwelling time for the venous catheter systems amounts to 96 690 patient days (or 265 patient years); the system being in place for 517 patient days on average range from 8 days to almost 7 years. An average operation time of 33 min was needed for the surgical procedure. Today 108 venous systems are still in use, 22 have been removed for various reasons, and 51 patients have died.

In 179 patients (93.7%) implantations have been performed without any intraoperative problems. Complications during surgery occurred in 12 cases, in 9 of which the Port-a-Cath was inserted without any further problems by changing the site of vascular access. Technical problems related to the catheter system arose in 3 cases due to inappropriate handling of the apparatus. Only one (0.5%) pneumothorax occurred.

In the postoperative period a total of 17 (8.9%) complications occurred: 11 in patients using cytostatic agents and 6 in patients being treated with antibiotic agents (Table 1). Two catheters had to be removed, on days 172 and 174 after implantation respectively, because of a suspected superinfection, both times in patients treated with antibiotics; one of these was suffering from osteitis with

Table 1. Postoperative complications in 191 patients with an implanted venous catheter

No complications	174
Complications	17 (8.9%)
Infection	5 (2.6%)
positive culture (day 514, 43, 96)	3 (1.6%)
negative culture (day 172, 174)	2 (1.0%)
Catheter dislocation	6
Irreversible occlusion	1
Hematoma	1
Blood sampling impossible	2
Mechanical phlebitis (P.A.S.Port)	2

septic complications, the other from aplastic anemia. However, no pathogenic organisms were cultured from swabs from these patient subsequently.

In three other patients bacterial contamination was detected, the catheter systems being removed on day 514, 43, and 96 respectively. The first patient was a 60-year-old lady suffering from bowel occlusion due to metastatic gastric carcinoma; this patient needed long-term parenteral nutrition. One and a half years after implantation, she began to puncture the system herself. After only a short period of self-manipulation the infection occurred. The other two patients had a P.A.S.Port implanted; they were suffering from AIDS and osteosarcoma respectively. The AIDS patient too was using the system himself. After the systems were removed, the septicimia disappeared, and in two patients a new system could be implanted 2 weeks later.

One case of irreversible occlusion was observed, caused by thrombosis of the subclavian vein. The catheter dislocated six times, necessitating two reoperations. The remaining complications were divided into impossibility of blood sampling, hematoma in patient receiving anticoagulation therapy, and abacterial phlebitis in two patients with a peripheral access device. However, these complications should be related to the total indwelling time of all catheter systems: over a total of 96 690 patient days, for every 1000 days a device was in place, overall 0.18 complications and 0.03 infections occurred.

Discussion

From 1983 to 1990 we implanted 191 venous Port-a-Cath devices for a variety of diseases, mostly of an oncological or infectious origin. The advantages of a fully implantable catheter system are convincing. The most important is the low rate of complications compared to percutaneously implanted venous catheters; this can be attributed to the intact skin barrier. An infection rate of 30%–50% (Weeling et al. 1986; Landoy et al. 1984) is reported in the literature for percutaneous venous catheters and one of 20%–30% (Landoy et al. 1984; Pessa and Howard 1985; Ready et al. 1985) for the Hickman and Broviac catheters. Totally implantable devices show the significantly lower infection rate of 0%–10% (Laffer et al. 1989; Bloch et al. 1990; Fuchs et al. 1987; Bothe et al. 1984; Meurette et al. 1985; Kondi et al. 1988).

In our own patients, in 191 venous Port-a-Cath systems we saw three cases of bacterial superinfection. Two other systems had to be removed due to suspected infection, but no pathogenic organisms were found in the subsequent bacterial investigation. Most of the reported complications, such as dislocation or occlusion, were not related to the catheter system itself, but were attributable to an inadequate implantation technique or insufficient care.

Only an accumulation of practical experience in the implantation technique and conscientious nursing care can keep down the complication rate, as a comparison of our initial 22 implantations with the next 26 implantations has shown. With increased surgical skill and intensive nursing training, the complication rate could be reduced from 1.0 to 0.2 per 1000 patient days in the second observation period (Ludwig et al. 1988).

Summary

The introduction of totally implantable catheter device has provided a simple, permanent and safe access to the vascular system. They have greatly improved the quality of life of the patients involved, whose activities, daily hygiene and bodily attractiveness remain practically unrestricted.

To gain the greatest freedom from complications in the use of fully implantable catheter devices, the following requirements are important in to our experience:

1. Experience with only *one* kind of catheter system, irrespective of whether it is claimed to be the best, the simplest, or the cheapest. Various companies offer a variety of totally implantable catheter devices. Every system has its advantages and its disadvantages. However, each system also requires a considerable degree of surgical experience and experience in postoperative care and management to keep the complication rate as low as possible. Frequent changing to other systems does not enlarge the experience obtained.
2. The experience of the *surgical team*. In Basel catheter systems are implanted by three surgeons only. We are convinced that this contributes to our relatively low rate of complications. Brothers et al. (1988) also show that the rate of complications is inversely related to the experience of the surgeon involved.
3. The experience, commitment and training of the *nursing staff* responsible for the care and maintenance of the implanted catheter device. This care and

maintenance of the implanted catheter device should start immediately after the surgical procedure. In Basel the Port-a-Cath systems are the responsibility of two members of the nursing staff of the Oncology Department, who also continue to be responsible for the training of nurses and patients in the hospital, in the patient's home, and in the general practitioner's office.

If these requirements are fulfilled, we believe that fully implantable catheter systems will remain a valuable instrument not only for the nursing staff and physicians, but also for the patients.

References

Bloch HR, Laffer U, Dürig M, Landmann J (1990) Venöser Port-a-Cath. Chirurgische Erfahrungen mit 147 implantierten venösen Port-a-Cath-Systemen. In: Dürig M, Laffer U (eds) Tumorchirurgie und Lebensqualität. Karger, Basel, pp 123–128 (Basler Beiträge Chirurgie, vol 2)

Bothe A, Piccione W, Ambrosino J, Benotti P, Lokich J (1984) Implantable central venous access system. Am J Surg 147: 565–569

Brothers TE, von Moll L, Niederhuber J, Roberts J (1988) Experience with subcutaneous infusion ports in three hundred patients. Surg Gynecol Obstet 166: 295–301

Fuchs R, Leimer L, Koch G, Westerhausen M (1987) Klinische Erfahrungen mit bakteriell kontaminierten Port-a-Cath Systemen bei Tumorpatienten. Dtsch Med Wochenschr 112: 1615–1618

Kondi ES, Pietrafitta J, Barriola J (1988) Technique for placement of a totally implantable venous access device. J Clin Oncol 37: 272–277

Laffer U, Dürig M, Bloch HR, Zuber M, Stoll HR (1989) Implantierbare Kathetersysteme (Port-a-Cath): erste chirurgische Erfahrungen mit 205 implantierbaren Systemen. Dtsch Med Wochenschr 114: 655–658

Landoy Z, Rotstein C, Lucey J, Fitzpatrick J (1984) Hickman–Broviac catheter use in cancer patients. J Surg Oncol 26: 215–218

Ludwig R, Ludwig C, Laffer U, Stoll HR, Obrecht JP (1988) Vollständig implantierbares venöses Kathetersystem: vier Jahre Erfahrung bei onkologischen Patienten. Schweiz Med Wochenschr 118: 305–308

Meurette J, Depadt G, Meynadier J (1985) Vascular access. Eur J Surg Oncol 11: 295–298

Pessa ME, Howard R (1985) Complications of Hickman–Broviac catheters. Surg Gynecol Obstet 161: 257–260

Ready AR, Downing R, Fielding JWL, Temple J (1985) Venous access using the Hickman catheter. Eur J Surg Oncol 11: 155–157

Smith JL, Flanigan MJ (1987) Peritoneal dialysis catheter sepsis: a medical and surgical dilemma. Am J Surg 154: 602–607

Weeling RE, Hall JM, Meyer RL, Arbaugh JJ (1986) Implantable venous access devices: an alternative method of extended cancer care. J Surg Oncol 33: 73–75

Phase II Study of Intra-arterial Fluorouracil and Mitomycin-C for Liver Metastases of Colorectal Cancer

U. Metzger, W. Weder, M. Röthlin, and F. Largiadèr

Chirurgische Klinik, Triemli Spital, 8063 Zürich, Switzerland

Introduction

Hepatic metastases are present in approximately 20% of patients undergoing resection of primary colorectal cancer and subsequently occur in an additional 40% of patients, making the liver the most common site of metastatic disease. Survival of untreated patients with liver metastases ranges from a few months to approximately 2 years and is generally determined by the extent of hepatic disease at presentation (Wood et al. 1976). For patients with liver-only metastases, surgical resection offers the only possibility of cure, but it is not feasible in most patients because of the extent or location of disease. Conventional intravenous chemotherapy has generally produced responses in only 10%–20% of patients. Several recent phase II trials with systemic fluorouracil and folinic acid (leucovorin) have reported response rates ranging from 16% to 45% (Arbuck 1989).

With the introduction of fully implantable drug delivery systems in the early 1980s, the idea of administering chemotherapy into the hepatic artery to increase the drug concentration at the tumor site gained renewed interest (Niederhuber et al. 1984). Infusion of floxuridine into the hepatic artery resulted in response rates between 29% and 83% in metastatic colorectal cancer confined to the liver, with a median survival of 10–17 months. Randomized studies showed a significantly higher response rate to intrahepatic infusion than to systemic therapy, but this did not translate into a significant survival benefit, partly because of the crossover design in most of these trials (Chang et al. 1987; N. Kemeny et al. 1987; Hohn et al. 1989). The toxicity of intrahepatic floxuridine is dose-dependent but still considerable, with biliary sclerosis observed in up to 29% and drug-induced hepatitis in up to 80% of the patients; in more than half of the patients this led to termination of therapy because of drug toxicity rather than progression of the disease (Hohn et al. 1989). Toxicity and the high costs of fully implantable pumps prompted us to evaluate the effectiveness, toxicity, and feasibility of hepatic artery infusion of 5-fluorouracil (FU) and mitomycin-C (MMC)

Recent Results in Cancer Research, Vol. 121
© Springer-Verlag Berlin · Heidelberg 1991

administered by an external portable pump and a subcutaneous port system.

Patients and Method

Patients with measurable unresectable colorectal liver metastases without evidence of extrahepatic disease entered this study. Patients with far advanced disease (more than 75% of liver replaced by tumor), those unfit for laparotomy, and those who had previously undergone chemotherapy were excluded. Normal bone marrow and kidney function and the informed consent of the patient were required. Preoperative evaluation included blood, chemical and liver function tests, carcinoembryonic antigen (CEA) measurement, chest X-ray, colonoscopy, and a CT scan of the whole abdomen. The data for the 30 fully evaluable patients are given in Table 1. At laparotomy the abdominal cavity was carefully examined and patients with extrahepatic disease were excluded from the study. An intra-arterial hepatic catheter (Port-A-Cath, Pharmacia) was placed into the gastroduodenal artery with cholecystectomy and careful ligation of the right gastric and gastroduodenal arteries. The port was placed over the right lower chest wall. FU 2000–2500 mg in 100 ml normal saline with 5000 IU heparin was infused over 24 h on days 1–5 through an external portable pump (Deltec CADD, Pharmacia). MMC 10 mg/m^2 in 50 ml normal saline with 1000 IU heparin over a 2-h period was added at day 6 up to a maximum total dose of 60 mg. Treatment courses were repeated every 6 weeks until disease progression, severe side effects, or irreversible occlusion of the catheter occurred. The catheter was flushed with 5000 IU heparin every week, and a complete blood count, blood chemistry profile, CEA, and liver ultrasound scan were done before each treatment cycle. CT of the abdomen was performed every 6 months. All patients in this study had at least four consecutive cycles of chemotherapy and were evaluated after this period.

Table 1. Patient data ($n = 30$)

Age (years)	62.5 (42–75)
Sex (M/F)	23/7
Synchronous metastases	9
Metachronous metastases	21
≤25% Liver involvement	13
>25% Liver involvement	17
Pretreatment CEA level (ng/ml)	78 (2.5–2750)
ECOG performance status	
grade 0	12
grade 1	17
grade 2	1

Results

Of the 30 patients, 17 (57%) had a partial response and one had a complete disappearance of tumor signs on the CT scan, resulting in an overall response rate of 60% (95% confidence interval 40%–80%). In 8 patients (26%) the disease stabilized, and 4 patients (13%) were clear nonresponders to the intra-arterial chemotherapy. There was a more than 50% drop from the pretreatment CEA level in 22 patients (73%), although this was not considered an independent response criterion. The median time to progression in responding patients was 13 (5.8–20) months. Progression took place in the liver (54%), in the lung (16%), at the site of the primary tumor (12%) but also at such uncommon sites as the pericardium, the brain, the supraclavicular lymph nodes, and bone marrow.

The median overall survival from the start of intra-arterial chemotherapy was 18.2 (6.4–36.8) months; in the responding patients it was 25.5 months and in the nonresponders it was 15 months. The mean number of treatment courses was 9.2 (4–17) per patient. MMC was added to FU in 2.6 (2–5) courses per patient.

The treatment toxicity is shown in Table 2. The most important clinical side effect of chemotherapy was mucositis, with severe episodes in two patients leading to postponement of the subsequent therapy cycle for an additional 2–4 weeks. Nausea and vomiting were always controllable by the prophylactic oral administration of 4×10 mg domperidone (Motilium, Janssen) per day. Bone marrow toxicity was negligible and did not affect the planned chemotherapy dosage and schedule. Not a single case of chemical hepatitis or sclerosing cholangitis was observed in this series. Right upper quadrant abdominal pain was a precursor symptom of pending hepatic artery thrombosis and was an indication for emergency angiography.

Regarding technical problems, intra-arterial administration of urokinase and heparin succeeded in reversing catheter occlusion in eight instances. However, in six patients (20%) intra-arterial access occluded definitively after a median period of 12 months after the start of treatment. Catheter displacement (into the

Table 2. Treatment toxicity

	WHO grade	n	%
Nausea/vomiting	I	5	16
Mucositis	I+II	6	20
	III	2	7
Leukopenia	I+II	7	23
Thrombocytopenia	I	2	7
Abdominal pain	I+II	3	10

Table 3. Technical problems

	n	%
Catheter occlusion	6	20
Catheter displacement	1	3
Catheter rupture	1	3
Infection	2	7

duodenum), catheter rupture and two septic complications (pocket abscess, liver abscess) precluded another four patients from continuing intra-arterial chemotherapy (Table 3).

Discussion

This study was undertaken to evaluate the feasibility and effectiveness of intra-arterial FU and MMC chemotherapy directed against liver metastases of colorectal cancer. With one exception our patients were treated on a completely outpatient basis and were seen by the investigators every other day during chemotherapy courses for careful examination and monitoring of side effects and for refilling of the portable pump reservoir. With few exceptions, the side effects of treatment were mild and transient, only rarely impairing the quality of life or hindering the routine daily activities of the patients. No dose-limiting toxicity was observed with this regimen. The absence of any biliary toxicity is in sharp contrast to the floxuridine-containing regimens (N. Kemeny et al. 1984; Hohn et al. 1985; M. Kemeny et al. 1985; Haq et al. 1986). Continuous infusion of FU was shown to be efficient and safely administrable at a low dose over a prolonged period, with mucositis as the predominant side effect (Huan et al. 1989). In a nonrandomized comparison, of FU and floxuridine treatment, Rougier et al. (1989) found significantly different incidences of chemical hepatitis (2.3% of 42 FU-treated patients, 37.5% of 16 floxuridine-treated patients) and sclerosing cholangitis (0% vs. 25%). A possible solution to overcome floxuridine toxicity is to alternate hepatic intra-arterial administration of floxuridine and FU, as proposed by Stagg et al. (1988).

The major drawback of employing intra-arterial FU via an implantable port system are the technical, catheter-related problems which led to premature termination of treatment in one third of our patients. In a collective series comprising 647 patients, Hottenrott and Lorenz (1987) found a technical failure rate of 23% after 12 months. Catheter-related problems are minimized by the fully implantable pumps, most probably because of the permanent flow in the system.

Our response rate and survival data are comparable to those obtained in other phase II studies using floxuridine given via implantable pump systems (Table 4).

Table 4. Hepatic metastases of colorectal origin: results of intra-arterial therapy with floxuridine delivered by implantable pump

Authors	Year	Patients (n)	Reduction CEA by 30%	Objective tumor response (WHO)	Average survival (months)
Balch et al.	1983	81	88%	?	?
Weiss et al.	1983	17	71%	29%	13
Niederhuber et al.	1984	50	91%	83%	18
Kemeny N. et al.	1987	48	60%	50%	17
Shepard et al.	1985	40	—	20%	14
Johnson and Rivkin	1985	40	—	47%	13
Schwartz et al.	1985	22	74%	15%	10.5
Kemeny M.M. et al.	1986	31	—	52%	23
Rougier et al.	1989	16	88%	53%	18

The most important prognostic variable in patients with hepatic metastases from colorectal cancer is the percentage of tumor involvement of the liver, with a median survival of 24 months for patients with less than 30% liver involvement, vs. 10% if they had more than 30% involvement (N. Kemeny et al. 1989). Of our 30 patients, 17 had more than 25% liver involvement; the total median survival of 18.2 months is therefore not attributable to this patient selection factor. Patients in this series had had no previous systemic chemotherapy, which might have affected the response results, although it is well known that one third of patients with progressive disease receiving systemic chemotherapy will respond to intra-arterial treatment (N. Kemeny et. al. 1987; Hohn et al. 1989). The value of adding MMC to intra-arterial FU is yet unclear; it was done on the basis of an early report by Patt et al. (1980), who achieved a response rate of 83% with floxuridine and MMC. By limiting the maximum total dose to 60 mg MMC we observed no MMC-related side effects, in particular no hemolytic–uremic syndrome (Lesesne et al. 1989). Whether intra-arterial chemotherapy has a significant impact on the survival of patients with liver metastases is unknown. Compared to a "no treatment option" (Palmer et al. 1989) our patients did significantly better, with a median survival of 18.2 months (43% of patients with less than 25% liver involvement) vs. 12 months in Palmer's series (80% of patients with less than 25% liver involvement).

We conclude that intra-arterial 5-FU and MMC is a less toxic alternative to floxuridine in the treatment of metastatic colorectal cancer confined to the liver. Catheter-related technical problems are the most important treatment-limiting factors. The definitive impact on survival should be tested in proper phase III studies without a crossover design.

Summary

Effectiveness, toxicity and complications of 5-fluorouracil (FU) and mitomycin-C (MMC) treatment were analyzed in 30 patients with metastatic colorectal cancer confined to the liver. The treatment schedule was FU 2.0–2.5 g/day for 5 days followed by MMC 10 mg/m^2 every 2 h on day 6 to a maximum total dose of 60 mg. Treatment courses were repeated every 6 weeks and were given on an outpatient basis via external pump and arterial port systems. In 30 fully evaluable patients, one complete response, 17 partial responses (overall response rate 60%), and stabilization of disease in 8 patients (26%) were obtained for a median duration of 13 months. Median overall survival was 18.2 months (25.5 months for responding patients, 15 months for nonresponders). Grade 1–2 toxicity (WHO classification) consisted of leukopenia (23%), mucositis (20%), nausea/vomiting (16%), and abdominal pain (10%). Two patients (7%) developed severe mucositis. No life-threatening side effects were observed; in particular, there was no sclerosing cholangitis or chemical hepatitis. Catheter-related problems (occlusion, displacement, rupture, infection) occurred in 10 patients (33%) at a median follow-up time of 12 months.

We conclude that intra-arterial FU and MMC constitute an effective, safe, and nontoxic treatment in metastatic colorectal cancer confined to the liver. Catheter-related problems are the most important factors limiting treatment.

References

Arbuck SG (1989) Overview of clinical trials using 5-fluorouracil and leucovorin for the treatment of colorectal cancer. Cancer 63: 1036–1044

Balch CM, Urist MM, Soong SJ (1983) A prospective phase II clinical trial of continuous FUDR regional chemotherapy for colorectal metastases to the liver using a totally implantable drug infusion pump. Ann Surg 198: 567

Chang AE, Schneider PD, Sugarbaker PH, Simpson C, Culnane M, Steinberg SM (1987) A prospective randomized trial of regional versus systemic continuous 5-fluoro-deoxyuridine chemotherapy in the treatment of colorectal liver metastases. Ann Surg 206: 685–693

Haq MM, Valdes LG, Peterson DF, Gourley WK (1986) Fibrosis of extrahepatic biliary system after continuous hepatic artery infusion of floxuridine through an implantable pump (Infusaid pump). Cancer 57: 1281–1283

Hohn D, Melnick J, Stagg R, Altman D, Friedman M, Ignoffo R, Ferrell L, Lewis B (1985) Biliary sclerosis in patients receiving hepatic arterial infusions of floxuridine. J Clin Oncol 3: 98

Hohn DC, Stagg RJ, Friedman MA, Hannigan JF, Rayner A, Ignoffo RJ, Accord P, Lewis BJ (1989) A randomized trial of continuous intravenous versus hepatic intra-arterial floxuridine in patients with colorectal cancer metastatic to the liver: the Northern California Oncology Group Trial. J Clin Oncol 7: 1646–1654

Hottenrott C, Lorenz M (1987) Stellenwert der regionalen Chemotherapie der Leber. Z Gastroenterologie 25: 364–373

Huan S, Pazdur R, Singhakowinta A, Samal B, Vaitkevicius VK (1989) Low-dose continuous infusion 5-fluorouracil. Evaluation in advanced breast carcinoma. Cancer 63: 419–422

Johnson LP, Rivkin SE (1985) The implanted pump in metastatic colorectal cancer of the liver. Risk versus benefit. Am J Surg 149: 595

Kemeny MM, Battifora H, Blayney DW et al. (1985) Sclerosing cholangitis after continuous hepatic artery infusion of FUDR. Ann Surg 1202: 176–281

Kemeny MM, Goldberg D, Beatty D, Blaney D, Browning S, Soroshow J, Ganteame L, Hill RL, Kakal WA, Rihimaki DU, Terz JJ (1986) Results of a prospective randomized trial of continuous regional chemotherapy and hepatic resection as treatment of hepatic metastases from colorectal primaries. Cancer 57: 492

Kemeny N, Daly J, Oderman P, Shike M, Chun H, Petroni G, Geller N (1984) Hepatic artery pump infusion: toxicity and results in patients with metastatic colorectal carcinoma. J Clin Oncol 2: 595–600

Kemeny N, Daly JM, Reichmann B et al. (1987) Intrahepatic or systemic infusion of fluorodeoxyuridine in patients with liver metastases from colorectal carcinoma. Ann Intern Med 107: 459–465

Kemeny N, Niedzwiecki D, Shurgot B, Oderman P (1989) Prognostic variables in patients with hepatic metastases from colorectal cancer. Cancer 63: 742–747

Lesesne JB, Rothschild N, Erickson B, Korec S, Sisk R, Keller J, Arbus M, Woolley PV, Chiazze L, Schein PS, Neefe JR (1989) Cancer-associated hemolytic-uremic syndrome: analysis of 85 cases from a national registry. J Clin Oncol 7: 781–789

Niederhuber JE, Ensminger W, Gyves J, Thrall J, Walker S, Cozzi E (1984) Regional chemotherapy of colorectal cancer metastasis to the liver. Cancer 53: 1336

Palmer M, Petrelii NJ, Herrera L (1989) No treatment option for liver metastases from colorectal adeno-carcinoma. Dis Col Rect 32: 698–701 (1989)

Patt Y, Mavligit G, Chuang V et al. (1980) Percutaneous hepatic arterial infusion (HAI) of mitomycin C and floxuridine: an effective treatment for metastatic colorectal carcinoma in the liver. Cancer 46: 261–265

Rougier P, Lasser P, Elias D, Ghosn M, Ducreux M, Lumbroso J, Sidibe S, Droz JP (1989) Intra-arterial hepatic chemotherapy for metastatic liver from colo-rectal carcinoma origin. Select Cancer Ther 5: 47–54 (1989)

Schwartz SI, Jones LS, McCune CS (1985) Assessment of treatment of intrahepatic malignancies using chemotherapy via an implantable pump. Ann Surg 201: 560

Shepard KV, Levin BJ, Karl RC, Faintuch J, Dubrow RA, Hagle M, Cooper RM, Beschorner J, Stablein D (1985) Therapy for metastatic colorectal cancer with hepatic artery infusion chemotherapy using a subcutaneous implanting pump. J Clin Oncol 3: 161

Stagg RJ, Lewis BJ, Chase J et al. (1988) Alternating hepatic intra-arterial (IA) floxuridine (FUDR) and IA 5-fluorouracil (5-FU) for colorectal cancer metastatic to the liver: a rational approach to prolong the benefit of IA fluoropyrimidine therapy by minimizing biliary and systemic toxicity. Proc Am Soc Clin Oncol 7: 99

Weiss GR, Garnick MB, Ostreen RT (1983) Long-term hepatic arterial infusion of 5-fluorodeoxyuridine for liver metastases using an implantable infusion pump. J Clin Oncol 1: 337 (1983)

Wood CB, Gillis CR, Blumgart LH (1976) A retrospective study of the natural history of patients with liver metastases from colorectal cancer. Clin Oncol 2: 285–288 (1976)

Maintenance and Care of Patients with Drug Delivery Systems

N. Nadau

Santé Service, 15 Quai Dedion Bouton, 92800 Puteaux, France

First of all, to introduce myself: I have the privilege to represent 200 nurses who provide chemotherapy for more than 400 cancer patients a day and, more importantly, provide global supportive or palliative care for more than 600 cancer patients a day, involving pain management, nutritional and psychological support.

In this paper I would like to discuss the maintenance and care of the cancer patient with a drug delivery system at home. I will begin with a short description of Santé Service and then go on to discuss maintenance of a cancer patient with a drug delivery system from the specific viewpoint of home care, with special reference to a chamber port (Port-A-Cath).

Santé Service

Santé Service is a nonprofit association, affiliated with all the cancer centers in Paris and the Federation of nonprofit institutions, which represent 130 000 hospital beds in France, and finally, Santé Service works in conjunction with the Home Care Service of the Paris Medical University System.

Santé Service was created in 1958 and for the last 24 years has been directed by Mrs A.M. Candotti. Our primary objective is to provide a comprehensive home care program involving a multidisciplinary staff including nurses, nurse's aides, special ancillary staff, dieticians, occupational therapists, physical therapists, a quality care department, and a research department.

We are the largest home care service in France, and 80% of our patients are cancer patients. Santé Service aims to maintain optimal coordination with the referring hospital. Patients are therefore seen at the hospital by our own staff, working with the hospital staff. A home care program is intended to ensure the best possible specific and complementary care, not to compete with the hospital.

We only admit a patient to our program if the following requirements are met: the patient and his hospital physician must agree to the admission, there must be a satisfactory home environment, and an appropriate health insurance agreement must exist.

Maintaining a Patient with a Drug Delivery System at Home

Home care patients are not like hospital patients, and insufficient clinical observation may lead to major complications.

The preservation of the vascular capital of a cancer patient is perhaps one of the most essential tasks of cancer nursing. Once the patient has lost all vascular access, it is impossible to provide valuable chemotherapy or supportive drug therapy; the intravenous routes, whether natural (vein), catheter, or implantable chambers, must therefore be regarded as a major responsibility of the cancer nurse, followed by meticulous catheter care and management of chamber ports.

Nurses must also know how to use chemotherapy pumps. It is not acceptable for a nurse, particularly a home care nurse, not to know how to resolve all problems arising from this apparatus. Nurses can represent a key confidence figure to the patient and his family if they are knowledgable about the pump and catheter system used in chemotherapy. Today more than 50% of ambulatory chemotherapy at Santé Service is administered via pumps.

The development of catheters and implantable chambers does not allow the nurse to be less informed or less professional in intravenous perfusion. Santé Service provides special courses integrating medical nursing and industrial recommendations concerning apparatus and techniques in modern chemotherapy.

Santé Service covers the Paris region (a radius of about 50 km around Paris) through four satellite sectors. Each satellite assures home care for a section of the Paris region and is connected to the central office and the various in-hospital Santé Service offices. Each satellite has a complete multidisciplinary staff. The service is provided 24 h a day, every day.

The administration of cancer chemotherapy in a home care setting is a serious and complex nursing responsibility in which the nurse is alone with her patient. This condition is unique and probably the major difference between hospital cancer nursing and home care cancer nursing.

Santé Service employs only experienced nurses (at least 2 years' experience), who then undergo a special training program offered by Santé Service. This program is further complemented by continuous educational courses in coordination with a medical research department at Santé Service, a quality care department at Santé Service, and, most importantly, a particular nursing structure that allows nurses to work in teams in terms of their practical daily program and with weekly meetings. Nurses ensure supportive care to their patients, but they cannot and should not try to assume the total responsibility of that supportive care; they must seek help from all the medical and paramedical team. Burnout is a true problem in cancer nursing and requires supportive care training for the nurses. Santé Service has a voluntary program for nurses who want to attend.

The Chamber Port

Any injection through the port has to be done with a very strict sterile technique. The nurse must be familiar with the appropriate preventive techniques and the instruments. It is fundamental that she prepares the equipment before she begins. She uses a special kind of needle; she must be sure that it is in the chamber: there is a little resistance as she starts to push the needle, then she can feel a little metallic shock against the chamber. She will never leave the system open. Before any injection, she should inspect the skin carefully all around, looking for redness, ulceration, or infection, and palpating to see if the chamber is still in place.

The nurse will ask her patient to take his temperature at least once a day and she will report any changes. If all the conditions are not met, the nurse will *not perform the injection*. Any vascular leakage should be reported as soon as possible to the physician. *No* chemotherapy prescription should be administered without the appropriate antidote for extravasation leakage having been prepared first.

Flushing with heparin is done every 2, 3, 4 or 6 weeks, depending on the physician. The nurse must check that the prescription is written and signed by the physician and includes the name of the patient and the proper dosage of the heparin solution.

All this implies a good working relationship between the nurse and the physician. Records must be kept to aid the best medical decision. Santé Service keep its own medical and paramedical records. Nurses' observations are the key in all situations.

Conclusion

I would like to stress our role in the education of our nurses, using new drugs and new instruments for cancer patients. Home care nurses should work in constant cooperation with the hospital teams in order to provide successful management of the home care cancer patient.

Implantable Devices in Patients with Haematological Diseases

L. Schmid and A. Feldges

Medizinische Klinik C, Kantonsspital, 9007 St. Gallen, Switzerland

Introduction

The surgical implantation of catheters connected to subcutaneous reservoirs into a central vein in patients with malignant tumours has become a routine procedure in recent years [1–6]. In the past, many different methods of vascular access have been evaluated in patients suffering from acute leukaemia or other bone marrow-infiltrating malignancies. A number of specific problems exist, arising mainly from prolonged phases of bone marrow aplasia, such as catheter-induced bacteraemia or fungaemia, and insufficient flow capacity for simultaneous treatment with cytostatic drugs, antibiotics, blood transfusions and parenteral nutrition.

We therefore present the data of two controlled open studies evaluating the venuous Port-A-Cath system in patients receiving intensive chemotherapy for different haematological neoplasias. One study was conducted in children (Children's Hospital of St. Gallen), the other in adults (Kantonsspital of St. Gallen) [11].

Patients and Method

We analyzed the results after catheter implantation in 90 patients (50 children with a mean age of 8 years and 40 adults with a mean age of 38 years; overall age range 0.3–70 years). Forty percent of the children and 79% of the adults suffered from a haematological neoplasia (Table 1). Although the proportion is significantly higher in the adult group, it must be remembered that most of the children were being treated on intensive chemotherapy protocols irrespective of their diagnosis.

At the time of implantation, 5% of the adults and 8% of the children had fever. In 31% of the adults the granulocyte count was below $1.0 \times 10^9/l$ (Table 2). Only eight of the 40 children had a leucocyte count below $2.0 \times 10^9/l$ at

Table 1. Patients' diagnoses

	Children		Adults		All	
	n	(%)	n	(%)	n	(%)
Acute myelogenous leukaemia	2	(4)	12	(31)	14	(16)
Acute lymphoblastic/ undifferentiated leukaemia	14	(28)	11	(29)	25	(28)
Non-Hodgkin lymphoma	1	(2)	8	(19)	9	(10)
Hodgkin's lymphoma	3	(6)	3	(7)	6	(7)
Others	30	(60)	6	(14)	36	(40)
All	50	(100)	40	(100)	90	(100)

Table 2. Granulocyte count ($\times 10^9$/l) at time of implantation

	Children		Adults		All	
	n	(%)	n	(%)	n	(%)
Granulocyte count[a]						
<0.5	n.d.	n.d.	8	(19)	—	—
0.5–1.0	n.d.	n.d.	5	(12)	—	—
>1.0	n.d.	n.d.	29	(69)	—	—
Fever present	4	(8)	2	(5)	6	(7)
No fever	46	(92)	40	(95)	86	(93)
Antibiotics given	10	(20)	7	(17)	17	(18)
No antibiotics given	40	(80)	35	(83)	75	(82)

[a] Children's group: leucocyte count <1.0, 3 patients; 1.0–1.9, 5 patients.

Table 3. Platelet count ($\times 10^9$/l) at time of implantation

	Children		Adults		All	
	n	(%)	n	(%)	n	(%)
Platelet count						
<30	0		1	(2)	1	(1)
30–49	2	(4)	2	(5)	4	(4)
50–99	8	(16)	3	(7)	11	(12)
>99	40	(80)	36	(86)	76	(83)
All	50	(100)	42	(100)	92	(100)

the time of catheter implantation, and only two children and three adults had a platelet count below $50 \times 10^9/l$ (Table 3).

The surgical techniques used to implant the Port-A-Cath have been described elsewhere [3].

Results

Use of the Port-A-Cath

The mean time for which all 92 catheter systems in both groups were in place was 420 days (range 11–1512 days). In the children's group (mean 594 days, range 12–1512 days) the catheters remained in use significantly longer than in the adults (mean 212 days, range 11–563 days). However, some adult patients with leukaemia have now had their Port-A-Cath in place for more than 5 years.

To show that the Port-A-Caths were very intensively used, I will give three examples. The first is the use of antibiotics: more than 5100 infusions of antibiotics were administered through the 92 systems. Since most of the patients were severely immunocompromised, these were mainly combinations of β-lactams such as penicillins (974 short infusions) or cephalosporins (1352 infusions), combined with aminoglycosides (1955 infusions) or – more rarely – other types of antibiotics (887 infusions).

The second example is blood transfusions: 1020 units of blood were transfused. All types of blood products were given – erythrocyte concentrates (480) and platelet-rich plasma (114) – and 356 single-donor aphereses were carried out. The rate of transfusions was higher in the adult than in the children's group. All transfusions were performed without mechanical aids such as infusion pumps.

The third example is a critical point in the use of implantable devices: the possibility of blood sampling out of the port. In the adult group 1627 blood samples were taken out of the 42 implanted catheters. On about 8700 days out of the 8900 days of cumulative use in the adult group, blood samples could be taken. Over the whole observation time, on average 38 blood samples per Port-A-Cath were analysed. There are no data available for the children's group.

Complications

To judge whether the Port-A-Cath can be used routinely in patients with bone marrow insufficiency, one must look closely at the type and the incidence of complications that occur.

We divided all the unexpected events into "minor problems" and "true complications." In the adult patient group there were 13 minor events: four reversible blockages and nine needle displacements. The blockages were reversible after administration of streptokinase. No extravasation occurred during the displacements of the needle out of the port. No reversible blockage or needle displacement was documented in the children's group.

As to "true" complications, four venous thromboses occurred, one in the children's group and three in the adults' (Table 4). The seven cases of mechanical dysfunction involved two irreversible blockages, two catheter ruptures, one disconnection between the catheter and the port, and two cases of looping of the catheter.

The most striking complication in immunocompromised patients is infection. Five cases of local port infection led to explantation of the infusion system. The rate of true catheter infection cannot be exactly determined, because the Port-A-Cath was generally not explanted in cases of fever. In most cases aggressive antibiotic treatment including vancomycin was effective in controlling the systemic bacterial infection.

Tables 5 and 6 show the types of bacteria that were isolated from the blood of patients with an implanted Port-A-Cath during febrile neutropenia; as can be seen, bacterial isolates predominated over gram-negative at a rate of 26 to 11.

Table 4. "True" complications

	Children		Adults		All	
	n	(%)	n	(%)	n	(%)
Venous thrombosis	1	(11)	3	(25)	4	(19)
Mechanical dysfunction	2	(22)	5	(42)	7	(33)
Local infection	1	(11)	4	(33)	5	(24)
Catheter-related infection	5	(56)	0	(0)	5	(24)
All	9	(100)	12	(100)	21	(100)

Table 5. Types of gram-positive bacteria isolated

	Children		Adults		All	
	n	(%)	n	(%)	n	(%)
Staphylococcus epidermidis	13	(81)	5	(50)	18	(69)
Staph. capitis	0		1	(10)	1	(4)
Staph. aureus	0		1	(10)	1	(4)
α-Haemolytic streptococci	0		1	(10)	1	(4)
Viridans streptococci	3	(19)	1	(10)	4	(15)
Streptococcus pneumoniae	0		1	(10)	1	(4)
All	16	(100)	10	(100)	26	(100)

Table 6. Types of gram-positive bacteria isolated

	Children		Adults		All	
	n	(%)	n	(%)	n	(%)
Escherichia coli	2	(33)	3	(60)	5	(45)
Propionibacterium acnes	1	(17)	2	(40)	3	(27)
Corynebacterium	1	(17)	0		1	(9)
Fusobacterium	1	(17)	0		1	(9)
Bacillus cereus	1	(17)	0		1	(9)
All	6	(100)	5	(100)	11	(100)

Table 7. Incidence of complications

	Children ($n = 50$)	Adults ($n = 42$)	All ($n = 92$)
Cumulative time of use (patient days)	29 700	8 883	38 583
No. of complications per 1000 patient days	0.3	1.4	0.5

There was no difference between the results for children and adults. This fact has to be taken into account in the planning of antibiotic treatment in these patients.

The incidence of complications can be estimated as follows: if we consider only "true" complications, there were 1.4 complications per 1000 days of Port-A-Cath access in adults (Table 7). In the children's group the incidence was about 0.3 per 1000 days, a very low figure compared to those published in other studies [11].

Discussion

In cancer patients, access to peripheral or central veins is often a problem. Without prolonged, reliable and repeated vascular access, aggressive chemotherapy and intensive supportive care of malignant tumours are impossible.

The methods tried in the past all have some disadvantages. Bovine heterograft and arteriovenous fistulae showed a relatively high incidence of occlusion [12]. More commonly used were different types of silicone elastomer catheters, which were percutaneously introduced into central veins [8, 9]. Hickmann type catheters have also been intensively evaluated in the treatment of acute leukaemia [7, 13]. A number of studies have shown that the main problem of this method of venous access seems to be catheter-related infection.

More recently, different types of fully implantable systems have been used, especially in the treatment of solid tumours [1–6]. We have reviewed ten papers reporting on a total of 476 patients; the cumulative duration of use of all implanted systems was almost exactly 12 000 weeks [11]. The overall incidence of complications per 1000 days of access varied from 0.73 to 2.81.

Local infection of the port was the most common complication observed. In our experience, the rate of local infection is mainly dependent on the skill of the nurses and doctors using the implanted catheter. In most cases of local infection in our series in which the port had to be removed, there had been serious nonsterile manipulation of the apparatus by insufficiently instructed persons.

Venous thrombosis was the second most frequent complication observed. A detailed analysis of this type of complication has been presented elsewhere [11].

All the other types of complications were only occasionally observed [11]. Special attention must be paid to prevent extravasation of drugs or fluids [14].

One of the most crucial problems in the treatment of patients with prolonged bone marrow aplasia is the rate of *systemic infection* caused by indwelling venous catheters. There are different reports in the literature for bacteraemia, ranging from 4% to 25% [15–17]. Using percutaneous catheters, it is possible in our experience to reduce the infection rate to less than 10%. Our data suggest that there are no major differences in this respect between children and adults.

In cases of fever not related to blood transfusions or drugs, antibiotic therapy with a combination of a β-lactam plus an aminoglycoside was started immediately in our patients. If there was insufficient response after 3 days, or if there was a blood culture with gram-positive cocci, vancomycin was added. In our study, antibiotic therapy without removal of the implanted device effectively controlled systemic bacterial infection.

The high proportion of gram-positive cocci in our study has also been reported in patients with other types of catheters [18, 19]. There may be other causes for the increasing predominance of gram-positive cocci, e.g. changing strategies in the antibiotic treatment of granulocytopenic patients.

Conclusions

From the data presented here we conclude that implantable venous drug delivery devices such as the Port-A-Cath can be safely used in patients under intensive treatment for haematological diseases. There are no major differences in this respect between children and adults. The complication rate remains acceptably low, as long as manipulation of the implanted systems is restricted to skilled nurses and doctors.

References

1. Rothe A Jr, Piccione W, Ambrosino JJ, Benotti PN, Lokich JJ (1984) Implantable central venous access system. Am J Surg 147: 565–569

2. Gyves JW, Ensminger WD, Niederhuber JE, Dent T, Walker S, Gilbertson S, Cozzi E, Saran P (1984) A totally implantable injection port system for blood sampling and chemotherapy administration. JAMA 251: 2538–2541

3. Kessler W, Schmid L, Hoffmann R, Amgwerd R, Wicky B (1985) Erleichterung der Langzeit-Chemotherapie durch ein vollständig implantierbares Kathetersystem. Helv Chir Acta 52: 253–257

4. Starkhammer H, Bengtsson M (1985) Totally implanted device for venous access. Acta Rad 24: 173–176

5. Brincker H, Saeter G (1986) Fifty-five patient years' experience with a totally implanted system for intravenous chemotherapy. Cancer 57: 1124–1129

6. Lorenz M, Hottenrott C, Seufert RM, Kirkowa-Reimann M, Encke A (1986) Dauerhafter intravenöser oder intraarterieller Zugang mit einer subkutan liegenden implantierbaren Infusionskammer. Dtsch Med Wochenschr 111: 772–779

7. Hickmann RO, Buckner CD, Clift RA, Sanders JE, Stewart P, Thomas ED (1979) A modified right atrial catheter for access to the venous system in marrow transplant recipients. Surg Gynecol Obstet 148: 871–875

8. Blacklock HA, Pillai MV, Hill RS, Matthews J RD, Clark AG, Wade JF (1980) Use of modified subcutaneous right-atrial catheters for venous access in leukaemic patients. Lancet I: 993–994

9. Abraham JL, Mullen JL (1982) A prospective study of prolonged central venous access in leukemia. JAMA 248: 2868–2873

10. Reilly JJ, Steed DL, Ritter PS (1984) Indwelling venous access catheters in patients with acute leukemia. Cancer 53: 219–223

11. Schmid L, Walser K, Kessler W, Senn HJ (1990) Use of a fully implantable drug delivery system in the treatment of acute leukemias and disseminated lymphomas. Oncology (in press)

12. Wade JC, Newman KA, Schimpff SC, Van Echo DA, Gelber RA, Reed WP, Wiernick PH (1981) Two methods for improved venous access in acute leukemia patients. JAMA 246: 140–144

13. Reed WP, Newman KA, De Jongh C, Wade JC, Schimpff SC, Wiernick PH, McLaughlin JS (1983) Prolonged venous access for chemotherapy by means of the Hickman catheter. Cancer 52: 185–192

14. Lockich J, Moore C (1986) Drug extravasation in cancer chemotherapy. Ann Intern Med 104: 124

15. Tomford JW, Hershey CO, Mclaven ChE, Proter DK, Cohen DI (1984) Intravenous therapy and peripheral venous catheter-associated complications. A prospective controlled study. Arch Intern Med 44: 1191–1194

16. Wagman LD, Kirkemo A, Johnson MR (1984) Venous access: a prospective randomised study of the Hickman catheter. Surgery 95: 303–308

17. Cairo MS, Spooner S, Sowden L, Bennetts GA, Towne B, Hodder F (1986) Long-term use of indwelling multipurpose silastic catheters in pediatric cancer patients treated with aggressive chemotherapy. J Clin Oncol 4: 784–788

18. Wade JC, Schimpff SC, Nervman KA, Wiernick PH (1982) *Staphylococcus epidermidis*: an increasing cause of infection in patients with granulocytopenia. Ann Intern Med 97: 503–508

19. Davies AJ (1985) Coagulase negative staphylococcal infections. Br Med J 290: 1230–1231

Home Intravenous Antibiotic Therapy: New Technologies

D.N. Williams

Department of Medicine, Section of Infectious Disease, Methodist Hospital and Park Nicollet Medical Center, 5000 West 39th Street, Minneapolis, MN 55416, USA

Introduction

Over the past 15 years, an increasing variety of intravenous (IV) therapies have been administered to patients both at home and in the outpatient setting. Intravenous anti-infective and chemotherapeutic agents, analgesics, blood product and coagulation factor replacement, immunoglobulins, and even positive inotropic drugs [12] have been safely and effectively administered at home. All of these therapeutic modalities share a number of characteristics including the need for an integrated team approach (physicians, pharmacists, and nurses), careful inclusion and exclusion criteria, a structured follow up process, and increased responsibility on the patient's part for self-care. [17] In the United States, the increased interest in, and availability of, structured home care infusion services (both hospital- and home-based), new venous access devices, the increased emphasis on the economic aspects of health care provision, and the development of a variety of new infusion technologies, have enabled more patients to be appropriately and conveniently treated with home or outpatient IV antibiotics. In most instances, either the patient or someone in the home (parent, spouse, or other support person) administers the IV drug. In Europe, potential barriers to the implementation of home IV antibiotic services include such issues as who may legally administer IV drugs, the availability of trained staff, and financial reimbursement for such services. Structural and legal issues may differ between countries.

The main focus of this paper is a new development in the delivery of home IV antibiotics, namely the utility of new infusion devices. Our experience [18] with one such device (a computerized ambulatory drug delivery pump) is emphasized. It may be that these infusion devices will have a special niche in Europe, as they may satisfy regulatory and other concerns regarding self-administration of IV antibiotics.

Recent Results in Cancer Research, Vol. 121
© Springer-Verlag Berlin · Heidelberg 1991

Development of Outpatient or Home IV Antibiotic Therapy

In the United States, home IV antibiotic programs were initially developed by physicians in suburban community teaching hospitals [1, 9, 10, 13–16]. These early studies showed that home IV antibiotic therapy was safe, effective, and economical. Over the past decade, many models of home IV antibiotic therapy have emerged, with local variations. In Europe, Winter et al. [19], at the London Chest Hospital, and Baumgartner and Glauser [3], at Lausanne, Switzerland, have clearly demonstrated the utility of such approaches.

At Methodist Hospital, Minneapolis, USA, we have developed a hospital-based program with an emphasis on patients returning whenever possible to the outpatient area to be clinically evaluated, have their IV cannula site inspected, and pick up additional supplies of antibiotics. By way of contrast, all of the infusion companies (which now deliver most of the home IV antibiotic therapy in the United States) visit patients in their own homes. Methodist Hospital's home IV antibiotic therapy was initiated in 1974. To date, we have treated approximately 1000 patients with an average duration of home IV antibiotic treatment of 14 days, gaining a total experience of more than 14000 days of home IV therapy. Most of our initial experience [9, 10] with home IV antibiotics was dominated by the treatment of skin and soft tissue infections, septic arthritis, and osteomyelitis. During the 1980s, a much greater variety of infections were treated, including the infectious complications of both the Acquired Immune Deficiency Syndrome (AIDS) and various malignancies. During this same era, we saw the advent and use of the third-generation cephalosporins, with a concomitant reduction in the use of penicillins, particularly the antistaphylococcal penicillins.

The availability of an IV nurse team to manage venous access issues has enabled us to continue to favor the use of peripheral IV cannulae (in 84% of patients treated) for routine home IV antibiotic therapy. However, many of our oncology patients already have central lines in place, making this the obvious route for such therapy. As a result of careful patient selection criteria, education, and follow up, the home IV antibiotic program has been marked by low incidence both of drug and venous access complications and of hospital readmissions (less than 5%).

Recent Developments in Home (Outpatient) IV Antibiotic Therapy

Until relatively recently the "typical" patient discharged from hospital to home would self-administer the prescribed IV antibiotic by a gravity infusion method (usually using "minibags"). Depending on the antibiotic and the type of infection, this might mean drug administration from once to six times a day. For some patients, issues such as the frequency of drug administration or impaired manual dexterity or cognitive function impeded their ability to successfully self-administer IV antibiotics. The advent of new technologies has enabled patients hitherto considered ineligible for home IV antibiotic therapy to be successfully treated at home.

New Infusion Devices

The devices currently available for home IV antibiotic therapy range from elastomeric infusion devices (which are used for one-time administration) through to multi-channel, programmable, portable, syringe systems. Our experience has been primarily with computerized ambulatory drug delivery pumps (CADD-VT and CADD-PLUS; Pharmacia Deltec). Various criteria can be used to classify the infusion devices [11]. While some devices are designed to deliver large fluid volumes or multiple solutions at independent rates, the focus of this presentation will be on those devices designed for intermittent IV antibiotic administration in the home. It should be noted, however, that there has been a relative dearth of specific information on the utility of infusion devices in home IV antibiotic therapy [5, 6, 7, 18]; most of the currently available literature deals with devices for chronic pain control [8] and chemotherapy [4].

Elastomeric Infusion Devices

The simplest devices for home IV therapy employ an elastomeric design such that positive pressure is generated when the drug is infused into the bottle. There are now several devices in this category. The Intermate 100 and 200 (Baxter) are intended for antibiotic therapy. They both have a volume capacity of 105 ml and deliver the antibiotic solution at rates of 100 or 200 ml h, respectively. The "infuser" obviates the need for gravity infusion. The device is simple, has the advantage of reducing the time necessary for patient education, and circumvents problems with air entrapment. However, there are no alarms on the system and the patient has to use a new container for each antibiotic dose.

Syringe Pumps

The earliest syringe pumps were designed for intermittent infusion and delivered a single antibiotic dose at a single flow rate. The duration of the infusion was determined by the syringe size and the volume of the medication. More recent models can be programmed to deliver antibiotics at varying rates or times (for example, the 360 Infuser, Becton Dickinson, Lincoln Park, NJ, USA). Newer pumps, such as the Harvard 400 Mini-Infuser System (Bard Medical Systems, North Reading, MA, USA) can be programmed to deliver multiple doses from a single syringe at predetermined time intervals. These devices are ambulatory, lightweight, reliable, and have safety features such as an alarm mechanism. Disadvantages of the syringes include volume constraints (volumes are from

1–60 ml), stability issues (possible drug interaction with the plastic) and, with some antibiotics, an increased incidence of phlebitis.

The Intelliject IV drug delivery system (Intelligent Medicine Inc.) is a four-channel, programmable, portable, syringe system. The channels can be programmed separately to give different flow rates, and this may represent a convenient way of treating home IV antibiotic patients who require two or more IV antibiotics. This may have particular relevance to the oncology patient, who may be neutropenic and have a mixed infection or infection in more than one anatomic site. Note that one of the "free" channels can be programmed for heparinization and another for a fluid flush between antibiotic doses. The system is quite heavy, weighing just over 1.36 kg. Programming the pump requires interaction with a personal computer, so that when an alarm is triggered problem solving requires direct access to the computer.

Portable Programmable Infusion Pumps

There are several lightweight pumps available for home IV antibiotic therapy. The pumps most frequently used are the Provider Series (Pancretec Inc.), the CADD-VT and, more recently, the CADD-PLUS pumps. All employ a peristaltic pump action, are battery powered, and are capable of delivering a prescribed amount of drug intermittently over a 24-h period from a prefilled cassette or a reservoir. Drugs can be administered at any desired time interval, and between drug administration a "keep vein open" rate (usually 0.2 ml/h) can be used. Our initial experience was with the CADD-VT pump [18]. More recently, we have used the CADD-PLUS pump, which can utilize a remote reservoir for drug infusion. This feature obviates the volume constraints with the CADD-VT, in which the attached drug cassette had a volume of either 50 or 100 ml. The CADD-VT and CADD-PLUS are easily programmed and have several alarm devices to indicate problems, such as battery failure or elevated drug delivery pressure, as well as a "lock out" feature to prevent tampering.

The pump is programmed by entering the dosage (or volume) of antibiotic to be administered (infusion volume), the time over which the antibiotic will be administered (infusion) and the time between doses (infusion cycle). Treatment with a desired antibiotic is initiated using the infusion pump for at least 24 h, and usually 48–72 h before the patient's discharge. When infusion pumps are used, because of the duration of treatment or concern regarding drug-related phlebitis, central IV cannulae are frequently inserted.

Our experience with home IV antibiotic treatment using these infusion pumps includes patients with diagnoses such as osteomyelitis, septic arthritis, deep soft tissue infections, endocarditis, visceral abscesses, pneumonia, meningitis, and urinary tract infections. Antibiotics administered via the CADD pumps include penicillin, cefazolin, oxacillin, vancomycin, gentamicin, tobramycin, ticarcillin–clavulanic acid, ceftazidime, cefotaxime, and clindamycin.

Advantages and Disadvantages of New Technologies

Before infusion pumps became available, 10%–15% of the patients we now treat were felt to be ineligible for home IV antibiotic therapy. Most of these patients were unable to be discharged because of the frequency of their dosing regimens. Infusion pumps have enabled patients with potentially troublesome issues such as frequency of drug administration, lack of manual dexterity or of a support person, or aversion to needles, to be safely managed at home. Moreover, in patients in whom therapeutic compliance is an issue, infusion pumps insure programmed drug administration over a 24-h period and a "lock" feature on the infusion pump prevents "tampering." These patients can also be visited at home or asked to return to the outpatient facility on a daily basis to change their drug cassette. Home IV therapy using the infusion pump may prove to be especially appealing, not only in circumstances documented here, but also in the elderly patient who, for a variety of reasons, has difficulty with self-administration of IV drugs. Finally, the use of the infusion pump in the immunologically compromised host is advantageous in that the reduction in the number of times the IV cannula has to be manipulated lessens the likelihood of IV cannula-related infections.

As previously indicated, home IV antibiotic therapy requires a designated team approach with integration of medical, nursing, and pharmacy services. The use of new, technologically "sophisticated" devices makes this requirement mandatory. As with any new modality, we have encountered some problems:

1. When peripherally placed central lines are used, they may from time to time be compressed, so that the antibiotic infusion may "shut off" with changes in body position. This will set off an alarm and may require the pump to be reprogrammed. This problem, however, may be obviated by increasing the "keep vein open" volume flow rate to 0.5 ml/h.
2. Drug-induced phlebitis is a concern because of the increased antibiotic concentration, particularly when the 50-ml cassettes are used. However, with both the CADD-PLUS and the Pancretec series, larger fluid volumes can be used (via a remote reservoir), thus reducing the incidence of this problem. Drug-related phlebitis can be further reduced when central rather than peripheral IV access lines are used.
3. Some of our patients have objected to being "hooked up continuously" rather than being able to administer the drug intermittently. Others have commented adversely on the weight of the pump and the noise that the pump makes.

Pharmacological Considerations in Home IV Antibiotic Therapy

Certain antibiotics may be best avoided, or used only in specific situations in the home, irrespective of the precise means of drug administration. Such examples include:

1. IV administration of tetracycline, doxycycline, erythromycin, or vancomycin, because of their tendency to cause drug-induced phlebitis. When vancomycin and amphotericin are used on an outpatient basis, we invariably use a central venous access device to circumvent this problem.
2. Sulfamethoxazole–trimethoprim, imipenem–cilastatin, and ampicillin all present problems in terms of drug stability. This is particularly true at room temperature (at 22°–25°C they are stable for less than 8 h), and this makes it technically difficult to advocate these drugs for home IV use.
3. Metronidazole, as it is marketed in the United States, comes in a prepackaged container and is difficult to use with syringes or infusion pump systems.
4. Acyclovir is a problem from the standpoint of both drug stability and the volume required for solubility.
5. Amphotericin presents problems because of phlebitis, volume considerations, and stability. It is usually administered over a period of several hours, rather than over 30–60 min as most other drugs are.
6. Pentamidine presents the added hazards of acute or delayed hypoglycemia and hypotension.
7. When aminoglycosides are used with the CADD-VT and CADD-PLUS pumps, diluent should be normal saline rather than sterile water.

New Technologies in Perspective

The justification for favoring new infusion devices over traditional gravity infusion in the home needs to be analyzed from a number of standpoints.

Clinical Issues

In our program, the use of the programmable ambulatory infusion pump was prompted by clinical needs in selected patients. We have now demonstrated that many patients previously considered "ineligible" for self-administration of IV antibiotics in the home can be safely and effectively treated with the aid of infusion pumps. Antibiotic administration using the infusion pump is especially useful in those patients who:

1. Require frequent (every 4–6 h) IV drug administration.
2. Have impaired manual dexterity or cognitive function.
3. Are unwilling or unable to learn the necessary techniques.
4. Have an aversion to needles.
5. Lack a support person at home.
6. Are immunologically compromised (reduces the number of times the IV cannula has to be manipulated).

The use of pumps may also have the added safeguard of facilitating IV antibiotic therapy at home in situations where there are potential barriers, as a result of regulation or custom, to such use. However, the indications for IV anti-infective agents needs to be constantly reappraised because of the development and availability of effective oral agents such as the quinolones, the second- and third-generation cephalosporins, and fluconazole.

Economic Issues

A detailed analysis of the economics of home IV antibiotic therapy in the United States and Switzerland has reaffirmed the cost-effectiveness of this approach to medical care [2]. However, the use of infusion pumps also needs to be analyzed from a cost standpoint. The cost of the pump may be offset by savings generated from a reduction in pharmacy time in compounding the antibiotic doses, and the elimination of heparin flush kits, as well as by reductions in nursing time and visits, and by earlier hospital discharge.

Acknowledgements. The author acknowledges the support and enthusiasm of the medical, pharmacy, and IV nursing staffs at Methodist Hospital, Minneapolis, in the development of the Home IV Program. The author also wishes to thank Allan C. Kind, M.D., for his support, and Robin Doering for typing the manuscript.

References

1. Antoniski A, Anderson BC, Van Volkinburg EJ, Jackson JM, Gilbert DN (1978) Feasibility of outpatient self-administration of parenteral antibiotics. West J Med 128: 203–206
2. Balinsky W, Nesbitt S (1989) Cost-effectiveness of outpatient parenteral antibiotics: a review of the literature. Am J Med 87: 301–305
3. Baumgartner JD, Glauser MP (1983) Singe daily dose treatment of severe refractory infections with ceftriaxone. Arch Intern Med 143: 1868–1873
4. Finley RS (1987) The delivery of chemotherapy via continuous infusion. Highlights on antineoplastic drugs. November–December 5–20
5. Hola ET, Cronin CM, DeMonaco HJ, Franco ER, Pauley SY (1986) Evaluation of a multiple-dose syringe pump system for intermittent IV drug delivery. Am J Hosp Pharm 43: 2474–2478
6. Kamen BA, Gunther N (1985) Administering a 24-hour supply of antibiotics with a programmable, automated syringe. Am J Hosp Pharm 42: 2715–2716
7. Kane RE, Jennison K, Wood C, Black PG, Herbst JJ (1988) Cost savings and economic considerations using home intravenous antibiotic therapy for cystic fibrosis patients. Pediatr Pulmonol 4: 84–89
8. Kerr IG, Stone, M, DeAngelis C, Iscoe N, Mackenzie R, Schueller T (1988) Continuous narcotic infusion with patient-controlled analgesia for chronic cancer pain in outpatients. Ann Intern Med 108: 554–557
9. Kind AC, Williams DN, Persons G, Gibson JA (1979) Intravenous antibiotic therapy at home. Arch Intern Med 139: 413–415

10. Kind AC, Williams DN, Gibson JA, Person G (1985) Outpatient intravenous antibiotic therapy: 10 years' experience. Postgrad Med 77: 105–111
11. Kwan JW (1989) High-technology IV infusion devices. Am J Hosp Pharm 46: 320–335
12. Miller LW, Merkle EJ, Herrmann V (1990) Outpatient dobutamine for end stage congestive heart failure. Crit Care Med 18: S30-33
13. Poretz DM, Eron LJ, Goldenberg RI, Gilbert AF, Rising J, Sparks S, Horn CE (1982) Intravenous antibiotic therapy in an outpatient setting. JAMA 248: 336–339
14. Rehm SJ, Weinstein AJ (1983) Home intravenous antibiotic therapy: a team approach. Ann Intern Med 99: 388–392
15. Smego RJ, Gainer RB (1985) Home intravenous antimicrobial therapy provided by a community hospital and a university hospital. Am J Hosp Pharm 42: 2185–2189
16. Stiver HG, Telford GO, Mossey JM, Cote DD, Van Middlesworth EJ, Trosky SK, McKay NL, Mossey WL (1978) Intravenous antibiotic therapy at home. Ann Intern Med 89: 690–693
17. Williams DN, Gibson JA, Kind AC (1984) Outpatient intravenous antibiotic therapy. J Antimicrob Chemother 14: 102–104
18. Williams DN, Gibson JA, Bosch D (1989) Home intravenous antibiotic therapy using a programmable infusion pump. Arch Intern Med 149: 1157–1160
19. Winter RJD, Deacock SJ, George RJD, Shee CD, Geddes DM (1984) Self-administered home intravenous antibiotic therapy in bronchiectasis and adult cystic fibrosis. Lancet I: 1338–1339

Socioeconomic Aspects of an Implantable Drug Delivery Device

B. Horisberger, M. Sagmeister, and L. Schmid

Interdisciplinary Research Centre for Public Health, Rorschacherstraße 103c, 9000 St. Gallen, Switzerland

Introduction

The surgical implantation of a catheter, establishing a connection between a subcutaneous reservoir and a large vein or the hepatic artery, has become a routine modality for long-term chemotherapy in cancer patients. The development of programmable pumps linked to cassettes containing 50–100 ml of the drug has enabled patients to receive outpatient instead of inpatient treatment [1].

The pumps have also been successfully employed as a means for palliative pain control with outpatients [2].

Various types of drug delivery devices (DDD) have already been developed and further technological development is in progress. With the experience accumulating and the many data available, it seemed timely to examine the relative costs of applying this relatively new technology in patients (a) for chemotherapy in cancer treatment and (b) for palliative pain control.

Aim and Type of Study

The purpose of this study was to calculate the costs of using the implantable DDD and pump compared with an equally effective alternative therapeutic modality not involving these devices. Both procedures are standard in the hospital departments where the study was carried out. The product used in the patients we studied was the Port-A-Cath system.

The study was conducted from the perspective of all the direct economic costs to society incurred in hospital care and outpatient care, regardless of who actually pays the bills. In Switzerland, where hospital care is heavily subsidized, hospital costs are often of lesser interest to a third-party payer (e.g., to the medical insurance company than the costs of ambulatory care, where costs have to be covered by the insurers on a fee-for-service basis within a system of tariffs.

Recent Results in Cancer Research, Vol. 121
© Springer-Verlag Berlin · Heidelberg 1991

Methods

The study was a cost-minimization analysis. This approach can be used when it can be assumed that treatments are identical in their effectiveness and that only difference lies in the costs of the modalities compared [3]. Only those cost data that varied according to the treatment modality used were collected. The costs of the drugs were assumed to be equal.

The direct costs for treatment were assessed in detail on the basis of a retrospective chart review of both inpatients and outpatients and of the records of the accounting department in two Swiss hospitals (Kantonsspital St. Gallen and Ospedale San Giovanni Bellinzona). Data from three groups of patients treated between 1984 and 1989 were analyzed (Table 1).

The alternative pathway of clinical management, using a complementary type of treatment without permanent vascular access (via the implantable DDD) and without a portable pump was defined by clinical experts highly experienced in the management of cancer patients. The direct costs of using the implantable DDD or the portable pump were then compared to those of the complementary technology without the device, i.e., the comparison was made between clinical practice under normal operating conditions and a hypothetical scenario. In the case of chemotherapy, it was assumed that the alternative to permanent vascular access with the Port-A-Cath would be intermittent access via a vascular catheter.

For continuous therapy of more than 1 day's duration it was assumed that the patient would have been hospitalized had the DDD not been used. In the case of pain treatment it was assumed that patients without the pump would have remained hospitalized.

Direct Costs

To assess the *direct costs* related to the use or nonuse of the DDD we considered the changes in resource utilization associated with and without the use of the

Table 1. Analysis of patients treated with DDD

Clinical condition	No. of patients (n)	Modality of DDD used	Average duration of use of DDD per patient (days)
Acute myeloid leukemia	15[a]	Central venous system with/without pump	873
Liver metastasis	6[a]	Hepatic artery with pump	316
Intractable pain	9[b]	Subcutaneous pump	24

[a] Patients of the Kantonsspital St. Gallen.
[b] Patients of the Ospedale San Giovanni Bellinzona.

device. In outpatient charges, additional visits with a private doctor were not included, since all therapy was performed at the outpatient department of the hospital. Extra visits were assumed to be equal in both groups of patients.

Patients Receiving Chemotherapy

In patients receiving i.v. or i.a. chemotherapy the following inputs were included in the analysis:

Costs with DDD	Costs without DDD
1. Implantation of device for permanent vascular access (hardware and costs of surgical procedure)	1. Provision of intermittent vascular access (material and costs of alternative option, e.g., central venous catheter)
2. Hospital care – Nursing – X-ray – Treatment complications – Hospital days	2. Hospital care – Nursing – X-ray – Treatment complications – Hospital days
3. Outpatient Care – visits – Maintenance of DDD – Cassettes – Treatment complications	3. Outpatient Care – visits – Maintenance of alternative device – Nil – Treatment complications
4. Infusion pump – Capital costs (assuming a lifetime of 3 years)	4. – Nil

The costs for implantation and maintenance of the DDD (including the costs for treatment of complications) were based on detailed costing studies and were compared to average costs of the alternative option (e.g., subclavian catheterization and maintenance costs per session of therapy [4, 5]; complications [6]). Hospital costs were calculated as average costs incurred in the particular hospital department [7, 8].

The costs for outpatient care were assessed on the basis of fees for individual acts. Diagnostic procedures were added as extras (as billed). The costs for the medication (chemotherapy) were not taken into account since they were considered identical in the patient groups studied. However, the costs for additional therapy as a consequence of complications (e.g., infection) were included.

Patients in the Pain Treatment Program

In the opinion of the treating medical experts, patients in this group ($n = 9$) experienced intractable pain as a consequence of advanced tumors. Frequent and regular injection of a pain-relieving drug was therefore necessary. Experience showed that with the use of a programmable pump some of the patients who would otherwise have been kept hospitalized could be discharged.

In the patients with intractable pain a slightly simplified list was used to compare costs:

Costs with pump	Costs without pump

1. Outpatient care
  – Visits
  – Cassettes
  – Capital costs for pump
  (assuming a lifetime of 3 years)
	1. Outpatient care
	  – Visits
	  – Nil
	  – Nil

2. Hospital care
  – Hospital days
	2. Hospital care
	  – Hospital days

Indirect Costs

Indirect economic costs of the changes in productivity were not compared since we noticed that the patients under scrutiny had no earnings that could be lost or gained as a result of using the device (phases of chemotherapy; advanced malignant disease). The effectiveness of the treatments was considered to be equal. Experience showed that during treatment episodes patients did not work even when not hospitalized. "Free" costs (e.g., patient time) were not included.

Results

Acute Myeloid Leukemia (AML). The estimated cost differences between the two treatments for 15 AML patients, are outlined in Table 2. The distribution of additional costs and savings related to the use of DDD is shown in Fig. 1.

Table 2. Cost items and average cost differences for 15 AML patients with an implantable DDD compared to the costs of a hypothetical patient-management pathway without the device

Cost factor	Average cost differences per patient between DDD and alternative treatment (SFr)
Implantation	+ 420
Maintenance	+ 400
Outpatient care	+ 300
Hospital days	− 6 700
Treatment complications	+ 490
Other items	+ 430
Total	− 4 660
With pump	− 20 740
Without pump	− 182

+ additional expenses with the DDD; −, savings.

Gains(-)/Losses(+) per Patient

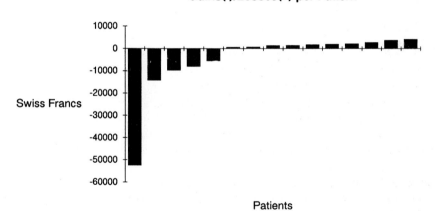

Fig. 1. Distribution of gains and losses in 15 AML patients with DDD compared to hypothetical patient management without the device

Liver Metastasis. The average cost differences between the two treatments, for six patients suffering from liver metastasis are outlined in Table 3. The distribution of additional costs and savings related to the use of DDD is shown in Fig. 2.

Table 3. Cost items and average cost differences for six patients with liver metastasis treated with an implantable DDD compared to the costs of a hypothetical patient-management pathway without the device

Cost factor	Average cost differences per patient between DDD and alternative treatment (SFr)
Implantation	− 1 400
Maintenance	− 2 600
Outpatient care	+ 1470
Hospital days	− 12 800
Treatment complications	− 520
Other items	− 1 750
Total	− 17 600
With pump	− 17 600
Without pump	—

+, additional expenses with the DDD; −, savings.

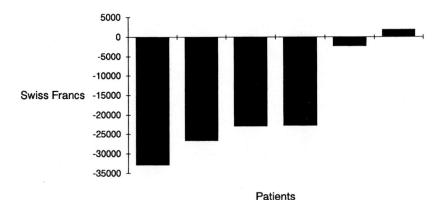

Gains(-)/Losses(+) per Patient

Fig. 2. Distribution of gains and losses in six patients with liver metastasis treated with DDD and compared to hypothetical patient-management without the device

Intractable Pain. The estimated cost differences between the two treatments for nine patients with intractable pair are outlined in Table 4. The distribution of additional costs and savings related to the use of the pump is shown in Fig. 3.

Table 4. Cost items and average cost differences for nine patients with intractable pain treated with programmable pump compared to the costs of hypothetical pain relief without the device

Cost factors	Average cost differences per patient between DDD and alternative treatment (SFr)
Pump	+130
Outpatient care	+150
Hospital days	−2 640
Other items	−60
Total	−2 420

+, additional expenses with the DDD; −, savings.

Gains(-)/Losses(+) per Patient

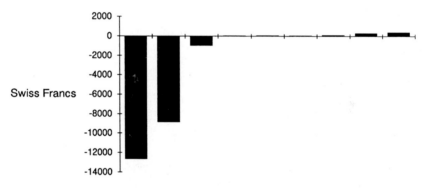

Fig. 3. Distribution of gains and losses in nine patients with intractable pain treated with a programmable pump and compared to hypothetical patient-management without the pump

Sensitivity Analysis

Because precise data on the hypothetical cases were unavailable for this socioeconomic evaluation, the hospital costs had to be assumed on the basis of "best estimate." In order to evaluate the impact of changes in the number of hospital days avoided by using the DDD we performed a sensitivity analysis to test the assumptions made.

Together with the clinical expert, we examined the quality and number of outpatient episodes that could only be performed on an outpatient basis with the use of implantable DDD. The number of hospital days thus avoided was

Table 5. Average number of hospital days avoided per patient in the clinical expert's opinion

Clinical condition	Patients (n)	Average number of hospital days avoided
AML	15	17.5
Liver metastasis	6	43.5
Intractable pain	9	6.2

Table 6. Sensitivity analysis under three different assumptions regarding expected number of hospital days avoided

Clinical condition	Benefit calculated under different assumptions (SFr)		
	Hospital days saved 100%	Hospital days saved 50%	Hospital days saved 0%
AML	− 4660	− 1310	+2040
Liver metastasis	−17600	−11200	−4800
Intractable pain	− 2420	− 1100	+ 220

considered a beneficial effect of the DDD (Table 5). The averted costs were calculated per patient on the basis of the average costs per hospital day in the respective year.

In the sensitivity analysis we reduced the expected number of hospital days avoided by 50% and 100%. The results of the calculations performed on the basis of these assumptions are shown in Table 6.

Discussion

This retrospective study is characterized by the analysis of data collected previously in two Swiss hospitals. Because of the detailed hospital records it was possible to calculate costs. Detailed costing data had been obtained from the accounting departments of the two hospitals, using data sets from insurance claims and other attributable sources.

Although retrospective studies are limited in the extent to which statements about the absent "noncases" (that is, patients without the use of DDD) can be made the sensitivity analysis allowed us to test the uncertainty associated with this type of analysis by varying the key assumption in the analysis, namely hospitalization avoided.

Table 7. Complications observed during 14 696 days of use

Complication	Number
Occlusion	4
Infection	3
Disconnection	2
Leakage	0
Other	2
Total	11

The safety of the device is illustrated by a low complication rate. In a total of 14 696 days of use (corresponding to about 40 years), a total of 11 complications were reported. The frequency of complications was therefore 0.75/1000 days of use (Table 7).

Conclusion

Appropriate use and maintenance of the Port-A-Cath system and the portable pump resulted in savings of between 2 420 and 17 600 Swiss francs in the 30 cancer patients studied. Even if the key assumption, in the opinion of clinical experts, is reduced by 50%, the direct economic gain lies between 1 100 and 11 200 Swiss francs per patient.

The implantable DDD can be considered to be a cost effective and reliable tool for management of tumor patients in need of repeated phases of chemotherapy. A pump program for subcutaneous morphine infusion enables the patient to quit the hospital and was cost effective in the cases we studied. Substantial savings of up to 15 000 Swiss francs per patient or more can be expected when the DDD and pump are combined. The Port-A-Cath system and comparable devices represent promising advance in the management of cancer patients.

Acknowledgement. The first debt that the authors have is to Elia Milazzo from the oncology department and to Luca Borner, director of the Ospedale San Giovanni in Bellinzona. Without their support the analysis of pain therapy patients would not have worked out.

Secondly, we owe a less visible – but not less deserved – debt to Erika Girardet from the accounting department of the Kantonsspital St. Gallen, whose assistance in assigning costs to the individual components of the Port procedure proved to be invaluable at the practical level of this study.

References

1. Schmid L, Walser K, Kessler W, Senn HJ (1990) Use of a fully implantable drug delivery system in the treatment of acute leucemias and disseminated lymphomas. Oncology (in press)
2. Hay L (1987) A hospital-community pump program for subcutaneous narcotic infusion. In: Enge V (ed) New concepts in drug delivery. Medicöpea, Toronto, pp 23–26
3. Luce BR, Elixhauser A (1990) Types of socioeconomic evaluation. In: Culyer AJ (ed) Standards for socioeconomic evaluation of health care products and Services. Springer, Berlin Heidelberg New York, pp 30–43
4. Paritätische Kommission (eds) (1988) Spitalleistungskatalog. Lucerne
5. Report of the Expert Committee of the Paritätische Kommission, 1989 (unpublished)
6. Eerola R, Kaukinen L, Kaukinen S (1985) Analysis of 13 800 subclavian vein catheterizations. Acta Anaesthesiol Scand 29: 193–197
7. Kantonsspital St. Gallen, Accounting department, St. Gallen, Switzerland, 1989
8. Ospedale San Giovanni Bellinzona, Administrative Center, Bellinzona, Switzerland, 1989
9. Luce BR, Elixhauser A (1990) Decision Analysis. In: Culyer AJ (ed) Standards for socioeconomic evaluation of health care products and services. Springer, Berlin Heidelberg New York, pp 117–123

Nutrition and the Cancer Patient

Strategies and Needs for Nutritional Support in Cancer Surgery

P. Schlag and C. Decker-Baumann

Section für Chirurgische Onkologie, Klinikum der Universität Heidelberg,
Im Neuenheimer Feld 110, W-6900 Heidelberg, FRG

In tumor patients who have to undergo surgery, the rate of postoperative complications and recovery after surgery depend on various factors, such as the nature and duration of the surgical intervention, preoperative nutritional status, age, and additional preoperative therapies (chemo- and radiotherapy).

Surgical treatment can contribute to poor nutritional status in many ways. In the preoperative phase, the alimentation can be considerably restricted by long periods of fasting required for detailed diagnosis and during and immediately prior to surgery. Without artificial feeding, important deficiencies in energy and protein can occur. Further nutritional problems arise when the site of operation directly includes the organs involved in food intake and digestion.

The objectives of alimentary therapy are

- To keep the patient in as good a nutritional state as possible
- To eliminate preoperative nutritional deficiencies
- To prevent complications resulting from malnutrition, such as those due to lowered resistance to infection
- To improve the patient's tolerance of ensuing radical therapies (chemo- and radiotherapy).

An accurate nutritional history is necessary to attain these objectives. This should cover present nutritional status, medical history, eating and dietary habits, and exploration of all related problems. The rationale for nutritional therapy on the basis of this collection of data is illustrated in Fig. 1.

Recording the Nutritional Status

Recording the nutritional status allows diagnosis and quantification of malnutrition, and preoperative dietary therapy can be initiated. Anthropometric, immunologic, and chemical laboratory methods are used or multivariable indices are calculated to assess the nutritional status.

Recent Results in Cancer Research, Vol. 121
© Springer-Verlag Berlin · Heidelberg 1991

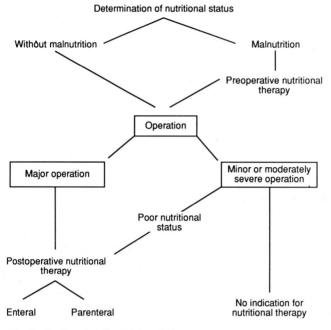

Fig. 1. Rationale of nutritional therapy

Mullen et al. (1980) developed a prognostic nutritional index (PNI; Table 1) especially for cancer patients undergoing surgery. This index calculates the postoperative risk of complications on the basis of serum albumin and transferrin concentrations, triceps skinfold thickness, and retarded immune reactivity to standard antigens.

PNIs were determined in a cohort of 159 patients undergoing elective, curative, or palliative surgery. Patients with PNI scores exceeding 40% had a sixfold higher risk of postoperative mortality than patients with scores below 40%.

Table 1. Prognostic Nutritional Index (PNI; Mullen 1980; Smale et al. 1981)

PNI % = 158 − (16.6 Alb + 0.78 TSF + 0.20 TFN + 5.8 DH)
  Alb = serum albumin (g/100 ml)
  TSF = triceps skinfold (mm)
  TFN = serum transferrin (mg/100 ml)
  DH = skin test with three ubiquitous antigens
      0 = no induration
      1 = induration < 5 mm
      2 = induration > 5 mm

Table 2. Nutritional Index (NI; Müller et al. 1986)

Nutritional Index: 1.9579
$$-0.0017 \times IgM \; (mg/dl)$$
$$+0.0188 \times prealbumin$$
$$-0.0075 \times complement \; factor \; C3 \; (mg/dl)$$
$$-0.0066 \times fibrinogen \; (mg/dl)$$
$$+0.003 \times cholesterol \; (mg/dl)$$
$$-0.1858 \times vitamin \; A \; binding \; protein \; (mg/dl)$$
$$+0.6636 \times thyroxine \; binding \; globulin \; (mg/dl)$$

Another index, the nutritional index (NI) of Müller et al. (1986; Table 2), was developed on the basis of step-by-step discrimination analysis.

Prospective evaluation of this index in 211 cancer patients showed that greater malnutrition, corresponding to a lower index score, resulted in higher rate of postoperative complications and mortality after resection of the carcinoma (Müller et al. 1986).

The diagnostic value of individual parameters, as against composite indices, is the subject of some controversy (Christou et al. 1989; Debonis et al. 1986; Dempsey et al. 1988; Brenner et al. 1987; Leite et al. 1987; Cafiero et al. 1989). Some groups (Brenner et al. 1987; Leite et al. 1987; Puchstein et al. 1989) consider the specificity, sensitivity, and validity of pathologic serum albumin parameters to be of equal value to that of multivariable indices. Other authors question this statement, in particular because of the 20-day biological half-life of albumin (Dempsey et al. 1988; Ollenschläger 1987).

A relatively new method of recording the nutritional status is bioelectrical impedance analysis (BIA) for the determination of body composition (Fig. 2). An 800 μA alternating current is sent through the body via electrodes at hand and foot. Ohmic and capacitive resistance, which vary with the composition of the body, are measured. On the basis of these, together with the basic anthropometric parameters (sex, age, body weight, and size), the body fat, the lean body mass, total body fluid, and the basal metabolic rate are calculated by a microprocessor. These data yield further information on the nutritional status.

In a prospective study, the clinical and prognostic value of this method was investigated in 115 unselected cancer patients undergoing surgery (Table 3; Fritz et al. 1990). All postoperative complications were recorded until discharge from hospital. To minimize other factors, we took only patients treated by the same surgeon according to standardized operative techniques and perioperative therapy.

The incidence of severe postoperative complications was in clear correlation to the relative lean body mass (LBM). Thus, a risk group was defined comprising patients whose lean body mass was below their "functional normal weight," i.e. the LBM according to the standard tables for age and sex in relation to the Broca weight (Table 4). This risk group had a 31% rate of severe complications,

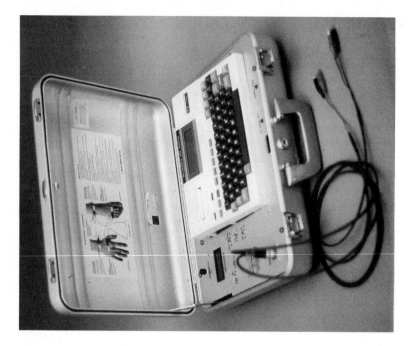

Date : 02/01/90
Time : 09: 21: 24

Name : H.Z.
Age : 48
Sex : F
Weight : 50.0 kg
Height : 158.0 cm
Level of activity : inactive
Resistance : 608 ohm
Reactance : 65 ohm

Total body fat :
24.1 %, 12.1 kg

Total lean body mass :
75.9 %, 37.9 kg

Ratio lean mass / fat : 3.1

Recommended weight range :
48.2 - 51.4 kg

Estimated basal metabolism :
1267 cal

Total body fluid :
58.5 %, 29.3 l

Fig. 2. Apparatus for bioelectrical impedance analysis

Table 3. Patients' clinical data

Patients: $n = 115$
M 60 (52%), F 55 (48%)

Diagnosis:

Esophageal carcinoma	10 (9%)
Gastric carcinoma	31 (27%)
Colorectal carcinoma	38 (33%)
Carcinoma of the liver	16 (14%)
Others	20 (17%)

Operation:

Esophagectomy	8 (7%)
Gastrectomy	17 (15%)
Partial gastrectomy	7 (6%)
Hemicolectomy	17 (15%)
Anterior proctectomy	12 (11%)
Proctectomy	5 (4%)
Hemihepatectomy	7 (6%)
Whipple's operation	3 (3%)
Others	39 (33%)
Total: Major operation	$n = 81$ (70%)
Minor operation	$n = 34$ (30%)

Table 4. Normal LBM (as percentage of total body weight)

	Age (years)				
	< 30	31–40	41–50	51–60	> 60
Men	86%	85%	84%	82%	81%
Women	77%	76%	75%	74%	73%

Table 5. Complications in the risk and nonrisk groups

	Patients (n)	Complications		
		Total	Minor	Major
Total (20%)	115	34 (30%)	11 (10%)	23 (20%)
Risk group (31%)	55	21 (38%)	4 (7%)	17 (31%)
Non risk group	60	13 (22%)	7 (12%)	6 (10%)

significantly higher than the 10% rate of the non risk group (Table 5; $p = 0.02$, Wilcoxon rank sum test). Thus, the relative lean mass, which indirectly represents the functional reserves of the body, proved to be a sensitive indicator for identifying patients at risk for postoperative complications.

Preoperative Nutritional Therapy

A correlation having been demonstrated between nutritional status and postoperative complications (Fig. 3), the positive influence of preoperative alimentary therapy on postoperative progress in malnourished patients was confirmed. The question of indication, duration, and type of nutritional therapy still had to be investigated.

Preoperative improvement of nutritional status by oral feeding often fails because of tumor-related food aversions, lack of appetite, gastrointestinal

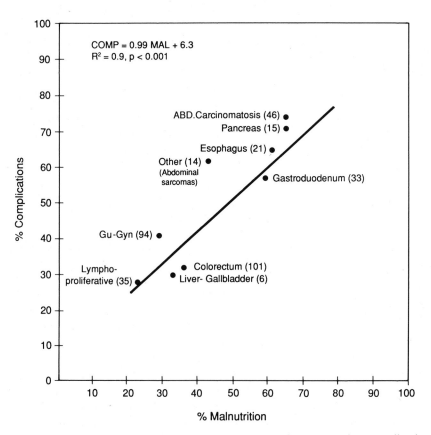

Fig. 3. Correlation between malnutrition and rate of postoperative complications in different malignancies. (From Meguid and Meguid 1985)

obstructions, and the periods of fasting necessary for detailed preoperative diagnostic procedures. Parenteral feeding is therefore frequently the method of choice.

To institute appropriate alimentary therapy, the energy requirement of the patient has first to be calculated. The basal metabolic rate is calculated using BIA, as stated above, or alternatively using the Harris–Benedict equation. Multiplication of this parameter by activity, stress and injury factors yields the energy requirement (Höllwarth and Schlag 1990).

As a rule, the energy required amounts to about 30–40 kcal/kg b.w., but it can be as high as 60 kcal/kg b.w., depending on the optimal body weight (OBW). The OBW is calculated according to the equation OBW (kg) = Broca weight − $(a \times b)$, where Broca weight = body size in cm − 100, a = Broca weight − 52, and b = 0.2 for males, 0.4 for females.

The daily protein requirement is covered by giving 1–1.5 g amino acids/kg b.w. Where malnutrition is severe, up to 2–3 g amino acids/kg b.w. can be given. The maximum glucose requirement is 5 g/kg b.w; the remaining energy should be substituted by fat emulsions. The reason for the addition of fat emulsions in parenteral feeding is the tumor metabolism: tumors favor glucose as an energy source, and increased glucose intake may enhance tumor growth. The formation of endogenous protein requires 120–200 kcal per gram nitrogen. We thus avoid having amino acids metabolized to provide energy and therefore being unavailable for protein synthesis. Electrolytes and trace elements should be infused in accordance with control blood counts. Vitamins also have to be substituted as required; the B vitamins especially are important as coenzymes in the protein, carbohydrate, and fat metabolism. To avoid vitamin deficiencies, the substitution of water-soluble and fat-soluble vitamins is necessary.

While relatively uniform recommendations have been established for the composition of parenteral nutrition, there is still discussion going on with regard to the duration of effective preoperative parenteral feeding. Several studies have investigated the influence of preoperative parenteral feeding on the rate of postoperative complications and mortality in cancer patients. The results showed a reduction of postoperative complications and consequently an improvement in prognosis. Bellantone et al. (1988) provided parenteral support of oral feeding in 49 malnourished patients for 7 days. They found significant differences between the control and the therapy group only in the cases of malnourished cancer patients; no significant differences were observed for benign diseases. They concluded nevertheless that suitable preoperative alimentary therapy can reduce postoperative complications, especially in cases of major gastrointestinal intervention with evidence of malnutrition.

Starker et al. (1983) examined 32 malnourished patients who had been fed exclusively parenterally for 5–14 days before undergoing major abdominal surgery. During this period two different reactions to completely parenteral feeding were observed. In some patients the extracellular fluid volume, which had increased due to the malnutrition, dropped, resulting in loss of weight and increased serum albumin concentrations. The other patients gained weight and

Table 6. Studies on preoperative nutritional therapy

Author	Randomized controlled	n	Criteria for inclusion	Criteria for malnutrition	Disease	PE + oral feeding	TPE Preop.	Postop.
Bellantone et al. 1989	Prospective	100	Major resection in GIT	Serum albumin <3.5% and/or total lymphocytes <1500/mm³	Benign + malignant disease in GIT	Yes	7 d	—
Starker et al. 1983	No randomization, prospective	32	Malnutrition, major abdominal operation	Serum albumin <3.5%, loss of weight >10%	Benign + malignant disease	TPE	5–14 d	Until oral food intake
Fan et al. 1989	Prospective	40	Esophageal cancer, dysphagia to solid and liquid food	Loss of weight >10%	Esophageal carcinoma	Yes	14 d	7 d until Gastrografin X-ray
Smith and Hartemink 1988	Prospective		PNI >30%	PNI >30%	Predominantly malignant disease in GIT	TPE	10 d	

TPE, total parenteral feeding; GIT, gastrointestinal tract; PE, parenteral feeding.

their serum albumin levels remained steady or dropped, owing to fluid retention and expansion of extracellular volumes. The postoperative progress was different between the two groups: there were a significantly higher numbers of postoperative complications in the group of patients with fluid retention (predominantly tumor patients). Patients in another study who reacted to exclusively parenteral feeding with fluid retention had a lower rate of postoperative complications after a prolonged period (3–4 weeks) of exclusively parenteral feeding than patients who retained fluid after 1 week of parenteral nutrition. The authors conclude from the reduced risk of complications that 1 week of exclusively parenteral feeding will suffice if diuresis is initiated there-

Composition of PE nonprotein calories	Protein	Preoperative effect of nutritional therapy	Postoperative progress
30 kcal/kg b.w. per day –70% glucose –30% lipids	200 mg N/kg b.w. = 1.25 g AS/kg b.w.	—	Significant difference between infections in malnourished patients in the treatment and control group
Calorie intake 1.5 × basal metabolic rate – 50% glucose – 50% lipids	1.5–2 g AS/kg b.w.	Loss of weight and increase in serum albumin or weight gain and decrease in serum albumin or unchanged serum albumin	Significant difference in postoperative complications comparing groups with or without fluid retention
40 kcal/kg b.w. per day – glucose – lipids	250 mg N/kg b.w. = 1.6 g AS/kg b.w.	Loss of weight, increase in N, decrease or increase in serum albumin; skinfold thickness, arm circumference unchanged	Significant difference in postoperative complications comparing groups with increase or decrease in serum albumin
42–50 kcal/kg b.w. per day glucose	1.9–2.5 g AS/kg b.w.	Weight gain, increase in skinfold thickness and cellular immunity	Less complications in control group, statistically not significant

after; otherwise the duration has to be individualized for every patient, because fluid retention is a high operative risk and the cause of this response has to be identified.

Fan et al. (1989) reported on different reactions to 2-week preoperative parenteral feeding in patients with esophageal cancer. In this study, patients of both groups gained weight and their serum albumin levels changed (increased or decreased). Patients with decreased serum albumin experienced a significantly higher incidence of postoperative complications compared to the group of patients with increased serum albumin. These authors too state that the efficacy of prolonged parenteral feeding in patients with fluid retention still has to be examined. They do not recommend any optimal duration of parenteral feeding.

Smith's group (Smith and Hartemink 1988) investigated the effect of 10-day preoperative exclusively parenteral feeding on the rate of postoperative complications. During the course of the nutritional therapy they observed significant increases in weight, triceps skinfold thickness, and cellular immunity, while the changes in serum albumin and transferrin concentrations were not significant. Comparison of the control and the therapy group showed only a trend towards a reduction in postoperative complications. Like Müller et al. (1982), these authors attach high importance to the immune status as an indicator of the nutritional status and in their opinion 10-days of preoperative parenteral feeding can improve this parameter. They recommend determination of the immune status and plasma protein levels after 10 days and that, if there are pathological values, alimentary therapy should be continued further.

In view of their different patient groups and the different criteria by which nutritional status is defined and results evaluated, the studies are not comparable, but the general tendency is identical: the risk–benefit relationship for preoperative parenteral feeding in definitely malnourished patients and patients who have to fast preoperatively (e.g., because of preoperative diagnostic procedures, obstructions), is favorable (Detsky et al. 1987; Heberer 1989; Table 6).

Postoperative Nutritional Therapy

The characteristics of "postaggression" metabolism must be taken into consideration during the postaggative phase. The reactions of the body to an "aggression" can be divided into three phases (Fig. 4, Altemeyer et al. 1984; Hartig 1987). This discussion will focus on nutritional therapy in the "postaggression" phase when oral feeding is not possible. The main question is whether the catabolic condition can be corrected during this phase by appropriate nutrition regimens. Hypocaloric vs. hypercaloric, parenteral vs. enteral nutritional regimens will be discussed.

The idea of hypercaloric alimentation is based on the assumption the patient's energy requirement is considerably increased after major surgery. According to Altemeyer et al. (1984), however, measurement of the energy metabolism in polytraumatized intensive-care patients yielded values between 2000 and 3000 kcal/day: far below the assumed energy requirement of 4000–6000 kcal/day. Another argument against hypercaloric feeding concerns the metabolic imbalances caused by disturbed hormone regulation during the postoperative period, which require complicated laboratory monitoring. Comparing hypocaloric and hypercaloric feeding, Mory and Wehner (1989) found that the rate of complications was higher in patients on a hypercaloric regimen.

In general, a gradual building up of the infusion regimen is indicated. The values required should be calculated in relation to the patient's nutritional status. A hypocaloric regimen is recommended for patients with a good

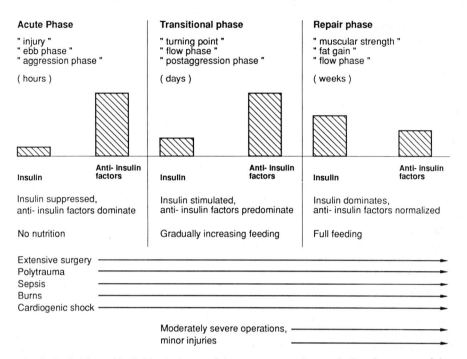

Fig. 4. Definition of individual phases of the post-traumatic metabolism by means of the relationship between insulin and anti-insulin hormones. (From Altemeyer et al. 1984)

nutritional status after minor to moderately severe operations (Hartig 1987; Scieszka et al. 1986). In addition to the calculated amino acid requirement (1.5–2 g As/kg b.w.), 10 kcal/g amino acid also have to be infused (Hartig 1987).

A normocaloric regimen should be chosen for patients with preoperative malnutrition and after major surgical interventions. The following factors have to be taken into consideration when establishing the infusion regimen:

1. For the above reasons, the maximum capacity of the glucose metabolism is reduced, i.e., glucose has to be administered in small doses not exceeding 2–5 mg/kg b.w. per minute (Vogel et al. 1987; Scigalla and Hahn 1986).
2. The energy supply has to correspond to the energy required to support the synthesis of protein from parenterally administered amino acids (see preoperative infusion regimen).
3. 1.5–2.0 g As/kg b.w. should be administered to take the protein catabolism into account.
4. Starting on day 4 after surgery (perhaps earlier), fat emulsions can be infused.

The aim of nutritional therapy, to reduce protein catabolism, is best achieved by concomitant administration of carbohydrates and amino acids. The excretion of nitrogen is reduced by 25% after administration of carbohydrates alone, by 50%

after administration of protein alone, and by 75% when protein and carbohydrates are administered concomitantly (Dietzke 1987).

In recent times enteral feeding has increasingly came into consideration as an alternative to parenteral feeding. The previously postulated concept of gastrointestinal atonia has to be abandoned (Bruining et al. 1981; Moss 1981). Enteral probes are to be recommended since peristalsis starts earlier in the small intestine than in the stomach. Arguments in support of this type of nutritional therapy include the physiological nature of the feeding, risk reduction, and reduction of costs (Höllwarth and Schlag 1990).

Studies on this type of nutritional therapy yielded positive results. Mona et al. (1983) fed 20 patients who had undergone surgery in the gastrointestinal tract by jejunal probe as early as 1–12 h postoperatively. The nutrient-defined diet for gavage was administered at doses increasing gradually every day according to the patient's tolerance. This type of feeding was very well tolerated, although 30% of the patients developed diarrhea. This side effect was eliminated by reducing the gavage or changing to a chemical diet. Positive results were also reported by Pasurka's group (1984). They fed colorectal carcinoma patients via a nasojejunal tube for 2 days preoperatively and started again only 8 h postoperatively. The calorie intake was increased from 500 kcal on the day of operation to 3000 kcal on postoperative day 3. The enteral administration was without complications. Bruning et al. (1988) also regarded this type of feeding positively. In their study of patients with carcinoma of the ear, nose, and throat, the nutritional therapy was also without complications.

As with parenteral feeding, it is not possible to avoid protein catabolism with enteral feeding. Laboratory controls showed decreasing values of plasma protein which gradually normalized (Pasurka et al. 1984; Bruning et al. 1988).

The positive results of postoperative enteral feeding presented in Table 7 cannot be generalized. In an ongoing study of gastrectomized patients in our hospital, the good tolerance of this nutritional therapy has not been confirmed so far: starting feeding on the 1st postoperative day led to intolerance reactions, so that in our opinion, feeding can only be started on the 2nd postoperative day at the earliest (Buhl et al., in preparation). It remains to be investigated whether tolerance can be improved by starting enteral feeding later and increasing considerably slower.

In sum, we find that postoperative nutritional therapy starting on day 2 or 3 is indicated after extensive surgery in the gastrointestinal tract, in order to reduce protein catabolism, which has a deleterious effect on the complication rate in tumor patients with poor nutritional status.

As stated above, which parameters are most useful in determining nutritional status is a matter of some controversy. Recent studies have found body composition to be more sensitive and more specific than anthropometric or laboratory data (Tellado et al. 1989). The analysis of the body composition yields data on the metabolically active body cell mass or lean body mass, the body fluid content, and the fat mass. Injury, fasting, and infection cause changes in the body cell mass which should be included into the evaluation of the

Table 7. Studies on postoperative enteral feeding

Author	n	Type of gavage	Enteral diet	Postoperative enteral feeding			Complications	Patients
				Onset	Length	Dosage		
Mona et al. 1983	20	Catheter jejunostomy, jejunal probe	NDD	1–12 h postop.	No data	10 ml/h in first 12 h, increased to 100 ml/h on day 3 postoperatively	30% diarrhea; change from NDD to CDD or reduction of intake led to improvement	Operation in GIT
Pasurka et al. 1984	14	Nasojejunal probe	CDD	8 h after operation	2 d pre-op., op day, 5 d postop.	1 kcal on day 1 postop. to 3 kcal from day 3 postop. + Ringer's solution on day 2 postop.	None	Colonic cancer
Bruning et al. 1988	20	Nasogastric probe	NDD	Day 1 postop.	3 weeks	32 kcal/kg or 43 kcal/kg b.w.	Nausea; eliminated by reduction of dose	Carcinoma in ear, nose and throat
Buhl et al. (manuscript in preparation)	20	Catheter jejunostomy, jejunal probe	CDD	Day 1 postop.	6 weeks	20 ml/h in first 24 h, increase to 100 ml/h on day 7 postop. then 21 kcal/kg b.w.	Diarrhea, vomiting, pain; symptoms partially reduced by reduced intake	Total gastrectomy (gastric cancer)

NDD, nutrient-defined gavage nutrition; CDD, chemically defined gavage nutrition.

nutritional status (Tellado et al. 1989). Most of the methods for determining the body composition, such as densitometry, and new methods, such as natural whole-body potassium counting, isotope dilution, and neutron-induced radioactivity, are suitable only for clinical research (Heberer and Günther 1988); they are too complicated and expensive to be used routinely. One alternative is bioelectrical impedance analysis (BIA). This method allows an approximate estimate of the body composition without much expenditure of time and financial resources. Our findings show it is possible to identify patients at risk of postoperative complication using BIA. The prognostic value of this technique needs, however, be confirmed by further studies; whether BIA is more valuable than conventional methods for determining nutritional status has yet to be clarified.

Another issue for discussion is the length of time for which preoperative parenteral feeding should be provided in order to be effective as an adjuvant therapeutic measure to reduce postoperative complications. Previous studies have shown its efficacy in selected risk patients, but criteria for indication, duration, type of nutritional therapy, and follow-up need to be developed. In weighing up risk and benefit, the possible complications inherent in parenteral feeding have to be taken into account.

In postoperative nutritional therapy, too, there are no proven guidelines, geared to achieving a favorable risk–benefit relationship, in regard to the use of infusion schemes in parenteral feeding. Postoperative enteral feeding, which we have just been discussing, requires further investigation. Since our negative findings on this type of early postoperative feeding do not agree with results from other studies, it may be possible that the achievement of positive results depends on the surgical intervention, the time enteral feeding is started, and the details of the nutritional regimen. Further studies will be needed to clarify for which operations enteral is equal or superior to parenteral feeding. A generally accepted plan for enteral feeding will be necessary if it is to be practised routinely.

Since postoperative feeding cannot correct the metabolic changes in the "postaggression" phase, it will be necessary to find drugs which can minimize the protein catabolism. Recent investigations by Manson and Wilmore (1986) demonstrated a protein-saving effect of growth hormone in combination with hypocaloric nutritional regimens. Controlled clinical studies on this treatment mode are still pending.

Summary

Nutritional therapy in tumor patients undergoing surgery should be regarded as a supportive therapy. They render the operation tolerable or even feasible, and they have a positive effect on postoperative progress and wound healing. Malnourished patients definitely profit from nutritional therapy. However, the effectiveness of a nutritional regimen should not be overestimated: postoperative progress, wound healing, and complication rate depend not only on nutritional status but also on the nature of the operation, age, and preoperative treatment. As a rule, parenteral feeding is superior to enteral feeding directly after surgery. Enteral nutritive regimens are to be favored when long-term feeding is indicated: in this case the advantages of this type of feeding prevail.

References

Altemeyer K-H, Seeling W, Schmitz JE et al. (1984) Posttraumatischer Stoffwechsel – Grundlagen und klinische Aspekte. Anaesthesist 33: 4–10

Bellantone R, Doglietto GB, Bossola M. et al. (1988) Preoperative parenteral nutrition in the high risk surgical patient. JPEN J Parenter Enteral Nutr 12: 195–197

Brenner U, Müller JM, Keller HW et al. (1987) Der Vergleich prognostischer Ernährungs indizes zur Präoperativen Erfassung von Risikopatienten. Infusionstherapie 14: 215–221

Bruining HA, Schattenkerk ME, Obertrop H. (1981) Early postoperative feeding by needle jejunostomy as an alternative to total parenteral nutrition. World J Surg 5: 436

Bruning PF, Halling A, Hilders FJM et al. (1988) Postoperative nasogastric tube feeding in patients with head and neck cancer: a prospective assessment of nutritional status and well-being. Eur J Cancer Clin Oncol 24: 181–188

Buhl K, Decker-Baumann C, Schlag P (1990) Postoperative enterale Ernährung nach Gastrektomie. (to be published)

Cafiero F, Gipponi M, Moresco L et al. (1989) Selection of pre-operative haematobiochemical parameters for the identification of patients at risk of infection undergoing surgery for gastro-intestinal cancer. Eur J Surg Oncol 15: 247–252

Christou NV, Tellado-Rodriguez J, Chartrand L et al. (1989) Estimating mortality risk in preoperative patients using immunologic nutritional and acute-phase response variables. Ann Surg 210/1: 69–77

Debonis D, Pizzolato M, Zamboni M et al. (1986) Quantitative nutritional assessment of 102 consecutive patients admitted to a general surgery ward in Buenos Aires, Argentina. Nut Int 2 (3): 168–171

Dempsey DT, Mullen JL, Buzby GP (1988) The link between nutritional status and clinical outcome: can nutritional intervention modify it? Am J Clin Nutr 47: 352–356

Detsky AS, Baker JP, O'Rourke K et al. (1987) Perioperative parenteral nutrition: a meta-analysis. Ann Intern Med 107: 195–203

Dietze GJ (1987) Prinzipien der künstlichen parenteralen und enteralen Ernährung In: Peter K, Dietze GE, Hartig W, Steinhardt HJ (eds) Differenzierte klinische Ernährung. Zuckschwerdt, Munich, pp 1–5 (Klinische Ernährung, vol 25)

Fan ST, Lau WY, Wong KK et al. (1989) Pre-operative parenteral nutrition, randomized clinical trial. Clin Nutr 8: 23–27

Fritz T, Höllwarth I, Romaschow M, Schlag P (1990) The predictive role of bioelectrical impedance analysis (BIA) in postoperative complications of cancer patients. Eur J Surg Oncol 16: 326–331

Hartig W (1987) Postoperative Ernährung. In: Peter K, Dietze GE, Hartig W, Steinhardt HJ (eds) Differenzierte Klinische Ernährung. Zuckschwerdt, Munich, pp 16–26 (Klinische Ernährung vol 25)

Heberer M (1989) Trends der Stoffwechselforschung und der perioperativen Ernährungstherapie. Dtsch Ges Chir Mitt 5: 39–42

Heberer M, Günther B (1988) Praxis der parenteralen und enteralen Ernährung in der Chirurgie. Springer, Berlin Heidelberg New York, pp 314–316

Höllwarth I, Schlag P (eds) (1990) Kompendium Künstliche enterale Ernährung. Kohlhammer, Stuttgart (in press)

Leite JFMS, Antunes CF, Monteiro JCMP et al. (1987) Value of nutritional parameters in the prediction of postoperative complications in elective gastrointestinal surgery. Br J Surg 74: 426–429

Manson JM, Wilmore DW (1986) Positive nitrogen balance with human growth hormone and hypocaloric feedings. Surgery 100: 188–197

Meguid MM, Meguid V (1985) Preoperative identification of the surgical cancer patient in need of postoperative supportive total parenteral nutrition. Cancer 55: 258

Mona D, Geroulanos S, Uhlschmid G (1983) Die frühe postoperative enterale Ernährung mit der Jejunalsonde. Helv Chir Acta 50: 31–38

Mory M, Wehner W (1989) Die hypokalorische Ernährung in der frühen postoperativen Phase bei Patienten nach kolorektalen Eingriffen. Infusionstherapie 16/1: 41–43

Moss G (1981) Maintenance of gastrointestinal function after bowel surgery and immediate enteral full nutrition. JPEN J Parenter Enteral Nutr 5: 215–220

Mullen JL, Buzby GP, Matthews DC et al. (1980) Reduction of operative morbidity and mortality by combined preoperative and postoperative nutritional support. Ann Surg 192: 604–613

Müller JM, Brenner U, Dienst C et al. (1982) Preoperative parenteral feeding in patients with gastrointestinal carcinoma. Lancet i: 68–71

Müller JM, Keller HW, Brenner U et al. (1986) Adjuvante künstliche Ernährung in der Tumorchirurgie. Infusionstherapie 13 (3): 126–132

Ollenschläger G (1987) Indikationen und Methoden der klinischen Ernährung bei onkologischen Patienten. In: Peter K, Dietze GE, Hartig W, Steinhardt HJ (eds) Differenzierte klinische Ernährung. Zuckschwerdt, Munich, pp 177–188 (Klinische Ernährung, vol 25)

Pasurka B, Filler D., Kahle M (1984) Enterale Ernährung nach Colonresektionen. Chirurg 55: 275–279

Puchstein C, Mertes N, Nolte G (1989) Erfassung des Ernährungszustandes. Infusionstherapie 16: 222–228

Scieszka S, Kampa U, Scigalla P. (1986) Postoperative parenterale Ernährung mit glucosehaltiger Komplettlösung. Wehrmedizin 4: 64–66

Scigalla P, Hahn B (1986) Möglichkeiten und Grenzen des Einsatzes von Glucose bei der vollständigen parenteralen Ernährung in der postoperativen Phase. In: Peter K, Dietze GE, Hartig W, Steinhardt HJ (eds) Klinische Ernährung im Gespräch II. Zuckschwerdt, Munich (Klinische Ernährung, vol 20)

Smale BF, Mullen JL, Buzby GP et al. (1981) The efficacy of nutritional assessment and support in cancer surgery. Cancer 47: 2375–2381

Smith RC, Hartemink R (1988) Improvement of nutritional measures during preoperative parenteral nutrition in patients selected by the prognostic nutritional index: a randomized controlled trial. JPEN J Parenter Enteral Nutr 12: 587–591

Starker PM, Lasala PA, Askanazi J et al. (1983) The response to TPN. Ann Surg 198: 720–724

Tellado JM, Garcia-Sabrido JL, Hanley JA et al. (1989) Predicting mortality based on body composition analysis. Ann Surg 209: 81–87

Vogel WM, Guttmann J, Krieg N (1987) Parenterale und enterale Ernährung bei Polytraumatisierten. eds In: Peter K, Dietze GE, Hartig W, Steinhardt HJ (eds) Differenzierte klinische Ernährung. Zuckschwerdt, Munich, pp 27–39 (Klinische Ernährung, vol 25)

Tumor Anorexia: Causes, Assessment, Treatment

G. Ollenschläger[1], B. Viell[2], W. Thomas[3], K. Konkol[1], and B. Bürger[1]

[1] Klinik II und Poliklinik für Innere Medizin, Universität Köln, Josef-Stelzmann-Straße 9, 5000 Köln 41, FRG
[2] Z. Chirurgischer Lehrstuhl, Universität Köln, Josef-Stelzmann-Straße 9, 5000 Köln 41, FRG
[3] Institut für Psychosomatik und Psychotherapie, Universität Köln, Josef-Stelzmann-Straße 9, 5000 Köln 41, FRG

Introduction

The major cause of death in patients with cancer is the generalized body wasting known as cancer cachexia (Lawson et al. 1982; S. Warren 1932). This syndrome is characterized by a mixture of metabolic abnormalities which lead to weight loss through accelerated wasting of host tissue mass together with failure of adequate nutrient intake (Kern and Norton 1988).

The cachexia–anorexia syndrome is variably expressed depending on tumor type and stage, and may differ from host to host bearing the same tumor type. Its prevalence in cancer patients was intensively studied by the Eastern Cooperative Oncology Group (DeWys et al. 1980): more than 50% of about 3000 patients had lost weight before the initiation of cytostatic treatment, and 15% had lost more than 10% of their premorbid weight. Tumors of nonvisceral organs, such as breast cancer, rarely resulted in significant host weight loss, in strong contrast to cancers of the gastrointestinal tract. Nonetheless, this study indicated that cachexia is not only caused by disfunction of the digestive organs, as patients with lung cancer also showed weight loss.

The true prevalence of cancer cachexia is difficult to determine and will depend upon the sensitivity of nutritional assessment and the patients groups studied. Taken together, most studies indicate that over 40%–50% of cancer patients suffer from clinically detectable malnutrition (Buzby et al. 1980; Nixon et al. 1980; Ollenschläger and Sander 1985; Smale et al. 1981; Bozzetti et al. 1989), and many groups now regard anorexia as the primary event for the onset of undesired weight loss of tumor patients (Lindmark et al. 1984; Ollenschläger et al. 1989).

Because of the well-known prognostic significance of tumor-associated weight loss (Nixon et al. 1980; Warnold and Lundholm 1984), early diagnosis and adequate treatment of anorexia are highly relevant to the care of tumor patients. Furthermore, the inadequate food intake resulting from anorexia correlates highly to the impaired subjective well-being ("quality of life") of tumor patients

Recent Results in Cancer Research, Vol. 121
© Springer-Verlag Berlin · Heidelberg 1991

(Brunig et al. 1985; Lanham and Digiannantonio 1988; Ollenschläger et al. 1990a,b).

Causes of Anorexia

Anorexia in the cancer patient is a difficult problem to study, since the clinical picture varies greatly (DeWys 1977). Furthermore, since the regulation of appetite is a very complex process (Silverstone 1976; Sullivan and Gruen 1985), anorexia in the tumor patient may be of multiple origins (Ollenschläger et al. 1987). All the various pathogenetic factors in tumor anorexia can be summarized into three groups: tumor-induced anorexia, therapy-induced anorexia, and psychogenic anorexia.

Tumor-Induced Anorexia

Hypophagia (anorexia) and cachexia are in general late features of cancer, but anorexia may also be a major complaint during early tumor stages.

Lack of interest in food is a common depressive symptom of a patient suffering from a severe and perhaps life-threatening disease. Unrelieved pain, disturbances in taste, dysphagia, nausea, and constipation all lead to decreased food intake, while hepatomegaly, abdominal tumors, or ascites can compress the stomach and thereby affect intake. Electrolyte imbalances such as hyponatremia and hypercalcemia, as well as liver failure and uremia, are also associated with depressed appetite.

Beside these clinical causes, lots of mechanisms have been discussed in order to explain the early satiety and impaired appetite of the tumor patient, e.g., the influence of tumor toxins, taste changes, and amino acid imbalances on the central feeding control (DeWys 1979; Ollenschläger et al. 1984; von Meyenfeldt and Soeters 1985). All these hypotheses, however, have remained more or less unproven causes or unspecific concomitants of human tumor anorexia. More interesting are recent data suggesting that tumor anorexia can be interpreted as a consequence of a chronic acute-phase response of the cancer-bearing host (Brennan 1977).

Anorexia combined with increased hepatic protein synthesis and loss of muscle mass is a frequent sequela to most inflammatory states, and is mediated by cytokines such as interleukin-1 and cachectin/tumor necrosis factor (Fong et al. 1989; Moldawer et al. 1988a, Tracey et al. 1988). It was recently proposed that many of the host changes that occur in cancer cachexia could also be explained by increased synthesis and release of cytokines (Moldawer et al. 1987; R.S. Warren et al. 1987; Moldawer et al. 1988b; Sherry et al. 1989). So far these hypotheses are based upon data from animal models, and further studies are necessary to clarify the interactions of cytokines and feeding behavior.

Table 1. Nutrient intake, nitrogen balances, and creatinine height indices of cancer patients during 7 days' oncological polychemotherapy. (Ollenschläger et al. 1989)

Parameter (medians/ ranges)	Patients		Controls (n=12)
	with (n=7) weight loss	without (n=8) weight loss	
Energy intake (kcal/kg IBW/day)	16.5 (2.2–22.4)	37.2 (28.7–52.1)	36.9 (32.1–48.5)
Protein intake (g/kg IBW/day)	0.6 (0.1–1.0)	1.3 (0.9–1.5)	1.2 (0.8–1.9)
N balance (g/day)	−8.4 (−6.3−−34.3)	+0.6 (−0.1−+9.5)	−0.1 (−1.3−+1.2)
CHI after therapy/ sampling period (% ref.)	73 (54–87)	99 (99–105)	101 (90–116)
Weight change (% init. body weight)	98.1 (91.7–99.9)	100 (100–102)	100 (99.5–100.7)

Therapy-Induced Anorexia

The therapy of cancer often induces anorexia. Narcotic analgesics can cause nausea and therefore contribute to anorexia if not given with concomitant antinauseant medications. Many chemotherapeutic drugs induce nausea, vomiting, mucositis, leukopenia with fever and sepsis, or gut dysmotility syndromes, leading to acute and chronic reductions of food intake – especially in cases of combined therapy. Radiation therapy may also be associated with similar side effects such as pain, nausea, and vomiting, leading to anorexia, especially in cases of head and neck or abdominal irradiation (Pezner and Archambeau 1985). Chemotherapy-associated malnutrition is primarily a consequence of diminished spontaneous food intake (Merritt et al. 1981; Ollenschläger et al. 1988, 1989; Ollenschläger 1989; deVries et al. 1982), resulting from anorexia (see Tables 1, 2).

In contrast to other results (DeWys and Walters 1975), we did not find abnormalities of taste in leukemic patients to correlate with impaired food intake (Ollenschläger 1989); we also could not find any significant deviation of the usual ratios of protein, fat and carbohydrates in this study group.

Surgical therapy can be another reason for anorexia, as is known from the chronic eating problems of gastrectomized patients (Raab et al. 1988). Furthermore, if anorexia is an integral part of the stereotypic postoperative acute-phase reaction (Shenkin et al. 1980), impaired appetite may be more or less unavoidable in every surgical patient.

In order to gain information on the perioperative course of appetite, we evaluated prospectively the subjective assessment of patients with (18 males, 14 females) and without (16 males, 24 females) malignant disease who underwent

Table 2. Coefficients of correlations between weekly reported weight changes, nutrient intake, self-assessed items of subjective well-being for 13 acutely leukemic patients during 220 weeks of induction treatment. (Ollenschläger 1989)

Subj. items (LASA score)	Energy intake (kcal/kg IBW)	Weight changes (% BW of previous week)
Anorexia	−0.4655**	−0.3767**
Nausea	−0.3146**	−0.2404*
Emesis	−0.3715**	−0.2310*
Taste change	−0.2975**	—
Stomatitis	—	—
Pain	—	−0.2583**

IBW, ideal body weight.
$*p < 0.05$; $**p < 0.0001$.

Table 3. Perioperative LASA scores for appetite of surgical patients with benign and malignant gastrointestinal diseases. (B. Viell, unpublished results)

Diseases/ immobilization periods	Appetite scores[a] – medians (1st–3rd quartiles)			
	1 d preop.	7 d postop.	14 d postop.	21 d postop.
Colorectal cancer				
1 week (n=9)	98 (93–99)	73 (32–81)		
2 weeks (n=6)	95 (94–95)	78 (51–95)	73 (51–94)	
3 weeks (n=4)	99 (60–99)	32 (4–88)	54 (21–86)	72 (49–78)
Upper GI tract cancer				
1 week (n=6)	77 (52–97)	40 (37–91)		
2 weeks (n=3)	97 (20–99)	10 (2–18)	52 (31–72)	
3 weeks (n=4)	49 (23–76)	2 (0–3)	34 (21–47)	50 (16–90)
Upper GI tract, benign disease				
1 week (n=24)	90 (58–97)	79 (47–93)		
2 weeks (n=9)	93 (29–96)	90 (36–93)	96 (91–97)	
3 weeks (n=6)	88 (43–97)	41 (37–60)	55 (9–74)	70 (50–90)

[a] 0, no appetite; 100, good appetite; GI, gastrointestinal.

curative surgery of the gastrointestinal tract over a period of 3 weeks (see Table 3). From these preliminary data we deduced that the incidence, intensity, and duration of early postoperative anorexia depend highly on the severity of the disease and postoperative complications. All patients with colorectal cancer and benign diseases of the upper gastrointestinal tract with 3 weeks' immobilization were anorectic at week 1 after surgery – regardless of preoperative nutritional status. This was in contrast to persons in the same groups but with an immobilization period of less than 3 weeks. As expected, patients with malignant tumors of the upper gastrointestinal tract had much worse pre- and postoperative appetite scores than those of the other groups.

Psychogenic Anorexia

One feature of cancer anorexia which was studied in both man and the rat is the occurrence of "learned food aversions." A learned food aversion is acquired via the unconscious association (by a person or an animal) of consumption of a particular food with a concurrent or subsequent unpleasant reaction (Levine and Emery 1987). One possible explanation for anorexia in patients receiving treatments with severe and unpleasant side effects – such as chemotherapy and radiotherapy – is that the patients may have acquired learned food aversions

(Bernstein 1978; Smith et al. 1984). Furthermore, chronic unpleasant symptoms of tumor growth may also be an unconditioned stimulus of tumor-associated anorexia (Bernstein and Sigmundi 1980). In order to prevent learned food aversions arising, therefore, tumor pain and the side effects of antitumor therapy should be prevented or treated as intensively as possible, using individually planned regimens (Aulbert and Niederle 1990; Thiel 1987).

Appetite can be influenced by mental stress (Padilla 1986), and it is often assumed that tumor anorexia may derive from anxiety and depression. However, it was found that depression was in fact no more frequent in tumor patients than in nontumor patients (Holland et al. 1977; Lanham and Digiannantonio 1988). In the case of acute leukemic patients during induction polychemotherapy, too, we could not see any correlation between either nutritional behavior or weight changes and the subjective factor "psychological distress". (Table 4). Thus, psychogenic anorexia of tumor patients seems to be more often a learned food aversion and not depression-associated. Cancer patients at higher risk of depression are those in a poor physical condition, in an advanced stage of illness, with inadequately controlled pain, and with a preexisting depressive syndrome (Lesko and Holland 1988).

Table 4. Coefficients of correlations between weekly reported weight changes, nutrient intake, self-assessed items, and factors of subjective well-being (LASA/factor analysis) for 13 acutely leukemic patients during 220 weeks of induction treatment. (Ollenschläger 1989)

Parameter/ subj. items	Factors of subjective well-being		
	Weakness (malaise)	Dysphoria (psychol. distress)	Side effects of tumor therapy
Weight loss (% body weight of previous week)	0.3985**	—	—
Energy intake (kcal/kg IBW)	−0.2412*	—	−0.3989**
Anorexia (LASA score)	0.4926**	—	0.6350**
Nausea (LASA score)	—	—	0.8699**
Emesis (LASA score)	—	—	0.8298**
Taste change (LASA score)	—	—	0.5301**

IBW, ideal body weight; LASA, Linear Analogue Self-Assessment.
$*p < 0.01$; $**p < 0.001$.

Assessment of Anorexia

In different studies the diagnosis of anorexia has been variously based on patient's subjectively complaining of lack of appetite or on objective measurements of spontaneous oral food intake. To our mind, the differentiation between "subjective" and "objective" anorexia (Bozzetti et al. 1989; von Meyenfeldt et al. 1988) is misleading: anorexia (from the Greek "without appetite") is by definition subjective. Instead of a so-called "objective" anorexia we recommend use of the term "inadequate oral nutrient intake" (IONI), as proposed by Meguid and Meguid 1985.

Measurements of individual appetite can be made using visual analogue scales, e.g., the Linear Analogue Self-Assessment (LASA) scales (Aitken 1969; Priestman and Baum 1976; Table 5). Further instruments for measuring the subjective well-being or "quality of life" of cancer patients were recently discussed in detail by van Knippenberg and de Haes (1988).

Although the definition of subjective anorexia is relatively vague, the appetite scores of tumor patients and quantified food intakes are in quite high correlation, as was demonstrated by Bozzetti et al. (1989) ($r = 0.71$) and by our own results (Tab. 3). Nevertheless, subjective anorexia and measured inadequate oral intake are only partially concordant, since patients may deny changes in appetite but may nonetheless have a reduced caloric intake (DeWys 1977). Therefore, exact quantification of the daily food intake is necessary, both for verification of the subjective complaints and for planning nutritional strategies. Retrospective diet histories are invalid methods: total omission of some food types and incorrect recall about the frequency of intake may lead to underestimation of all nutrients (Krall and Dwyer 1987). Thus, meals eaten less frequently or not so recently would tend not to be remembered, and foods believed to be socially acceptable might be reported in larger quantities than foods the individual feels he or she should avoid (Jensen 1981). Another bias might be introduced by the patient's expectation: malnourished HIV-infected patients, who were aware of the correlation between nutritional status and individual outcome, highly overestimated their usual nutrient intake (Bürger et al. 1990), as proven by the recall-to-record comparison (Adelson 1960).

In order to estimate food intake correctly, a (prospective) dietary record over a period of more than 6 days (Beaton 1985) is necessary, using food composition tables or computerized nutrient data bases (Hoover et al. 1985).

Table 5. Linear Analogue Self-Assessment scale for items of subjective well-being. (Ollenschläger 1989)

During the last week, I was

not   x   -------------------- x   *very intensely*

suffering from anorexia.

Treatment of Anorexia

The management of anorexia depends on the control of all potentially reversible underlying factors.

Pharmacologic stimulation of appetite has been only marginally successful. The usage of corticosteroids has resulted in appetite stimulation in some anorectic patients (Hanks et al. 1983), but its use only for correction of anorexia remains controversial and should be limited to selected patients. Further drugs, which – outside controlled studies – have been used as appetite stimulants are antiserotoninergic agents (cyproheptadine) and anabolic steroids (Levy and Catalano 1985). Recently it was suggested that the gestagen megestrol acetate can possibly cause appetite stimulation in tumor patients (Aisner et al. 1988). Whether the weight gain of megestrol acetate-treated patients results from an antianorectic effect of the drug, or from gestagen-induced fluid retention, is now under investigation.

Antidepressants, tranquilizers, and antiemetics may be indirectly effective as antianorectics in patients whose anorexia is of predominantly psychologic or emotional origin or due to a learned food aversion.

Nonspecific dietetic measures for stimulation of the patient's appetite have been discussed in detail elsewhere (Padilla 1986; Ollenschläger et al. 1988; Ollenschläger 1990; Sauer and Thiel 1987). With the help of thorough dietetic care ("intensified oral nutrition": daily nutrition interview, continuous nutrition education, meals of choice, etc.), effective oral nutrition is possible for the majority of nonsurgical tumor patients even during the highly anorexigenic induction therapy of acute leukemias (Fig. 1).

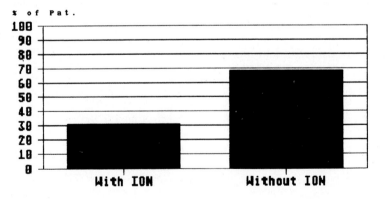

Fig. 1. Malnourished patients with acute leukemia (% patients in each group) after induction therapy (LAM-6, TAD, Ulm protocols) with ($n = 16$) and without ($n = 16$) "intensified oral nutrition". Median treatment periods: LAM-6: 9 weeks; TAD: 8 weeks, Ulm: 13 weeks. All patients of both groups obligatory lost 8% (mean) of the initial weight during the first month after the begin of chemotherapy. (Ollenschläger 1989)

References

Adelson SF (1960) Some problems in collecting dietary data from individuals. J Am Diet Assoc 36: 453–461

Aisner J, Tchekmedyian NS, Tait N, Parnes H, Novak M (1988) Studies of high-dose megestrol acetate: potential applications in cachexia. Semin Oncol 15: 68–75

Aitken RCB (1969) Measurements of feelings using visual analogue scales. Proc R Soc Med 62: 989–993

Aulbert E, Niederle N (1990) Die Lebensqualität des chronisch Krebskranken. Thieme, Stuttgart, pp 71–101, 131–164

Beaton GH (1985) Nutritional assessment of observed food intake: an interpretation of recent requirement reports. In: Draper HH (ed) Advances in nutritional research, vol 7. Plenum, New York, pp 101–127

Bernstein IL (1978) Learned taste aversions in children receiving chemotherapy. Science 200: 1302–1303

Bernstein IL, Sigmundi RA (1980) Tumor anorexia: a learned food aversion? Science 209: 416–418

Bozzetti F, Agradi E, Ravera E (1989) Anorexia in cancer patients: prevalence and impact on nutritional status. Clin Nutr 8: 35–43

Brennan MF (1977) Uncomplicated starvation versus cancer cachexia. Cancer Res 37: 2359–2364

Brunig PF, Egger RJ, Gooskens AC et al. (1985) Dietary intake, nutritional status and well-being of cancer patients: a prospective study. Eur J Cancer Clin Oncol 21: 1449–1459

Bürger B, Ollenschläger G, Fätkenheuer G, Salzberger B, Moll H, Schrappe-Bächer M (1990) Pilotstudie zu Ernährungsdiagnostik und Ernährungshalten von Patienten mit HIV-1-Infektion. Infusionstherapie 17 (Suppl 1): 51

Buzby GP, Mullen JF, Matthews DC et al. (1980) Prognostic nutritional index in gastrointestinal surgery. Am J Surg 139: 160–167

deVries EGE, Mulder NH, Houwen B, deVries-Hospers C (1982) Enteral nutrition by nasogastric tube in adult patients treated with intensive chemotherapy for acute leukemia. Am J Clin Nutr 35: 1490–1496

DeWys WD (1977) Anorexia in cancer patients. Cancer Res 37: 2354–2358

DeWys WD (1979) Anorexia as a general effect of cancer. Cancer 43: 2013–2019

DeWys WD, Walters K (1975) Abnormalities of taste sensation in cancer patients. Cancer 36: 1888–1896

DeWys WD, Begg C, Lavin PT (1980) Prognostic effect of weight loss prior to chemotherapy in cancer patients. Am J Med 69: 491–497

Fong Y, Moldawer LL, Marano M et al. (1989) Cachectin/TNF or IL-1a induces cachexia with redistribution of body proteins. Am J Physiol 256: R659–R665

Hanks GW, Trueman T, Twycross EG (1983) Corticosteroids in terminal cancer – a prospective analysis of current practice. Postgrad Med J 59: 28–32

Holland JCB, Rowland J, Plumb M (1977) Psychological aspects of anorexia in cancer patients. Cancer Res 37: 2425–2428

Hoover LW, Dowdy RP, Hughes KV (1985) Consequences of utilizing reduced nutrient data bases for estimating dietary adequacy. J Am Diet Assoc 85: 287–304

Jensen OM (1981) Dietary diaries and histories. In: Newell GR, Ellison NM (eds) Nutrition and cancer: etiology and treatment. Raven, New York, pp 111–121

Kern KA, Norton JA (1988) Cancer cachexia. J Parenter Enteral Nutr 12: 286–298

Krall EA, Dwyer JT (1987) Validity of a food frequency questionnaire and a food diary in a short-term recall situation. J Am Diet Assoc 87: 1374–1377

Lanham RJ, DiGiannantonio F (1988) Quality-of-life of cancer patients. Oncology 45: 1–7

Lawson DH, Richmond A, Nixon DW et al. (1982) Metabolic approaches to cancer cachexia. Annu Rev Nutr 2: 277–301

Lesko LM, Holland JC (1988) Psychological issues in patients with hematological malignancies. Recent Results Cancer Res 108: 243–270

Levine JA, Emery PW (1987) The significance of learned food aversions in the etiology of anorexia associated with cancer. Br J Cancer 56: 73–78

Levy MH, Catalano B (1985) Control of common physical symptoms other than pain in patients with terminal disease. Semin Oncol 12: 411–430

Lindmark L, Bennegard K, Eden E et al. (1984) Resting energy expenditure in malnourished patients with and without cancer. Gastroenterology 87: 402–408

Meguid MM, Meguid V (1985) Preoperative identification of the surgical cancer patient in need of postoperative supportive total parenteral nutrition. Cancer 55: 258–262

Merrit RJ, Ashley JD, Siegel SS, Sinatra F, Thomas DW, Hays DM (1981) Calorie and protein requirements of pediatric patients with acute nonlymphocytic leukemia. JPEN J Parenter Enteral Nutr 9: 303–306

Moldawer LL, Georgieff M, Lundholm KG (1987) Interleukin 1, tumour necrosis factor-alpha and the pathogenesis of cancer cachexia. Clin Physiol 7: 263–274

Moldawer LL, Andersson C, Gelin J, Lundholm K (1988a) Regulation of food intake and hepatic protein synthesis by recombinant-derived cytokines. Am J Physiol 254: G450–G456

Moldawer LL, Lowry SF, Cerami A (1988b) Cachectin: its impact on metabolism and nutritional status. Annu Rev Nutr 8: 585–609

Nixon DW, Heymsfield SB, Cohen AE et al. (1980) Protein-calorie undernutrition in hospitalized cancer patients. Am J Med 68: 683–690

Ollenschläger G (1989) Diagnostik und Therapie der Mangelernährung onkologischer Patienten während aggressiver Tumortherapie. Habilitationsschrift, University of Cologne

Ollenschläger G (1990) Ernährungstherapie des chronisch Krebskranken. In: Aulbert E, Niederle N (eds) Die Lebensqualität des chronisch Krebskranken. Thieme, Stuttgart, pp 117–130

Ollenschläger G, Sander F (1985) Indikationen und Ergebnisse der enteralen Ernährung in der Onkologie. Z Gastroenterol [Suppl] 23: 64–76

Ollenschläger G, Lang R, Fekl W et al. (1984) Imbalanzen neutraler Plasma-Aminosäuren als pathogenetischer Faktor der Anorexie. Klin Wochenschr 62: 1102–1107

Ollenschläger G, Jansen S, Fischer H, Mödder B (1987) Zur Pathogenese und klinischen Bedeutung der Anorexie onkologischer Patienten. In: Sauer R, Thiel HJ (eds) Ernährungsprobleme in der Onkologie. Zuckschwerdt, Munich, pp 12–24 (Aktuelle Onkologie, vol 35)

Ollenschläger G, Konkol K, Mödder B (1988) Indications for and results of nutritional therapy in cancer patients. Recent Results Cancer Res 108: 172–184

Ollenschläger G, Konkol K, Wickramanayake PD, Schrappe-Bächer M, Müller JM (1989) Nutrient intake and nitrogen metabolism in cancer patients during oncological chemotherapy. Am J Clin Nutr 50: 454–459

Ollenschläger G, Thomas W, Konkol K (1990a) Nutrition therapy and subjective well-being during induction regimens of acute leukemias. J Cancer Res Clin Oncol 116 (Suppl, Part I): S 355

Ollenschläger G, Konkol K, Sander F et al. (1990b) Orale Ernährungstherapie des internistischen Tumorkranken – ein integraler Bestandteil der supportiven Behandlungsmassnahmen. Akt Ernährungsmed 15: 66–71

Padilla GV (1986) Psychological aspects of nutrition and cancer. Surg Clin North Am 66: 1121–1135

Pezner R, Archambeau JO (1985) Critical evaluation of the role of nutritional support for radiation therapy patients. Cancer 55: 263–267

Priestman TJ, Baum M (1976) Evaluation of quality of life in patients receiving treatment for advanced breast cancer. Lancet i: 899–901

Raab M, Stützer H, Kotthoff G (1988) Nutrition analysis after complete gastrectomy due to malignant tumour. Aktuel Ernährungsued 13: 10–14

Sauer R, Thiel HJ (1987) Ernährungsprobleme in der Onkologie. Zuckschwerdt, Munich (Aktuelle Onkologie, vol 35)

Shenkin A, Neuhäuser M, Bergström J et al. (1980) Biochemical changes associated with severe trauma. Am J Clin Nutr 33: 2119–2127

Sherry BA, Gelin J, Fong Y et al. (1989) Anticachectin/tumor necrosis factor – a antibodies attenuate development of cachexia in tumor models. FASEB J 3: 1956–1962

Silverstone T (1976) Appetite and food intake: report on the Dahlem workshop on appetite and food intake. Abakon, Berlin

Smale BF, Mullen JL, Buzby GP et al. (1981) The efficacy of nutritional assessment and support in cancer surgery. Cancer 47: 2375–2381

Smith JC, Blumsack JJ, Bilek FS et al. (1984) Radiation-induced taste aversion as a factor in cancer therapy. Cancer Treat Rep 68: 1219–1227

Sullivan AC, Gruen RK (1985) Mechanisms of appetite modulation by drugs. Fed Proc 44: 139–144

Thiel HJ (1987) Ernährungstörungen durch Strahlentherapie. Ursachen – Prophylaxe – Therapie. In: Sauer R, Thiel HJ (eds) Ernährungsprobleme in der Onkologie. Zuckschwerdt, Munich, pp 65–102 (Aktuelle Onkologie, vol 35)

Tracey KJ, Wei H, Manogue KR et al. (1988) Cachectin/tumor necrosis factor induces cachexia, anemia, and inflammation. J Exp Med 167: 1211–1227

van Knippenberg FCE, de Haes JCJM (1988) Measuring the quality of life of cancer patients: psychometric properties of instruments. J Clin Epidemiol 41: 1043–1053

von Meyenfeldt MF, Soeters PB (1985) Anorexia in cancer. In: Bozzetti F, Dionigi R (eds) Nutrition in cancer and trauma sepsis. Karger, Basel, pp 54–67

von Meyenfeldt MF, Visser G, Buil-Maassen R, Soeters PB, Wesdorp RIC (1988) Food intake and nutritional status in patients with newly detected gastric or colorectal cancer. Clin Nutr 7: 85–91

Warnold I, Lundholm K (1984) Clinical significance of preoperative nutritional status in 215 noncancer patients. Ann Surg 199: 299–305

Warren RS, Starnes HF, Gabrilove JL, Oettgen HF, Brennan MF (1987) The acute metabolic effects of tumor necrosis factor administration in humans. Arch Surg 122: 1396–1400

Warren S (1932) The immediate causes of death in cancer. Am J Med Sci 184: 610–615

Nutritional Support of Patients with Advanced Cancer

V.F.P. Souchon

The Royal Marsden Hospital, Downs Road, Sutton, Surrey SM2 5PT, United Kingdom

Introduction

Advanced cancer is a condition which may last for weeks, months, or even years. The extent of nutritional support required therefore varies from patient to patient. The aim of nutritional support is to maintain or restore health through nutrition (Boisaubin 1984). In the context of advanced cancer, it is evident that the emphasis is on maintenance of the present state of health.

Major Nutritional Difficulties Experienced by Patients with Advanced Cancer

Anorexia

Appetite loss is very common in advanced cancer and can contribute to severe emaciation and muscle weakness. There are many contributing factors and it is important that the underlying cause of anorexia is treated at the same time as dietary changes are attended to.

Small attractive meals or snacks, high in energy but low in bulk, should be served frequently to tempt the appetite. Regular mealtimes need not be adhered to, as this in itself may become a source of stress for the anorexic patient. Relatives of hospitalised patients may be encouraged to bring favourite foods into the hospital. Nutritional supplements in the form of high-protein, high-energy drinks and desserts can be helpful to supplement or replace meals. Because appetite comes and goes, the patient should be encouraged to make the most of the time when he or she can eat. Some people find that their appetite is best at breakfast and then deteriorates as the day progresses.

Nausea and Vomiting

Nausea and vomiting are also common complaints of patients with advanced cancer. A study of terminally ill cancer patients in the United Kingdom in 1986 revealed that 62% of the patients studied experienced nausea and vomiting during their last 6 weeks of life. High incidences were seen in patients with stomach or breast cancer, female patients and the younger patients studied (Reuben and Mor 1986).

Dietary advice should be discussed with the patient and care givers in order to establish which foods are found nauseating. The smell of food may contribute to the nausea, and for this reason patients may be advised to take food and drinks cold, chilled or even frozen. Dry toast or crackers taken before meals can be helpful. Some patients find fizzy drinks help to alleviate nausea by making them "burp". Drinks taken through a straw will ensure that the patient drinks more slowly, and in addition the smell of the drink will be reduced. Patients may be advised to avoid the smell of cooking, and eat in a well ventilated room. Low-fat foods, high in carbohydrate are tolerated best.

Weight Changes

Weight loss is common in advanced cancer and is a source of concern for both patient and care giver. It is a constant reminder of the disease and often represents a deterioration in general health. The aim of nutritional support should be to prevent further weight loss; it is often difficult for the patient to gain weight in the advanced stages of cancer (Fearon and Calman 1987).

Dietary advice should again be discussed with the patient and care givers, and should include practical suggestions on fortifying favourite food and drinks. High-protein, high-calorie nutritional supplements, often served in the form of flavoured milk drinks or soups, can be taken with or between meals. "Little and often" is the general rule. Alcohol can be of value here, both as a source of energy and as an appetite stimulant.

Although we are interested in preventing weight loss, it is not always advisable to weigh the patient regularly. Watching a person lose weight when there is little or nothing that can be done to prevent it can be demoralising, to say the least (D'Agostino 1989).

Obesity

Obesity can also occur in advanced cancer, especially as a result of sudden inactivity. Although eating may be one of the few remaining pleasures in life, problems may occur when a patient with, for example, hemiplegia becomes too heavy to lift. Simple advice on reducing calories may be appropriate for a patient with a longer term prognosis.

Constipation

Constipation is a common problem which may be a direct result of physical inactivity, inadequate intake of fluid and fibre, and the use of analgesics (Cushman 1986). Constipation itself reduces the appetite and can cause discomfort and pain. A high-fibre diet including plenty of fluid may be recommended, but often such regimes are inappropriate when the patient cannot manage a large volume of food. In such cases it is easier to administer laxatives.

Diarrhoea

Diarrhoea is less common, but some malignancies such as the carcinoid syndrome can contribute to severe diarrhoea, which is debilitating and distressing. Dietary advice would be to reduce dietary fibre and perhaps lactose in the diet. Predigested formulas or digestive enzymes may be indicated if malabsorption is a cause of diarrhoea. Control of symptoms using appropriate medication can be effective.

Taste Changes

An alteration in the sensation of taste is not uncommon among cancer patients. This may be a lasting side effect of recent chemotherapy or radiotherapy or may be caused by the tumour itself. Oral infections can also affect the sense of taste, so oral hygiene is recommended prior to meals. Common taste aberrations include mouth blindness, a bitter or metallic taste in the mouth and a decreased threshold for salty and sweet flavours. Patience, understanding and imagination when cooking is necessary here. Taste changes can be very frustrating for patients and their care givers.

Mouth Infections

Stomatitis and oral infections as a result of poor oral hygiene and/or recent treatment may reduce nutritional intake. Xerostomia as a result of decreased saliva production can make swallowing very difficult. Here it is important to consider altering the texture of food to soft or liquid, to advise against salty and acidic foods, and to serve food cold or chilled.

Points to Consider When Planning Nutritional Support (Wojtylat 1984)

1. *Is nutritional support appropriate?*
   Here for instance, one would consider medical prognosis and long-term rehabilitation plans before suggesting aggressive therapy.

2. *Can the patient afford it?*

It is important to be aware that the patient and the patient's family may have financial difficulties. This may be as a result of hospital expenses, medical fees and a reduction of family income due to the patient and/or care giver leaving employment. A detailed dietary history taken while counselling the patient can give one an idea of what the patient normally eats and, hopefully, what he or she can afford.

3. *Will it be acceptable?*

Nutritional support should be planned with the patient, taking personal likes and dislikes into account. It is also important to consider the family's lifestyle, eating habits, and the cultural or religious aspects of their diet.

4. *Is the advice practical and easy to carry out?*

For example, the care giver may not be accustomed to cooking, and will already have a busy day caring for the patient. Quality time with the patient should not be thrown away by spending hours in the kitchen. It is also important to ensure that any nutritional supplements recommended are easy to obtain.

An individualised approach is always important in order that realistic, achievable goals may be set. Otherwise nutritional support can be a source of stress and frustration (D'Agostino 1989).

Methods of Nutritional Support

There are three alternative means of nutritional support available: oral, enteral and parenteral nutrition.

Oral Nutrition

Oral nutrition is always the first method of choice. Here foods will need to be chosen to agree with personal preferences, and texture may need to be adjusted to help the patient cope with chewing or swallowing difficulties. Catering for advanced cancer may require a lot of imagination, and it may be necessary to enroll the support of the hospital catering department and other disciplines such as Speech Therapy or Occupational Therapy.

Enteral Nutrition

Enteral feeding by means of nasogastric, nasojejunal, jejunostomy, gastrostomy or oesophagostomy tubes is usually the second route of nutritional support available to the patient. It may be recommended for patients with oesophageal tumours or fistulae, dysphagia for neurological reasons, or simply prolonged anorexia and weight loss. The variety of equipment available ensures that enteral feeding can be carried out safely with minimal discomfort to the patient. It is a simple procedure which may be continued at home, with feeding regimens planned to fit in with family routines. People can choose to receive their nutrition overnight when asleep, which allows them greater freedom during waking hours. This has proved particularly useful with terminally ill paediatric patients.

Enteral feeding has its advantages and disadvantages. Some patients dislike the idea of such a feeding method, and it should not be forced upon them. Others find that it is helpful because it reduces the responsibility on them to eat and drink. Relatives and care givers may find it a great relief not to be constantly encouraging the patient to eat.

It is important to remember that enteral feeding should not be used to prolong life in the absence of quality. This must be carefully considered before starting such a regimen, which may be difficult to stop, or may not benefit the patient in the long term. The following example should help to illustrate this point:

A 97-year-old man was admitted to our continuing care unit with dysphagia as a result of cancer of the glottis. He already had a tracheostomy tube for breathing purposes. His nutritional problems included dysphagia for solid foods and he aspirated anything he tried to drink. Nasogastric feeding was discussed by the multi-disciplinary tream because despite his advanced age he was self-caring and enjoying a good quality of life. It was, however, decided not to feed him enterally, because by prolonging his life through aggressive nutrition we would be allowing his tumour more time to grow. This would have resulted in more discomfort and pain for the future, and the possibility of death through haemorrhage. Instead we decided to continue with oral nutrition, and he was taught "safe swallowing" techniques by the speech therapist. This allowed him to swallow again without the danger of aspirating his drinks. He returned home after he and his daughters who cared for him were given suggestions for a liquid diet.

He was readmitted to hospital 2 months later when his dysphagia deteriorated further. By this time he was having difficulty with fluids causing him to choke and coming out of his nose and tracheostomy. When we presented his fluids in the form of frozen ice lollies he found he was able to swallow again. The frozen lollies melted slowly, allowing him to swallow small amounts more safely. This provided the added psychological comfort of being able to "eat" again. He died peacefully in hospital 3 weeks later.

Parenteral Nutrition

Parenteral nutrition is usually the last method of nutritional support offered to patients with advanced cancer. The disadvantages, however, usually outweigh the advantages of such a feeding method in this instance. The solutions are hypertonic and require the insertion of a central line into a major blood vessel. There is a high risk of sepsis, and the patient also requires regular biochemical monitoring. Parenteral nutrition is expensive and difficult to maintain at home, and this may limit quality time at home with the family.

Both parenteral and enteral nutrition are methods which are often easier not to start at all than to start and then stop after a period of time. For this reason it is very important to consider the risks, benefits and ethical aspects involved before beginning such a regimen.

Conclusion

Nutritional support of patients with advanced cancer is a challenging task. Knowledge of the patient as a whole is vital in order to give appropriate advice. Nutritional support should aim at improving the quality of life, not the length, and this should be remembered when planning care.

References

Boisaubin EV (1984) Ethical issues in the nutritional support of the terminal patient. J Am Diet Assoc 84 (5): 529–531

Cushman KE (1986) Symptom management: a comprehensive approach to increasing nutritional status in the cancer patient. Semin Oncol Nurs 2 (1): 30–35

D'Agostino NS (1989) Managing nutrition problems in advanced cancer. Am J Nurs 89 (1): 50–56

Fearon KCH, Calman KC (1987) Anorexia and cachexia. Ballieres Clin Oncol 1 (2): 291–303

Reuben DB, Mor V (1986) Nausea and vomiting in terminal cancer patients. Arch Intern Med 146: 2021–2023

Wojtylak FR (1984) The patient-centered approach to the terminally ill cancer patient. Nutr Support Serv 4 (7): 47–48

Food Service Provisions for the Cancer Patient

A. Millard

Lewisham Hospital, High Street, London SE13 6LH, United Kingdom

The nutritional difficulties experienced by patients with cancer are all too often not addressed by the person responsible for the food service provision in hospital, namely the catering manager. My personal view, as one responsible for the overall food service in the hospital where I work, is that any patients who are experiencing difficulties in eating should have *what* they want, *when* they want it. If someone wants, for example, an avocado with prawns because they just fancy it, provision should be made for this. By giving someone what they want, they are more likely to accept what they need nutritionally. If nutritional status is low, treatment acceptance and patient morale can also be low.

Food can be and is a very important part of a patient's day. The importance of the provision of patients' food is very often forgotten and the catering department sometimes has a rather low status. Hospitals tend to have regimented meal times that seem to be determined by staff working practices rather than patient needs. A limited choice is available, particularly at breakfast time, which is when some people – depending on the treatment they are undergoing find their appetite is best.

Problems encountered by the cancer patient include nausea, vomiting, constipation, taste changes, and chewing and swallowing difficulties, caused by radiotherapy, chemotherapy or surgery. All can lead to loss of appetite. These difficulties need to be recognised, addressed and, most importantly, solved by all those responsible for the care of the patient. This cannot occur unless a team approach is adopted. The catering manager, nurse, dietitian, medical and domestic staff, pharmacist and all other professions, along with the patient's relatives, can help to overcome these problems by sharing information and advice and maintaining good communications.

"Education" is an important word to use when trying to achieve this aim. Knowledge of each discipline's role in caring for the patient can help to change attitudes. No-one can work in isolation if a good food service is to be achieved.

The person closest to the patient should coax, encourage, and suggest foods that are available. Someone who is feeling unwell very often will eat something if the thought is suggested by someone else; it may only be a piece of dry toast or a sandwich, but at least some oral stimulation will occur. The food service providers must have the ability and commitment to respond to these additional needs as and when they occur. So often, a break in the communication chain can be traced to poor liaison between disciplines.

A great deal of emphasis is put on the cost of providing a food service in any hospital.

In England, the average daily allowance is around £1.88 (around DM5.50). This normally has to supply at least seven beverages a day, three cooked meals, any alcohol, and some food supplements. This can cause concern when planning any food service. It is therefore very important that food preparation and waste are kept to a minimum. The team of carers can ensure this happens through good liaison and communication.

Those responsible for any food service must bear in mind the following criteria when planning:

Patient Menu Choice

Meals should be as varied and offer as much choice as possible. There will obviously be some financial restraints, particularly in hospitals, but if patients can be provided with *what* they want to eat *when* they want to eat, this will go a long way in encouraging and stimulating their appetite, and, most importantly, will raise their calorie intake.

A variety of foods low in fat, high in carbohydrate, are well tolerated by those with advanced cancer, and also reflect the changing diet in society today. Foods high in fibre are often too bulky for patients, but should be available within the choices offered.

The menu should also take into account the problems associated with taste changes, and should not include food that is highly seasoned. It is easier to add condiments to stimulate taste at the point of service. It is a good idea to have additional salt, pepper, onion/garlic salt, nutmeg, paprika and other seasonings available for those who want it, rather than to add in bulk an estimated amount, for it is impossible for any-one other than the patient to know what is required at any particular meal time. This point can also be borne in mind by the carer preparing food at home.

Texture is very important for those with chewing and swallowing difficulties. Anything minced, puréed or liquidised can be very bland, and will soon become monotonous. Consideration could be given to prepared baby foods, which vary in taste and texture and also have the advantage of being in small portions, easily available and cheap.

If food has to be changed in texture, e.g. puréed, the food should be presented if at all possible in its "whole" shape to the patient, so that a visual picture remains which can help to make the puree more palatable. It is also vital that each part of the meal is puréed individually; the thought of a "mash" of meat, potato and two vegetables is enough to put a healthy person off their food, let alone some one who has a problem eating.

The menu should include variety of cold foods, again in small portions. Sandwiches with crusts removed and soft fillings are good snacks and can be eaten between and instead of meals. Some patients are deterred from eating just by the smell of the food put in front of them; cold food tends to have less smell and is therefore more acceptable. A word of warning, however: cold food *must* be kept cold and not allowed to rise in temperature, particularly if the food item is a high-risk protein dish containing, for example, eggs or meat. Food poisoning bacteria multiply quickest at room temperature, and with cancer patients particularly at risk from infection, the danger of food poisoning must be absolutely eliminated.

Appetite and Taste Stimulants

Appetite and taste stimulants must be included in any cancer patient's diet. Alcohol can be used to stimulate the appetite. Cocktails containing alcohol, and often dietary supplements, could also be prepared and presented in "cocktail glasses". A cocktail menu by the patient's bedside is a very successful way of stimulating taste buds.

Other foods can also be used, e.g. grapefruit and other citrus fruits, again in small, prepared, appetising portions. Frozen yoghurt in ice-cube trays or iced lolly containers can be very refreshing for those with mouth problems.

Presentation of Food

Provisions must be made for the patient to indicate the size of portion they wish to eat. Nothing is more off-putting to some one who is ill than a plate of food piled high. Small portions, attractively presented, with garnishes and good colour, are automatically more appealing. Often a successful way of ensuring this is to present food on smaller than average dinner plates.

Good presentation of food takes time, but can pay dividends in tempting patients to eat.

Conclusion

A good food service plays a vital role in aiding patients to tolerate and recover from treatment, as well as improving morale and general wellbeing.

The provision of all I have mentioned relies very heavily on not just the catering department, but all those involved in caring for the patient with cancer. Money is too often used as an excuse for poor service. I suggest attitude and communication are the major contributing factors to the difference between a good food service and a bad one.

Percutaneous Endoscopically Guided Gastrostomy in Patients with Head and Neck Cancer

R. Fietkau, H. Iro, D. Sailer, and R. Sauer

Strahlentherapeutische Klinik, Universität Erlangen-Nürnberg, Universitätsstraße 27, W-8520 Erlangen, FRG

Introduction

Before any therapy starts, 25%–50% of patients with tumors in the head and neck region have an already markedly reduced nutritional status [7, 10, 11, 26]. The causes are patient (life style etc.) as well as tumor specific [reviews in 6, 12, 26]. Nevertheless, these patients require aggressive multimodal tumor treatment, and the side effects of treatment [1, 3, 9–11, 18, 19, 27] induce further deterioration of the nutritional status.

In a prospective, partly randomized study starting in 1986, we studied the value of supplementary enteral feeding during and following radiotherapy. Since the nasogastric tube usually used until then was refused by the patients, owing to the associated stigmatization, we introduced for the first time percutaneous, endoscopically guided gastrostomy (PEG) [13] in tumor patients (Fig. 1). Gastroscopy is performed with the patient supine [15]. The stomach is inflated by continual air insufflation and the appropriate puncture site determined by diaphanoscopy. Following local anesthetization of all layers of the abdominal wall, a plastic cannula is advanced percutaneously into the stomach. A thread introduced through this cannula is grasped by the endoscopic forceps and pulled through the mouth together with the endoscope, so that one end of the thread issues through the mouth and the other through the abdominal wall. The tube is fixed to the oral end of the thread and pulled, by traction on the other end of the thread, into the stomach. The inner plastic disc of the catheter keeps the tube in the stomach; an outside plate is applied to fix it to the abdominal wall.

Physicians and nurses of the radiotherapy and otorhinolaryngological departments (*Strahlentherapeutische und HNO-Klinik*) in association with a specially trained nutrition team of the Erlangen University Medical Hospital (*Medizinische Universitätsklinik Erlangen*) were responsible for the nutritional therapy of the patients.

Our original study protocol was as follows. The nutritional status of the patients before radiotherapy was to be defined using a schedule including body

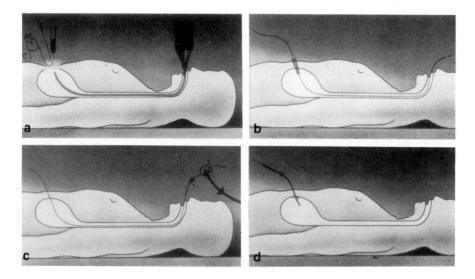

Fig. 1. a With the help of gastrostomy, diaphanoscopy is made and a plastic cannula is pulled into the stomach from the abdominal skin. **b** A thread, introduced through this cannula, is pulled out of the mouth, one end of the thread lying orally, the other on the abdominal skin. **c** Fixation of the tube at the oral end of the thread. The thread is pulled from the abdominal end of the thread through the upper digestive tract, the stomach, and the abdominal wall. **d** Tube fixed between abdominal skin and stomach by two plastic clises

measurements and biochemical and immunological parameters. The patients were to be divided up into three groups depending on nutritional status (good, intermediate, or poor). Patients with a good nutritional status were then to feed themselves orally, patients with a poor nutritional status were to receive PEG immediately for supplementary enteral feeding, while patients whose nutritional status was intermediate were to be randomized between oral food intake and PEG feeding. Assessment of objective indicators of nutritional status [2, 23] and quality of life as determined using the Padilla index [20] were to present the final criteria for comparison of the different nutritional regimens.

Only a short time after initiation of this study, however, we had to accept that the randomization was not going to be feasible. A large number of our colleagues were so impressed by the good results provided by enteral PEG feeding that they frequently carried out PEG before radiotherapy was started, so that proper, meaningful randomization became impossible. We therefore continued the study as an observation study.

Patients

A total of 212 patients with advanced tumors of the head and neck were included in this study performed from January 1986 until July 1988 (Table 1).

Table 1. Patient characteristics ($n = 212$)

Sex:		*Age:*	
Male	180 (84.9%)	22–79 years (median	54.8;
Female	32 (15.1%)	mean	54.9)
Primary tumor site:		*Staging (UICC):*	
Unknown primary	8 (3.8%)	Stage I	0
Larynx	37 (17.5%)	Stage II	20
Hypopharynx	30 (14.2%)	Stage III	64
Oropharynx	60 (28.3%)	Stage IV	109
Nasopharynx	8 (3.8%)	Staging unknown	19
Oral cavity	55 (25.9%)	or not possible	
Others (paranasal sinus, salivary glands etc)	14 (11.2%)		

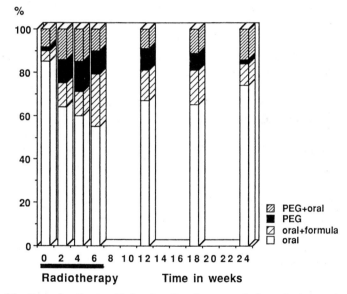

Fig. 2. Modalities of feeding of patients with head and neck tumors before, during, and after radiotherapy

Figure 2 shows how patients were fed before, during, and after radiotherapy. Before radiotherapy 90% of the patients fed themselves orally with a normal diet; only a few patients received supplementary oral formula diets. In approximately 10% of the patients PEG had already been performed before radiotherapy started. In the course of radiotherapy, the percentage of patients exclusively fed orally with a normal diet dropped to below 50%: 25% of the patients needed supplementary formula diets and another 25% required PEG. Roughly half of the PEG patients received supplementary oral nutrition; the others could only be fed via PEG.

During the observation period following the termination of radiotherapy the percentage of orally fed patients increased again, since some of the patients no longer needed the PEG and it could be removed without any complications.

The group of PEG patients were 47 in number. In accordance with the protocol, they received a PEG within 2 weeks after radiotherapy was started. Another 31 patients received PEG later than this and were therefore not taken into account. All patients taking food orally, with or without supplementary feeding, were included in the oral feeding group ($n = 134$).

Results

Anthropometric Parameters

Body weight was used as parameter for the body mass (Fig. 3). The initial weight of the orally fed patients (mean 73 kg) was on average clearly above that of the PEG patients. The orally fed patients experienced a mean weight loss of 3 kg during radiotherapy and after termination of the therapy the weight remained constant at this low level. Recovery of weight did not occur. By contrast, the patients with PEG gained on average 2 kg while therapy was still in progress.

Upper arm muscle circumference (Fig. 4) was taken as a measurement of lean body mass. Before the start of radiotherapy the values of the orally fed patients for this parameter were markedly above those of the PEG patients. In neither group did major alteration occur during or following radiotherapy. This means

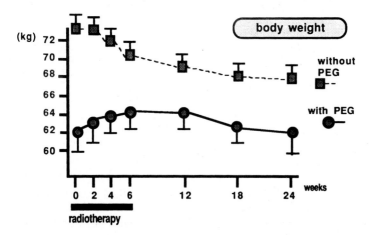

Fig. 3. Body weight as a measurement of body mass before, during, and after radiotherapy in patients with and without PEG

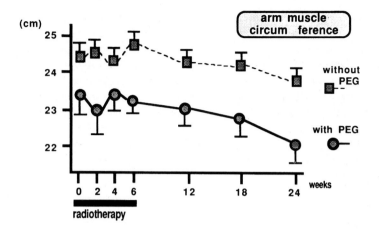

Fig. 4. Muscle circumference as a measurement of fat-free muscle mass before, during, and after radiotherapy in patients with and without PEG

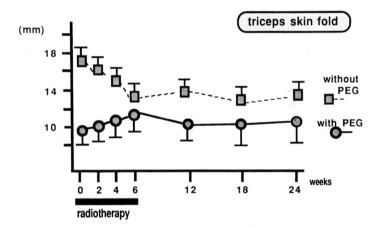

Fig. 5. Triceps skinfold as a measurement of fat reserves before, during, and after radiotherapy in patients with and without PEG

that the weight loss of the orally fed patients was not due to a decrease in muscle mass.

The triceps skinfold thickness was taken as an indicator of patients' fat reserves (Fig. 5). For this the orally fed patients had a markedly better preradiotherapy value than the PEG patients, but this dropped significantly during radiotherapy, while the values of the PEG patients increased clearly. We conclude from this that the weight loss in the orally fed patients is probably to be attributed to a decrease in their fat reserves. By contrast, the PEG patients began to replenish their low fat reserves while radiotherapy was still in progress.

Visceral Proteins

Further parameters investigated were the levels of different visceral proteins with a short half-life, for these react rapidly to alteration in the nutritional status of a patient. We used prealbumin (Fig. 6), cholinesterase (Fig. 7), and the retinol-binding protein (Fig. 8) as markers. The orally fed patients again had significantly better initial values than the PEG patients, but this ratio was reversed before radiotherapy was finished: the PEG patients' values improved steadily during therapy, whereas the metabolism of the orally fed patients deteriorated significantly.

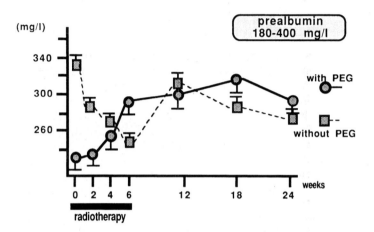

Fig. 6. Prealbumin before, during, and after radiotherapy in patients with and without PEG

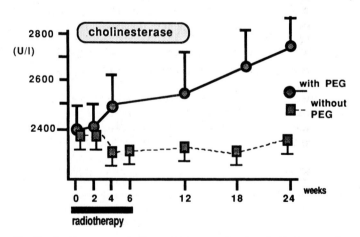

Fig. 7. Cholinesterase before, during, and after radiotherapy in patients with and without PEG

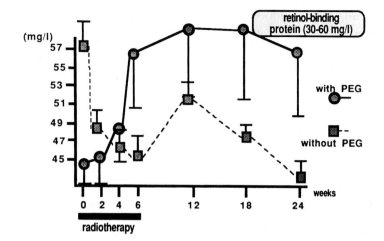

Fig. 8. Retinol-binding protein before, during, and after radiotherapy in patients with and without PEG

Proteins with a longer half-life, such as transferrin and albumin, remained constant in both groups during the observation period.

We were thus able to show that objective indicators of nutritional status can be improved by long-term enteral feeding.

Quality of life

We also studied the effects of enteral feeding via PEG on patients' quality of life. We are aware of the difficulties relating to the concept "quality of life." This term includes a large number of factors which vary in their importance to different patients in relation to the whole. Thus, they also depend on the status of the tumor and the success of therapy.

From the large number of questionnaires available [4, 14, 16, 20, 24, 25, 28], we chose the quality of life index developed by Padilla et al. [20]. For this, the patients answer the questions by marking a cross on a 10-cm, undivided line, with "normal condition for me" at one end (10 cm) and "worst condition" at the other (0). For the evaluation, you measure from the zero point to the cross in centimeters to one decimal. The higher the number, the better the patient feels. The total index is calculated from the mean value of the sum of the 12 questions. Using the index, three main spheres of life were studied (Table 2): general physical condition, normal human activities, and personal expectations regarding general quality of life. Of the originally 14 questions of the Padilla index, two were refused by our patients: those regarding sexual satisfaction and medical costs.

First we addressed the Padilla total index. Figure 9 shows that the orally fed patients had markedly better initial values than the PEG patients when radio

Table 2. Questions from the quality of life index [20]

I. *General physical condition*
  – How much *pain* do you have?
  – How much *nausea* do you have?
  – How frequently do you *vomit*?
  – How much *strength* do you feel?
  – How much *appetite* do you have?

II. *Important human activities*
  – Are you able to *work* at your usual tasks?
  – Are you able to *eat*?
  – Are you able to *sleep* well?

III. *General quality of life*
  – How good is your *quality of life*?
  – Do you have *fun*?
  – Is your life *satisfying*?
  – Do you feel *useful*?

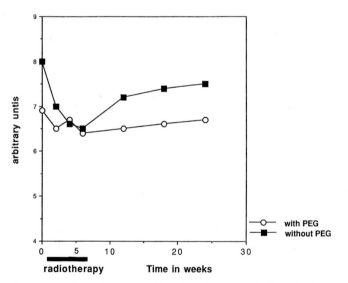

Fig. 9. Scores on Padilla quality of life index [20] before, during, and after radiotherapy in patients with and without PEG

therapy began. During therapy their total index dropped by 1–2 points to the level of the PEG patients and then subsequently recovered. The total indices of the PEG patients were lower before radiotherapy, but a further drop during and after radiotherapy was prevented. The individual curves were similar to those of the total index. As an example we take the question: "Are you able to work according to your usual requirements?" (Fig. 10).

For this, the score of the orally fed patients decreased; that of the PEG patients remained steady.

The question "How good is your appetite?" (Fig. 11) reveals a slightly different picture. Here, too, the scores in the PEG group were a little bit lower. From the first check onwards during radiotherapy, however, both curves ran parallel until the end of radiotherapy. The orally fed patients recovered very

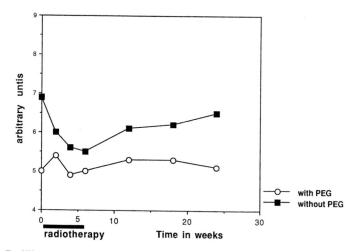

Fig. 10. Item from Padilla quality of life index [20]: "Are you able to work at your usual tasks?"

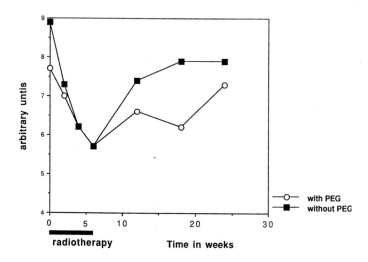

Fig. 11. Item from Padilla quality of life index [20]: "How good is your appetite?"

quickly until the first control after radiotherapy. The PEG patients, in contrast, recovered more slowly, but on last control attained scores closer to the original values than the orally fed patients. Thus, we can sum up by saying that patients' wellbeing could be stabilized by appropriate nutritional therapy via PEG. The quality of life of the exclusively orally fed patients, by contrast, decreased during radiotherapy.

Side Effects

No relevant side effects due to the performance of PEG were observed. In a total of 389 PEGs carried out in this hospital, approximately 10% of the patients ($n=42$) experienced a peritoneal irritation which caused transient pain. In only three cases did the tube have to be explanted. In six patients a local infection occurred in the further course, but this could in most cases be remedied with local or systemic antibiotic therapy.

Discussion

A qualitatively and quantitatively balanced diet is essential for tumor patients. Malnutrition results in increased morbidity and mortality and may ultimately jeopardize the success of therapy. Although studies comparing the value of oral vs. enteral feeding in radiotherapy of patients with tumors of the head and neck are rare, those that exist confirm our results. A randomized study [5] compared the nutritional status of 18 patients fed via nasogastric tube with that of 17 exclusively orally fed patients during and 1 month after radiotherapy. Although the radiation-induced toxicity in the enteral group was higher, the patients took in more calories, lost less weight, and showed a markedly better course as measured by albumin values and upper arm muscle circumference. In 17 patients who had prospectively received a feeding tube, Petzner et al. [22] found a loss of weight of only 4% compared to their initial body weight. The weight loss among the orally fed patients was 7.1%.

Most of the other prospective studies were performed in patients undergoing abdominal radiation. The studies showed a favorable influence of nutritional therapy on the weight loss and the gastrointestinal side effects of radiotherapy [21, 27]. Unfortunately, to date no controlled prospective randomized study has been able to show an advantage of either enteral or parenteral feeding in radiotherapy or chemotherapy [8, 17, 21] in relation to improvement of local tumor control, survival rate, or decrease of side effects of therapy.

On the basis of our experience we see an indication for PEG in the following situations:

1. If mastication or swallowing becomes impossible due to an advanced-stage tumor. Table 3 shows that the initial weight of the patients deteriorated with

Table 3. UICC stage, mean body weight before initiation of radiotherapy, and weight loss/gain after termination of radiotherapy in patients with and without PEG

	n	Average body weight before radiotherapy[a]	Average difference in body weight after 60 Gy	
			With PEG	Without PEG
Stage II	17	76.5 kg	—[b]	− 1 kg
Stage III	53	71.3 kg	+ 1.5 kg	− 2 kg
Stage IV	98	69.1 kg	+ 0.5 kg	− 3 kg

[a] Mean of all patients, with and without PEG.
[b] Not enough patients.

Table 4. Therapy modality initial weight before radiotherapy, and weight loss/gain after termination of radiotherapy in patients with and without PEG

Therapy	n	Average body weight before radiotherapy[a]	Average difference in body weight after 60 Gy	
			With PEG	Without PEG
Sim RCT	13	76.0 kg	—[b]	− 6.0 kg
Seq RCT	25	71.4 kg	+ 0.5 kg	− 3.5 kg
Additional iRT	43	68.0 kg	± 0 kg	− 3.5 kg
Radiotherapy	20	72.0 kg	—[b]	− 3.0 kg
Surg + radiother.	80	70.9 kg	+ 1.5 kg	−1.5 kg

[a] Mean of all patients, with and without PEG.
[b] Not enough patients.
Sim RCT, simultaneous radio-chemotherapy; Seq RCT, sequential radio-chemotherapy; iRT, interstitial radiotherapy; Surg, surgery.

increasing UICC stage. After termination of radiotherapy, the patients without PEG lost on average 1 kg in weight in stage II, 2 kg in stage III, and 3 kg in stage IV. With enteral feeding via PEG, patients were able to at least maintain their initial weight or even improve it. The other objective indicators of nutritional status showed a similar tendency.
2. If major weight loss due to aggressive tumor therapy is feared.

Table 4 shows the weight loss of patients in relation to therapy modality. Following surgery and radiotherapy – a procedure used mostly in the early stages of cancer – the mean weight loss of patients without PEG was 1.5 kg. Here the weight loss during previous surgery was not taken into account. If,

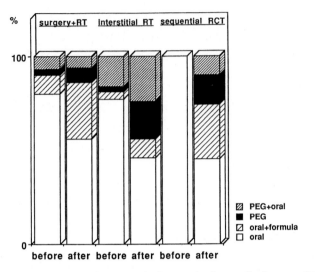

Fig. 12. Mode of feeding before and after radiotherapy (*RT*) in patients previously operated upon, or under going interstitial radiotherapy or sequential radiochemotherapy (*RCT*). It is interesting that the proportion of patients orally fed decreases whereas the proportion of patients fed enterally via PEG increases

additionally, interstitial radiotherapy was performed, the mean weight loss during radiotherapy without PEG was 3.5 kg. In simultaneous radio- and chemotherapy the patients without PEG lost 6 kg, in sequential radio- and chemotherapy the patients lost 3.5 kg. Patients with PEG at least kept their body weight constant.

The different influence of treatment modality on the patients is also shown by the following observations:

Correlation of mode of feeding upon termination of radiotherapy and the therapy performed shows that PEG became necessary in only 10–15% of cases after surgery and postoperative radiation, but in 25% of patients following sequential radio- and chemotherapy and in almost 50% of patients following interstitial radio- and chemotherapy (Fig. 12).

Summary

In 212 patients with tumors in the head and neck region the nutritional status prior to, during, and following radiotherapy, was determined by body measurements and biochemical and immunological parameters. In 165 orally fed patients the nutritional parameters deteriorated rapidly under radiation and afterwards recovered only slowly and incompletely, 31 patients requiring PEG during radiotherapy. By contrast, 47 patients with a poor initial status who had a prospectively performed percutaneous endoscopically guided gastrostomy

(PEG) experienced an amelioration of their nutritional status even before radiotherapy ended. The subjective status of the patients was assessed using the Padilla quality of life index [20]. Here, too, the PEG patients had significantly worse initial values than the orally fed patients. As with the objective indicators of nutritional status a significant deterioration was seen in the orally fed patients during radiotherapy, while the scores of the PEG patients remained constant.

We consider early institution of a carefully monitored enteral feeding by PEG useful for stabilizing the nutritional status of patients with tumors in the head and neck region, and therefore recommend, when aggressive multimodal therapy is planned – and particularly if primary malnutrition is already obvious – prophylactic performance of PEG prior to the start of therapy.

References

1. Aker SN (1979) Oral feedings in the cancer patients. Cancer 43: 2103–2107
2. Blackburn GL, Benotti PN, Bistrian BR, Bothe A, Maine BS, Schlamm HT, Smith MF (1979) Nutritional assessment and treatment of hosptial malnutrition. Infusionsther Klin Ernaehr 6: 238–250
3. Chencharik JD, Mossman KL (1983) Nutritional consequences of the radiotherapy of head and neck cancer. Cancer 51: 811–815
4. Clark A, Fallowfield LJ (1986) Quality of life measurements in patients with malignant disease: a review. JR Soc Med 79: 165–169
5. Daly JM, Hearne B, Dunaj J, LePorte B, Vikram B, Strong E, Green M, Muggio F, Groshen S, DeCosse JJ (1984) Nutritional rehabilitation in patients with advanced head and neck cancer receiving radiation therapy. Am J Surg 148: 514–520
6. Dickerson JWT (1984) Nutrition in the cancer patient: a review. J R Soc Med 77: 309–315
7. Donaldson SS (1977) Nutritional consequences of radiotherapy. Cancer Res 37: 2407–2413
8. Donaldson SS (1984) Nutritional support as an adjunct to radiation therapy. J Parenter Nutr 8: 302–310
9. Donaldson SS, Lenon RA (1979) Alterations of nutritional status: impact of chemotherapy and radiation therapy. Cancer 35: 2036–2052
10. Dwyer JT(1979) Dietetic assessment of ambulatory cancer patients. With special attention to problems of patients suffering from head–neck cancers undergoing radiation therapy. Cancer 43: 2077–2086
11. Fietkau R, Thiel H-J, Iro H (1987) Einsatzmöglichkeiten der perkutanen endoskopischen Gastrostomie (PEG) bei Patienten mit Tumoren im Hals-Nasen-Ohren-Bereich. Med Welt 38: 40–44
12. Fietkau R, Thiel H-J, Iro H, Richter B, Senft M, Rößler C, Kolb S, Sauer R (1989) Vergleich von oraler und enteraler Ernährung mittels perkutaner endoskopisch kontrollierter Gastrostomie (PEG) bei Strahlentherapie – Patienten mit Kopf – Hals – Tumoren. Strahlenther Onkol 165: 844–851
13. Gauderer MWL, Ponsky FL, Iznat RF Jr (1980) Gastrostomy without laparotomy: a percutaneous endoscopic technique. J Pediatr Surg 15: 872–875
14. Guyatt GH, Bombardier C, Tugwell PX (1986) Measuring disease-specific quality of life in clinical trails. Can Med Assoc J 134: 889–895

15. Iro H, Kachlik H-G, Fietkau R, Thiel H-J, Kolb S (1988) Erfahrungen mit der perkutanen endoskopisch kontrollierten Gastrostomie (PEG) bei HNO-Tumorpatienten. HNO 36: 111–114

16. Karnofsky DA, Burchenal JH (1949) The clinical evaluation of chemotherapeutic agents in cancer. In: McLeod CM (ed) Evaluation of chemotherapeutic agents in cancer. Columbia University Press, New York, pp 191–205

17. Klein S, Simes J, Blackburn GL (1986) Total parenteral nutrition and cancer clinical trials. Cancer 58: 1378–1386

18. Mossmann KL, Chencharik JD, Scheer AC, Walker WP, Ornitz RD, Rogers CC, Henkin RJ (1979) Radiation-induced changes in gustatory function. Comparison of effects of neutron and photon irradiation. Int J Radiat Oncol Biol Phys 5: 521–528

19. Mossmann KL, Shatzman A, Chencharik JD (1982) Long-term effects of radiotherapy on taste and salivary function in man. Int J Radiat Oncol Biol Phys 8: 991–997

20. Padilla GV, Presant C, Grant MM, Metter G, Lipsett J, Heide F (1983) Quality of life index for patients with cancer. Res Nurs Health 6: 117–126

21. Pezner RD, Archambeau JO (1985) Critical evaluations of the role of nutritional support for radiation therapy patients. Cancer 55: 263–267.

22. Pezner RD, Archambeau JO, Lipsett JA, Kokal WA, Thayer W, Hill LR (1987) Tube feeding enteral nutritional support in patients receiving radiation therapy for advanced head and neck cancer. Int J Radiat Oncol Biol Phys 13: 935–939

23. Schmoz G, Hartig W, Weiner R, Roick M (1982) Praxis der Ernährungsdiagnostik. Infusionstherapie 9: 130–143

24. Schuster D, Heim ME, Andres R, Queißer W (1986) Lebensqualität von Karzinom-Patienten unter Chemo- und Radiotherapie. Prospektive Studie bei Gastro-intestinal- und Bronchialkarzinom-Patienten. Onkologie 9: 172–180

25. Spitzer WO, Dobson AJ, Hall J, Chesterman E, Levi J, Shepherd R, Battista RN, Catchlove BR (1981) Measuring the quality of life of cancer patients. A concise QL-index for use by physicians. J Chron Dis 34: 585–597

26. Thiel H-J, Fietkau R, Sauer R (1988) Malnutrition and the role of nutritional support for radiation therapy patients. In: Senn HJ, Glaus A, Schmid L (eds) Supportive care in cancer patients. Springer, Berlin Heidelberg New York, pp 205–222 (Recent results in cancer research, vol 108)

27. Yatvin MB, Hinke DH (1986) Influence of host protein nutrition on the response of various tumours to ionizing radiation. Proc Soc Exp Biol Med 128: 200–206

28. Zubrod CG, Schneidermann M, Frei E (1960) Appraisal of methods for the study of chemotherapy of cancer in man: comparative trial of nitrogen mustard and triethylene thiophosphoramide. J Chron Dis 11: 7–33

Prevention of Radiogenic Side Effects Using Glutamine-Enriched Elemental Diets

S. Klimberg

College of Medicine, University of Florida, Box I/286, Gainesville, FL 32610, USA

In work from our laboratory we have demonstrated that the provision of a glutamine-enriched diet before or after whole abdominal radiation has a radioprotective effect. A major side effect of abdominal and pelvic radiation is injury to the bowel. Radiation enteritis affects a significant number of patients and is associated with complications such as bloody diarrhea, bowel perforation, and stricture whicy may increase mortality. The mucosal injury is characterized by destruction of proliferative crypt cells, a decrease in villous height, and ulceration of the gut mucosa. The morbidity, mortality, and cost associated with treatment of the complications of radiation enteritis are substantial, and thus any therapy that would protect the gut from radiation injury or accelerate healing of the radiated gut and/or decrease complications would be beneficial.

Glutamine is the principal fuel utilized by the intestinal tract but is absent from commercially available amino acid solutions and many enteral diets. Uptake of glutamine by the gut mucosa occurs from the gut lumen or from the blood stream.

The avid utilization of glutamine by the mucosal cells is due in large part to the high activity of the glutaminase enzyme, the first enzyme in a series of reactions that completely oxidize the carbon chain of glutamine to generate ATP for the mucosal cells. The amide nitrogen is also required for DNA biosynthesis, and recent studies suggest that glutamine may be required for the support of mucosal growth and function.

Therefore, we hypothesized that provision of oral glutamine following whole abdominal radiation would accelerate healing of the injured gut mucosa and improve outcome. The purpose of our studies was to examine the effects of oral glutamine on gut metabolism, structure, and function, and the acute complications associated with radiation enteritis.

Adult male Sprague-Dawley rats weighing 250 g were used for the first series of studies. After acclimation to the animal care facility at the University of Florida, the animals received a single dose of 1000 rads to the abdomen. The

Recent Results in Cancer Research, Vol. 121
© Springer-Verlag Berlin · Heidelberg 1991

thorax, head, gonads, and extremities were shielded. Previous studies with this model have shown the 10-day mortality to be approximately 50%.

Following radiation, the rats were randomized to a nutritionally incomplete liquid diet containing only 3% glutamine or an isonitrogenous diet containing glycine. One percent glucose was added for palatability. Rats were pair-fed for 4/8 days, during which time daily weights were obtained, the frequency of bloody diarrhea observed, and the number of deaths in each group tabulated. Autopsy was performed on all animals that died and the intestine carefully inspected for evidence of perforation. Control rats were not irradiated but were otherwise treated identically.

On day 4/8 following radiation, the animals underwent laparotomy and arterial and portal venous blood was taken for glutamine determination. The small intestine was removed for light and electron microscopy and determination of the enzyme glutaminase. The morphometric measurements taken in each specimen were mean villous height, villous number, and number of mitoses per crypt. The model included tracheostomy, cannulation of one of the carotids, and laparotomy with placement of a portal vein catheter.

Oral intake proved to be similar in all groups, as was weight loss during the 4-day study period.

In both irradiated and control rats bowel length, wet weight of the bowel, and mucosal weight were significantly increased when glutamine was provided in the diet.

In irradiated rats, the arterial glutamine in the glutamine group was 578, compared to 354 in animals provided the glycine diet. These levels were associated with normal or slightly increased gut glutamine extraction in the glutamine-fed animals, but a marked decrease in gut glutamine extraction in the glycine-fed animals. Similarly, provision of glutamine stimulated intestinal glutaminase-specific activity, which was nearly 10 in the glutamine-fed rats, compared to 6.5 in the glycine-fed rats. Similar but less dramatic effects were observed in rats that did not receive radiation.

Histologic evaluation of the gut mucosa using the light microscope demonstrated significant improvements in mucosal morphometrics when glutamine was added to the diet of the irradiated animals. There was a doubling in the villous height in animals receiving glutamine, who had a mean villous height of 0.54 mm compared to 0.29 mm in animals who did not receive glutamine. Similarly, there were 20% more villi per centimeter in the glutamine-fed rats than in those fed glycine. These improvements in villous height and number were associated with a raised number of metaphase mitoses per crypt (9 vs. 6).

Provision of glutamine to irradiated rats significantly influenced the morbidity and mortality associated with radiation injury to the bowel. The incidence of bloody diarrhea was estimated to be nearly double in rats fed the glycine diet. In rats who received glutamine following radiation treatment, the survival was 100%, and there no instances of bowel perforation were found at laparotomy. This is in marked contrast to the animals that did not receive glutamine in their diet, in whom the survival rate was only 45%, with a 30% incidence of bowel perforation. Although bacterial translocation was not examined in this particular study, similar studies in our laboratory with this animal model have shown that orally administered glutamine decreases the incidence of bacterial culture-positive mesenteric lymph nodes and blood.

An unexpected electron microscopic finding in all rats fed the glutamine-enriched diet was the presence of numerous small cells studding the villous surface. By transmission electron microscopy these small cells were found to be immature absorptive enterocytes not normally seen outside the crypts, where they first mature before migrating onto the villous surface. Their presence over the surface of the villi can be considered an epithelial left shift in an adaptive response to radiation injury. These immature absorptive cells were only rarely seen on the villi of those rats fed the glutamine-free diet.

Our next series of studies involved the feeding of glutamine prophylactically using a nutritionally complete diet. Again, weight loss was less in the glutamine-supplemented group. Mucosal morphometric studies revealed that villous number, villous height, and number of mitoses per crypt were doubled – even more markedly than in the previous series.

In a similar set of experiments, study of mucosal morphometrics demonstrated that glutamine gave superior results to glutamate or standard laboratory chow.

The studies described here demonstrate that the provision of oral glutamine either before or after radiation treatment accelerates healing of the irradiated bowel and decrease the·complications caused by abdominal radiation. The mechanism by which glutamine accelerates healing of the irradiated gut is nuclear but may be related to its ability to support mitoses in the proliferative zone of the villous crypts, since glutamine is an essential precursor for nucleic acid biosynthesis. We may be filling up the circulating glutamine pool. Clinical trials which examine the effects of glutamine-enriched diets on gut metabolism, structure, and function are in progress. The use of such specific nutritional therapy in the management of cancer patients who require multiple modality therapy may shorten hospital stays and, hopefully, improve outcome.

Diet to Prevent Gastrointestinal Cancer?

W.F. Jungi

Medizinische Klinik C, Kantonsspital, 9007 St. Gallen, Switzerland

Correlations between dietary habits and the occurrence of certain cancers have been known for a long time. There is abundant, impressive, if somewhat controversial epidemiological data on this topic (Diet, Nutrition and Cancer 1982). However, even the strongest statistically significant correlation between intake of a certain food and incidence or mortality of a certain tumor is no proof of a causal relationship. Epidemiological and preclinical research have clarified some possible causal connections, especially in the gastrointestinal tract, but in many instances it has still not been determined whether specific dietary components or habits really have an etiological role, are carcinogens or cocarcinogens, or are rather "innocent bystanders," i.e., markers, a consequence of malignant growth during the long phases of promotion and conversion (Fig. 1). Retrospective analyses are all of limited value and no substitute for the prospective trials which alone will bring definitive answers to which diet really enhances or hinders the development of a specific tumor and under what conditions.

Of interest in this respect are the so-called *macronutrients*, i.e., the basic components of our daily eating – carbohydrates, fat and protein – and the *micronutrients*, a collective term for vitamins, minerals, and other minor constituents of nutrition (Willett and MacMahon 1984). Contaminants and additives, feared and accused of every evil by laymen and the mass media, are of only minimal importance in carcinogenesis today; but as long as so much obscurity and uncertainty remain in the relationship between diet and cancer, there will be ample room for hypotheses, autistic thinking (Bleuler), and myths.

The dietary background of the two most important groups of gastrointestinal cancers can be simplified as follows:

High fat and protein   ⇒ colorectal cancer
low fiber, vitamin A

High salt, alcohol   ⇒ stomach cancer
low vitamins A, C, E, selenium

Recent Results in Cancer Research, Vol. 121
© Springer-Verlag Berlin · Heidelberg 1991

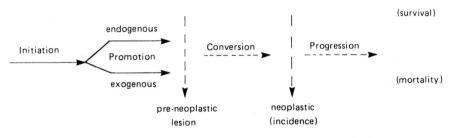

Fig. 1. Processes of tumor initiation and promotion. (From Micozzi and Tangrea, in Moon and Micozzi, 1989)

These patterns reflect our modern, unnatural eating and living habits, often labeled the "Western diet," and are in sharp contrast to the habits of so-called primitive, "uncivilized" peoples, who suffer much less from these highly malignant tumors in the stomach and large bowel. It must be therefore our goal to go "back to nature", or at least to correct our daily diet so as to reduce the risk of development of gastrointestinal cancer or the risk of recurrence after such a cancer has been detected and surgically removed.

Dietetic Possibilities for Prevention of Malignant Growth in the Gastrointestinal Tract

In principle there are three possibilities for cancer prophylaxis:

Primary: To avoid exposure to a carcinogen
Secondary: To prevent the consequences of carcinogen exposure
Tertiary: To arrest or reverse a premalignant lesion or prevent a recurrence

I will not deal with primary prevention. Secondary and tertiary prophylaxis can be practised by elimination of known or potential carcinogens or increasing the supply of anticarcinogens. The data gained from retrospective, mostly epidemiological analyses do not yet allow firm statements to be made on the preventive potential of certain macro- or micronutrients. This can only be determined by prospective intervention trials, and only a small number of such investigations have been performed so far, most of them in animals, few in man.

I have tried to collect all the available information on prospective trials of secondary and tertiary prevention of gastrointestinal cancer. I will concentrate on colorectal cancer, for which at least some data exist, whereas for gastric cancer almost no results of prospective trials can be found.

Anticancer Diet ("Krebsdiät")

Despite the uncertainty I have mentioned concerning the specific role of dietary constituents or habits in carcinogenesis, there are numerous advocates and promoters of sophisticated but entirely unproven dietary cancer therapies. They flourish above all in the German-speaking countries, and all refer to the "anoxia hypothesis" of Otto Warburg. Warburg claimed that irreversible damage of cell respiration was the sole and fundamental reason for malignant transformation of a cell. He himself and many of his epigones claimed and still claim to know ways and means of correcting this metabolic disturbance and improving cell oxygenation. These attempts to prevent or even treat cancer by dietary manipulations can be summarized under the promising epithet *"stoffwechselaktive krebsfeindliche Vollwertkost"* (metabolically active anticancer wholefood diet). There are many variants of this diet, linked to the names of Zabel, Kollath, Kretz, Kuhl, Gerson, Bircher-Benner, Schultz-Friese, Anemueller, and many others. They all recommend a diet rich in unrefined carbohydrates, rich in fiber and vitamins, and with little or no sugar, animal fat, and salt. None of these diets has ever been tested in a scientific trial worth mentioning. They have to be classified as unproven methods despite their broad acceptance and public promotion. Wholefood is healthy and to be recommended for everybody – but it has yet to be proven as a real anticancer diet.

Scientific Attempts at Dietary Prevention of Gastrointestinal Cancer

Candidates for dietary prevention of gastrointestinal cancer are listed in Table 1. Not all of them have been tested for this purpose, and very few have been given a trial in man. The greater number of studies in rat and mice colon tumors are summarized in Table 2. It is evident at first sight that there is no clear tendency, but considerable room for controversy. There is no clear-cut front runner which has been shown to reduce or prevent carcinogenesis in the colon reproducibly and safely. Vitamin C and selenium seem most promising, and possibly also butyrated hydroxyanisole (BHT), whereas the results with β-carotene are disappointing. β-Carotene and retinoids, however, still seem to be more

Table 1. Candidates for tertiary prevention of cancer in the gastrointestinal tract

---

Antioxidants:
Selenium, β-carotene,
α-tocopherol (vitamin E),
butyrated hydroxyanisole

Retinoids
Vitamin C
Fiber
Calcium, Vitamin D
Flavones, isothiocyanates, phenols, indoles
Prostaglandin inhibitors

Table 2. Dietary prevention studies in animals

Anticarcinogen tested	Animal	Effect[a]	Reference
Butyrated hydro-		↓	
xyanisole (BHT)	Mouse	±	Jones et al. 1981
Vitamin C		↓	
Vitamin C	Rat	±	Reddy et al. 1982
Vitamin C	Rat	↓	Colacchio and Memoli 1986
β-Carotene		−	
Vitamin C		↓	
β- Carotene	Mouse	−	Colacchio et al. 1989
α- Tocopherol		↓	
Canthazanthin		↑	
Cholesterin		−	
Cellulose	Rat	−	Tempero et al. 1988
Chol. + Cell.		↓	
Vitamin E	Mouse	↑	Toth and Patil 1983
Vitamin E	Mouse	↓	Cook and McNamara 1980
Selenium	Rat	↓	Jacobs 1983
Selenium	Rat	±	Birt et al. 1982

[a] ↓ reduction in tumor incidence; ↑ tumor increase; ± mixed or partial effect; − no effect.

promising than the preformed retinols. There is controversy about the effects of vitamin E (Cook and McNamara 1980; Knekht et al., 1988; Toth et al., 1983). Of interest is the study by Tempero et al. (1988), who showed that the mere addition of wheat fibre has no protective effect: this was seen only when cholesterol was added.

Tertiary Prevention Studies in Man

Intervention trials in the general population, although feasible, do not seem fruitful and advisable, because of the enormous number of probands and the long follow-up time that would be necessary to show even a small difference in expected events. Therefore, all studies so far have been performed in well-defined groups at high risk of developing manifest colon cancer from precancerous lesions or of recurrence after cancer surgery. They are summarized in Table 3.

Despite the limited number of trials and persons studied, the picture seems somewhat clearer than in animals: ascorbic acid, alone or in combination with

Table 3. Dietary prevention studies in man

	Anticarcinogen tested, dose	Effect[a]	Reference
Risk groups	Vitamin C, 3 g	↓ polyp area and labeling	Bussey et al. 1982
	Vitamin C, 4 g α-Tocopherol, 400 mg Wheat fiber, 22.5 g	↓	De Cosse et al. 1975, 1989
	Vitamin C, 400 mg Vitamin E, 400 mg	↓	McKeown-Eyssen et al. 1988
	Calcium, 1.25–1.5 g	↓ Labeling	Rozen et al. 1989
	Calcium, 1.5 g	↓ labeling	Buset et al. 1986
	Calcium, 1.25 g	↓ labeling	Lipkin and Newmark 1985
Adjuvant	γ-Linolenic acid	–	McIllmurray and Turkie 1987

[a] See footnote to Table 2.

vitamin E, can reduce the number, surface area, and proliferative activity of adenomatous colon polyps and may consequently delay recurrence, and hopefully also malignant transformation, of these polyps. The same effect may be achieved by an increased intake of calcium; calcium can revert the pathologically elevated enzyme ornithine decarboxylase – a hallmark of abnormal cellular proliferation (Newmark et al. 1984; Lipkin and Newmark 1985). At least two big intervention trials are under way in Europe (Heidelberg and Dijon), the results of which are eagerly awaited. Wargovich (cited in Moon and Micozzi 1989), however, points out that addition of calcium to the diet will not be a simple solution; calcium is bound by many dietary factors, including phosphate, fiber, phytate, and oxalates. Phytate itself stimulates colonic proliferation and may by its strong affinity to calcium lead to dietary insufficiency of this element. The interplay between ionic calcium and dietary lipids is also complex: the calcium transport facilitating agents (such as vitamin D) are critical. Unfortunately, selenium has hardly been studied prospectively at all so far. Calcium, vitamins C and E, and selenium would constitute a very easy and cheap means of reducing the incidence and mortality of one of the most frequent cancers in western countries, by retarding malignant transformation of well-defined and repeatedly examinable premalignant conditions. It may be crucial to apply tumor-inhibiting agents as early as possible, because the growth inhibiting effect disappears in manifest cancer (Buset et al. 1986). Anticarcinogens could also prevent recurrence of surgically removed colon cancer – a very promising venture, which could and should be studied prospectively as soon as possible.

Putting the Puzzle Together

The jigsaw puzzle is still in pieces, the picture not yet fully visible, but it can be imagined. I can only repeat Bresalier's and Kim's comments in their brilliant editorial on the subject (1985): "The role of diet in the genesis of colorectal cancer remains unclear. The complex nature of what we eat, and of our response to it, makes it difficult to define how individual dietary components affect us. Clinical trials are therefore essential in testing hypotheses generated by epidemiological and laboratory observations."

I have to leave you with the unifinished puzzle, with hypotheses, many experimental and few clinical data – which are not sufficient to make specific recommendations about how to change our undoubtedly cancer-promoting diet to a cancer-preventing one. But chemoprevention of cancer is possible in animals – why should it not be in man? We have to remind ourselves over and over again that carcinogens and anticarcinogens are species, tissue, organ, dose, and timing specific (Bertram et al. 1987) and operate over long periods of time. This implies that, even if laboratory studies are highly suggestive of a beneficial effect, only large, long-term intervention trials in humans with specific pathological alterations will provide definitive answers. There seems little doubt that, if chemoprevention works, it will be highly cost-effective and far more desirable than, for example, chemotherapy (Bertram et al. 1987). The goal is clear – to improve and to prolong the life of gastrointestinal cancer patients and those at risk of it. A high goal, but not unreachable!

References

Bertram JS, Kolonel LN, Meyskens FL (1987) Rationale and strategies for chemoprevention of cancer in humans Cancer Res 47: 3012–3031

Birt DF, Lawson TA, Julius AD, Runice CE, Salmasi S (1982) Inhibition by dietary selenium of colon cancer induced in the rat by *bis*-(2-oxopropyl)nitrosamine. Cancer Res 42: 4455–4459

Bresalier RS, Kim YS (1985) Putting the puzzle together. N Engl J Med 313: 1413–1414

Buset M, Lipkin M, Winawer S, Swaroop S, Freidman E (1986) Inhibition of human colonic epithelial cell proliferation by calcium. Cancer Res 46: 5426–5430

Bussey HJ, DeCosse JJ, Deschner EE, Eyers AA, Lesser ML, Morson BC, Ritchie SM, Thomson JPS, Wadsworth J (1982) A randomized trial of ascorbic acid in polyposis coli. Cancer 50: 1434–1439

Colacchio TA, Memoli VA (1986) Chemoprevention of colorectal neoplasms. Arch Surg 121: 1421–1439

Colacchio TA, Memoli VA, Hildebrandt L (1989) Antioxidants vs carotenoids. Arch Surg 124: 217–221

Cook MG, McNamara P (1980) Effect of dietary vitamin E on DMH-induced colonic tumors in mice. Cancer Res: 40: 1329–1331

DeCosse JJ, Adams MB, Kuzma JF, LoGerfo P, Condon RE (1975) Effect of ascorbic acid on rectal polyps of patients with familial polyposis. Surgery 78: 608–612

DeCosse JJ, Hille HH, Lesser ML (1989) Effect of wheat fiber and vitamins C and E on rectal polyps in patients with familial adenomatous polyposis. J Natl Cancer Inst 81: 1290–1297

Diet, Nutrition and Cancer (1982), National Academy Press, Washington

Jones FE, Komorowski FA, Condon RE (1981) Chemoprevention of DMH-induced large bowel neoplasms. Surg Forum 31: 435–437

Knekt P, Aromaa A, Maatela J, Alfthan G, Aaran RK, Teppo L, Hakama M (1988) Serum vitamin E, selenium and the risk of gastrointestinal cancer. Int J Cancer 42: 846–850

Lipkin ML, Newmark H (1985) Effect of added dietary calcium on colonic epithelial proliferation in subjects at high risk for familial colonic cancer. N Engl J Med 313: 1381–1384

McIllmurray MB, Turkie W (1987) Controlled trial of c-linolenic acid in Duke's colorectal cancer. Br Med J 294: 1260

McKeown-Eyssen G, Holloway C, Jazmaji V, Bright-See E, Dion P, Bruce WR (1988) A randomized trial of vitamins C and E in the prevention of recurrence of colorectal polyps. Cancer Res 48: 4701–4705

Moon TE, Micozzi MS (1989) Nutrition and cancer prevention. Karger, Basel

Newmark HL, Wargovich MJ, Bruce WR (1984) Colon cancer and dietary fat, phosphate, and calcium: a hypothesis. J Natl Cancer Inst 72: 1323–1325

Reddy B, Hirota N, Katayama S (1982) Effect of dietary sodium ascorbate on DMH or MH-induced colon carcinogenesis. Carcinogenesis 3: 1097–1099

Rozen P, Fireman Z, Fine N, Wax Y, Ron E (1989) Oral calcium suppresses increased rectal epithelial proliferation of persons at risk of colorectal cancer. Gut 30: 650–655

Tempero MA, Knott KK, Zetterman RK (1988) Relationship of dietary cholesterol and cellulose in the prevention of colon cancer. Cancer Detect Prev 13: 41–54

Toth P, Patil K (1983) Enhancing effect of vitamin E on murine intestinal tumorigenesis by DMH hydrochloride. J Natl Cancer Inst 70: 1107–1111

Willett WC, MacMahon B (1984) Diet and cancer – an overview. N Engl J Med 310: 633–638, 697–703

Alternative Dietary Therapies in Cancer Patients

M. Hunter

The Royal Marsden Hospital, Fulham Road, London, SW3 6JJ, United Kingdom

The term "alternative dietary therapy" refers to such unorthodox dietary modifications as claim to cure or treat cancer. The conditions and claims for such therapies are varied, confusing and often contradictory.

Most alternative dietary therapies originate from the eastern world, where diet and changes in diet have been used for many years to treat disease. These diets have often been suggested for most degenerative diseases, but nowadays their popularity and accredited success is mainly linked to patients with cancer. These diets – such as the Bristol Diet, Macrobiotics, Gerson Therapy, etc. – have in common the philosophy that bad diet can cause cancer and therefore a good diet can cure it. They also share the same basic dietary guidelines:

Strict vegetarian/vegan regimes
Large amounts of raw food
No sugar
Low salt
Juices
High dose vitamins and minerals

In more detail, this means:
No meat, fish or fowl
No dairy products
No animal protein
High doses of vitamin C
High doses of vitamin E
Pancreatic enzymes
Coffee enemas

These dietary regimes result in such problems as:

High bulk
Low energy content
Difficulty of preparation

Recent Results in Cancer Research, Vol. 121
© Springer-Verlag Berlin · Heidelberg 1991

High cost
Conflicting advice

In general, the harm that can result from these regimes far outweighs the benefits (Hunter 1988).

The success of and benefit to many patients following such diets is not, I believe, due to the nutritional content of the diet – a particular vitamin or mineral, for instance – but to their psychological effect. The so-called placebo effect has aroused interest in the medical world since the 1950s, when placebo-controlled trials were introduced as a means of testing the efficacy of drug treatments. It has been deduced since, in many studies, that significant placebo responses have been reported for at least a substantial majority of treated patients. It is in the area of pain control where the most extensive results have been obtained, many scientists claiming 35% or more patients responding to a placebo with relief from pain (Richardson 1989).

There also seems little doubt from research that the style of treatment administration can have an effect on the outcome of the treatment. The confidence and concern with which a treatment is administered appears to affect its strength of action. The behaviour of the therapist, be it doctor or dietitian, may have a subtle yet forceful influence on the patient's response to a placebo, and an important influence on patient satisfaction (Hovland et al. 1953; Richardson 1989).

My reason for stating this evidence is that it may substantiate the claims made for the beneficial effects alternative diets have on many patients. How?

1. *Expectancy effects.* The patient's expectation may be predictive of the outcome of treatment. The diets are extremely well presented – they appear credible. The therapist discusses outcome at a general level and then, more specifically, strange claims – for example, the suggestion that taking extra co Q 10 in tablet form may enhance metabolism – or relate evidence specifically to a particular cancer, e.g., colon cancer, breast cancer. The diets are presented logically, attractively and convincingly, often using scientific jargon to give substance or force. The patient therefore believes the treatment to be successful and it may be so.

2. *Cognitive dissonance.* The psychological theory of cognitive dissonance states that when a patient holds two or more beliefs which are inconsistent with each other, a state of tension (dissonance) arises which motivates the patient to reduce the inconsistency. The belief that no therapeutic change has occurred is potentially inconsistent with the knowledge of having received treatment. In the case of these diets, the facts that (a) the patient sought out the diet, (b) they cause discomfort/inconvenience, and (c) they are costly can be inconsistent with the idea that there is no benefit. The patient may therefore alter his or her perception of the occurrence of change, increasing the perceived benefits. There is much evidence of this happening in placebo research.

3. *Anxiety reduction.* That the reduction of anxiety may be responsible for certain placebo effects has been well documented. The influence of anxiety on symptom levels could be direct or may be via the influence of the perception of anxiety. Whichever it is, the most common reason why patients follow alternative diets is that it enables them to gain control. Gaining control→reduced anxiety→decreased symptoms→increased well being. (This obviously can have the opposite effect, however, where patients struggling with a diet actually increase their anxiety and so on.)

4. *Therapist effect.* These dietary regimes are usually advocated by very powerful individuals or groups, often with some background in psychotherapy – in fact, they are often referred to as counsellors. Those that I have met are single-minded and resolute and often very sincere and concerned. These factors increase the patient's expectation, confidence and belief in the regime.

What I am proposing is that alternative diets are in fact a form of psychotherapy – and not a nutritional therapy at all. I put it to you that if we devised a detailed, well-balanced nutritional regime and delivered it with the same consideration to the above factors as alternative practitioners do, we would achieve equal benefit, if not more, because we would not be inflicting any nutritional harm.

The individual nutrients or regimes are there as a structure on which to hang the psychotherapeutic interventions. The harmful effect of these diets is, I believe, related to the nutrients (or lack of nutrients). Their positive effect is due to the psychotherapeutic intervention. I hope that further research in this field will help to discover if what I propose is true. If it is, it would go a long way to explaining that which is already known: "If you don't believe it, it won't work!"

References

1. Hovland CI, Janis IL, Kelley HH (1953) Communication and pursuasion: psychological studies of opinion change. Yale University Press, New Haven
2. Hunter M (1988) Unproven dietary methods of treatment in oncology patients. In: Senn HJ, Glaus A, Schmid L (eds) Supportive care in cancer patients. Springer, Berlin Heidelberg New York, pp 235–238 (Recent results in cancer research, vol 108)
3. Richardson P (1989) Placebos: the effectiveness and modes of action. In: Broome A (ed) Health psychology. Chapman and Hall, London

Psychological Aspects of Malnutrition in Cancer Patients

R. Kreibich-Fischer

Goethestraße 33c, 1000 Berlin 37, FRG

The psychological problems of malnutrition in patients in the final stages of cancer are only a part of a series of psychological processes which revolve around the topic of nutrition during the entire illness. I would like to develop my topic with this in mind, as I describe the psychological aspects of nutrition, improper diet, malnutrition and weight control in connection with the development of the illness in the patient.

A breast cancer patient of mine recently remarked, "How could I have been living with cancer for so long already and not noticed anything? – I hadn't lost any weight at all." In this she betrayed a misconception held by many people about cancer: that its first signs are those of weight loss and emaciation. Actually, most patients nowadays (and this is partly due to early detection) arrive at the hospital for diagnosis in good general condition, without any signs of malnutrition.

The first phase of the illness (see Table 1) might be characterized by anger, helplessness, or resignation, depending on the individual patient. The patients have to deal with the question "Why me?", with the altered reality of their social realms, with fear and sorrow. They must learn to accept the day-to-day routine of the hospital, with its extensive diagnostic procedures and therapies and its impervious assimilation. During this time, psychotherapeutic intervention mainly involves translating the strange, new messages and signals for them as well as in reducing their fears. These are mainly fears of isolation due to the illness and fears of loss of personal integrity. However, patients are also afraid of being confronted with the possibility of an early death which is no longer someone's but may rather be their own. From the psycho-therapeutic point of view, then, this first phase of the illness is really more comparable to a crisis intervention. I, personally, have seldom had patients in this phase who were conscious of possible pathological factors like improper diet of psychological stress. The question of nutrition is often regarded as irrelevant to the illness and is usually dismissed as of negligible importance.

Recent Results in Cancer Research, Vol. 121
© Springer-Verlag Berlin · Heidelberg 1991

Table 1. Psychological phases in cancer in relation to nutrition

---

Phase I:
- Diagnosis shock
- "Why me?"
- Assimilation to hospital routine
- Changes in social realms
- Fear of illness and possible death
- Nutrition is not a topic of interest

Phase II:
- "What can I learn from this illness?"
- Development of a subjective theory of the illness
- Task of abandoning a passive attitude to the illness to allow for active strategies for coming to terms with it
- Change in attitude to diet as a possible factor in recovery from and cure of the cancer

Phase III:
- Fear due to progression of the illness
- Dependence on being free of pain
- Food intake becomes a central problem
- Weight control strongly influences psychological disposition

Phase IV:
- Frequent malnutrition
- Patient loses interest in regular food intake
- Interference in communication from excess attention by family/friends to food intake and weight of the patient
- Coming to terms with the reality of death between patient and family/friends

---

I would like to designate the next phase (phase II) as "Insight into what is necessary". Since I am concerned with psychotherapy as well as with research on social support in overcoming the illness and in the changing attitudes towards the meaning of life in cancer patients, this phase of the illness is especially important to me personally. It intersects with the topic at hand in that here the various aspects of the illness are being addressed intellectually and patients' subjective theories of illness are being developed. The question, "Why me?" is expanded to include that of "What can I learn from this illness?"

Let me illustrate this with an example. In a recent conversation, Mrs. M. told me, "Well, to tell the truth, I don't really know anything about myself. I've never actually thought about it before." We had been talking about two areas in her life: her physical and psychological needs and her habits, especially those of smoking and of diet. Mrs. M.: "I had already sometimes thought that I shouldn't be smoking so much, but I'd never thought there was anything wrong with my diet, I thought it was 'normal'." In answer to the question about what she considered "normal", she listed a number of food items which, from the nutritional, physiological point of view – in no way contributed to healthy maintenance of her body. She had never had any idea how her body processed the food it took in, or how it could utilize it or eliminate it because it contained too many harmful elements. About her needs, she was able to say it had always been important to her that things were going well with her family and that everyone was satisfied. "So does all this have anything to do with my cancer?" was her reply. She hesitatingly answered her own question by conceding a certain importance to smoking; she had read quite a bit about it.

In the following months, Mrs. M. entirely gave up her passive attitude to her illness, as indeed many patients eventually do. She sought information not only about the psychological aspects of having cancer but also about the role diet may play in the illness. This helped her a lot because she felt that, by doing this, she would not just be passively undergoing therapy, but be actively taking part in the healing process. In the meantime she read a lot about natural foods and then had become unhappy because she was not able to apply this new knowledge immediately to her eating habits, because her treatment would keep her in hospital for several weeks. Having to eat hospital food became a new burden. She often had her family bring her food which she considered to be more nutritious. This process was connected throughout with the development of a kind of mania. She refused to eat sugar and pork whenever she was especially hungry for them. Her initial enthusiasm for home-ground muesli had to be given up because it was just too inconvenient. Revamping her diet became the driving force for many other processes in the changing values in the life of Mrs. M. Nevertheless, she went to a lot of trouble to recognize her own needs and to fulfill them. Even after her release from the hospital, and in the years which followed, Mrs. M. continued to hold fast to the principles she had acquired from having been ill, and with great success.

The third phase in which diet has increasingly gained in importance for the cancer patient is medically characterized by the sudden progression in the illness through metastasis and the consequent spread of tumors throughout the body. During the time before this, in which the patient has been undergoing adjuvant chemotherapy, he may have lost weight owing to lack of appetite, but he recovers relatively quickly and can soon regain his normal size through regular eating habits. In the metastasizing phase, however, a condition is reached in which even during a break from therapy, or after having stopped therapy altogether, the patient continues to lose weight. The consumption of food becomes – second only to pain therapy – the standard of measurement for the entire illness. One example of this would be Mr. Z., a patient suffering from a pancreatic carcinoma, although I have recorded similar phenomena in many other patients. Mr. Z. had, against the wishes of his doctors, kept himself going quite well despite his tumor by eating a radically different diet, until he began to lose weight drastically and quickly arrived at a state of malnourishment. Mr. Z. was not willing to come to terms with this new turn in his illness. Preoccupation with food intake and weight control filled the last weeks of his life. He would sometimes weigh himself twice a day, and a variation of 300 g in weight loss or gain would significantly determine his moods.

The fourth phase, the final stage, is frequently characterized by malnutrition in the patient. Often his interest in food intake and weight control declines as the illness progresses. At the same time, however, friends and family are usually especially aware of them. The patients are often then badgered by them about eating. The less willing both sides are to talk, the more nutrition and weight control will become the main topic whenever they do. Instead of caring concern about the well-being of the patient and experiencing a quiet sharing of his fate, they are busy plying the patient with food. This is not only a burden for the patient but can also interfere painfully in his coming to terms with his approaching death, as well as increase his fear.

The phases of progression and continuing malnutrition constitute a psychologically extreme situation in which hopelessness increases. Family and friends as well as hospital staff often busy themselves with the diet of the patient as a pretext to avoid the talks and gradual leave-taking from both sides which are in fact more necessary. Patients feel they have been left alone if attention paid to them comes only in the form of food distribution and other superfluous activities which hinder a quiet sharing of time. As a psychotherapist I regret that the patients' chances to reflect on the stations of their lives and organize their thoughts are often lost. Family and friends also miss out on an important chance: to be able to become aware of the reality of their own deaths through the passing away of one near to them.

My therapeutic intervention consists in trying to stimulate a willingness to converse on both sides and to increase a sensitivity and heightened awareness of this unique situation. I can see, however, that this depends to a large extent on the quality of the relationship before the onset of illness and that changes in this are limited.

I would like to conclude with some general remarks. I am of the opinion that in future nutrition will continue to be increasingly important not only to cancer patients but also to all concerned people. The more people realize that the occurrence of tumors is neither to be explained nor treated monocausally but that everything is connected with everything else, and that medical research will not be able to offer a cure for cancer in the immediate future, the more a turn in the direction of additive therapies and a change in diet will take place. This, indeed, is already happening to a great extent. Through this the idea has been born that nutrition stands in direct relationship to the strengthening or weakening of the immune system. Foods low in nutritional value are a burden to the system; those high in it assist the body. Nutrition is therefore of great psychological importance, because it is here, with food intake, that people can feel they are directly doing something for their health. This reduces their feeling of helplessness and strengthens ability to deal with the illness. Demands for change within society, too, will appear in two areas: first, changes in the types of food eaten (e.g. cutting out excess fat, reducing the intake of sweets and altering processed foods), and, secondly, insistence on control of the food contamination caused by air and soil pollution and chemical treatment. Here, pressure from society will be necessary.

I myself am not a nutritionist, since I am solely concerned with the psychological condition of cancer patients. I am not indifferent, however, to the role which nutrition plays in the lives of my patients. Proper diet as instrumental in the prevention of cancer and other illnesses appears to me to be of utmost importance.

Nevertheless, I do not believe – and this has been confirmed in my past experience – that for for tumors of a certain size, diet can have a positive effect in bringing about their reduction. If we were to take the burden off the health system in our industrialized society through proper diet, this would have to start, in my opinion, in childhood. I feel the introduction of "Nutrition" as a school subject, in which psychological aspects of wellness could be considered at the same time, would be viable and meaningful.

Everyone has a shared responsibility for health. Proper diet contributes to illness prevention, and is therefore a manifestation of responsible behaviour.

Psychosocial Support in Oncology

A Model for the Development of Psychosocial Interventions

G.H. Christ

Department of Social Work, Memorial Sloan Kettering Center, 1275 New York Avenue, New York, NY 10021, USA

Introduction

I have been asked to describe the methods and approaches used to develop new psychosocial services and programs for cancer patients in the United States. I don't know whether the driving force that makes it possible for us to develop new programs in the US has similarities to the force that can be used for the development of such programs in Europe or Canada. The basic issue in the US in developing a new program is the response of the market economy. Two critical questions that we must answer are, "Is there a need or desire among consumers for this program?" and, "Will this program be paid for? – by the patient, by insurance, by donations, etc." The driving force for developing new programs in many European countries and Canada may be quite different. Since, unlike the US, the European system of health care is largely tax-supported, you may have to answer a different set of questions: "Is a new service essential?" and "Can it replace another service that may be less vital?"

Of the two systems, ours in the US is the less controlled. Many of you may have heard that in the US, the proportion of the gross national product going for the payment of health care is the highest in the world. One specific illustration of the problems associated with this is the car manufacturers' fight against increased medical insurance costs. They claim that these health care costs add $500 to the cost of every car, and that this is almost twice that of other countries. So, while on the surface it may seem more humane to develop programs on the basis of expressed need and desire on the part of patients, as you will hear, the patient without sufficient money to pay for these services or without prepaid health insurance may not have access to care without the intervention of the social services. Over 40 million people in the United States are without health insurance. In our system, the day of reckoning for excessive spending for health care generally comes after the services are developed and the available monies are spent, rather than before, as it does in the Canadian and European systems.

Recent Results in Cancer Research, Vol. 121
© Springer-Verlag Berlin · Heidelberg 1991

Despite these differences, Dr. Senn and the conference planning committee felt it might be of interest to you to hear how we go about thinking about, planning for, developing, and implementing psychosocial programs in the United States.

I will be drawing from my own experience which comes primarily from MSKCC, where I am the director of social work. Memorial Sloan-Kettering Cancer Center (MSKCC) is a 565-bed cancer research center. Our department has 35 social work clinicians whose job it is to provide psychosocial interventions for cancer patients and 15 research staff. We are responsible to assist in the process of identifying patients who are at greater risk for developing problems with cancer and its treatment at all stages of the illness. However, we must also develop intervention programs that provide support to all patients treated at the center who are experiencing stress at various points in the disease and treatment process.

Disease Stage Model and Associated Programs

In the past 10 years, I have evolved a practical way of schematizing patient needs for psychosocial services. We have called this the disease stages model. While the whole experience of cancer and its treatment is stressful to patients, we have found that there are certain nodal points or stages around which patients experience special stress. Each of these stages confronts the patient with a fairly predictable series of psychosocial tasks. These tasks may change over time as the treatment and disease processes change, altering the psychosocial consequences to the patient. This model represents a way of evaluating the comprehensiveness of services and identifying areas where new programs need to be developed. Specific interventions and intervention programs are designed to assist the patient in fulfilling these psychosocial tasks. We have developed a number of different programs for patients with different diagnoses at different illness phases [1].

Some of the stage such as diagnosis and terminal illness, are very familiar; indeed, until 10 years ago these were the only stages addressed by the mental health clinician.

On the other hand the stresses of treatment termination, of normalization, and of survivorship have more recently been understood to be times of significant stress for patients. These three have in common that they confront the patient with leaving intense medical surveillance and returning to a culture that expects them to quickly take up where they left off before the cancer developed.

We have responded to the increasing complexity of patients' needs by developing a series of treatment modalities that enable us to meet the broad range of their needs over the ever-lengthening course of the illness stages. Essentially these modalities represent important modifications and elaborations of traditional mental health interventions used with patients seeking help for psychological stress. These modalities of intervention include, but are not limited to, the following:

Individual counselling and/or therapy
Group therapy
Family therapy
Resource provision or case management
Patient education
Crisis intervention
Behavioral interventions such as hypnosis and relaxation
Supportive therapy
Insight-oriented therapy

And I might add:

Play therapy with young children with cancer
Patient advocacy

Before I describe the development of a new set of programs for the post-treatment or survivor stage, let me first illustrate the relationship of stage to interventions with the examples of the diagnosis and treatment effects stages.

Diagnosis

Although patients often experience social and emotional disequilibrium in response to a diagnosis of cancer, we find that few request counselling, supportive interventions, psychiatric consultation, or even join a self-help group on their own. Most patients are unable to request psychosocial support for a variety of reasons. Some are psychologically immobilized and cannot exert the emotional energy needed to get help. Others think a request for support indicates an inability to cope, a loss of independence, or an acknowledgement of the presence of mental illness. They do not perceive their needs clearly, in part because there is little approval for admitting such needs in our society. Furthermore, most patients are unaware that counselling may help assuage the existential terror that is evoked by a diagnosis of cancer or alleviate grief over the loss of body function or appearance, or that it may restore a sense of control. Because patients have difficulty requesting and using these services, it is often useful to have them prescribed by physicians, to have them universally available, and to have them easily accessible.

Before I continue describing the services for the diagnosis stage, however, there is an additional continuum to the illness stage we have found helpful in planning services: this is the mentally ill–vulnerable–resilient continuum. Patients may be viewed as being at different points along a continuum of need for counselling services, from those who are seriously mentally ill, to those who are psychosocially vulnerable, to those whom we have labelled as resilient. Although the majority of cancer patients can benefit from some form of counselling, others *must* receive it if they are to maintain their functioning and avoid social and emotional breakdown.

Mentally Ill Patients. Our experience has been that cancer patients with a history of mental illness or psychiatric treatment generally have an ongoing relationship with one or more mental health services in the community that may need information about their medical condition. Such patients are encouraged to communicate with their therapists or reinitiate communication with their previous therapists about their medical condition. A hospital staff member can additionally develop confidential, professional collaboration with the community therapist, a collaboration which also includes the patient's cancer physician. For example, the diagnosis of cancer may exacerbate a patient's preexisting mental illness or seriously affect his or her day-to-day functioning. Early intervention may be able to prevent a breakdown in functioning that can have lasting negative effects such as the loss of a job or the severance of important social relationships and the alienation of friends and relatives.

Vulnerable Patients. A much larger group of patients have a variety of social and psychological characteristics that place them at risk of emotional and social breakdown when confronting a diagnosis of cancer. They are not mentally ill, but their difficulty in coping may interfere with daily functioning and treatment compliance. Such vulnerable patients include, for example, those who are:

- Living alone or have few friends or relatives available to help them
- Over age 75
- Children or young adults
- Financially stressed, e.g., having no or very limited insurance coverage
- Parents of dependent children
- Multiply stressed – who have experienced a great deal of life stress or who are in the midst of other life crises, such as the recent loss of a job or a divorce
- Members of family situations characterized by high levels of conflict, for example, a previous history of violence or abuse
- Ill with other diseases or whose family members are ill, especially with cancer, which may lead them to have difficulty in being realistic about their own diagnosis and prognosis
- Subject to high levels of anxiety or depression or maladaptive coping behaviors such as treatment avoidance or substance abuse
- Very different culturally from the dominant culture of the health care staff or who have a different language than the health care staff

Often patients with these high risk characteristics are more difficult to identify than those with diagnosed mental illnesses. A system for early identification of such high risk patients, reinforced by physician recommendation for counselling services, can prevent major problems in treatment compliance.

Resilient Patients. At the other end of the continuum from patients with diagnosed mental illnesses are those who appear to be resilient, with good psychological and social resources. They may be considered "low risk" on the psychosocial continuum and therefore their psychological and support needs may be overlooked by professionals. Such individuals need to be informed of available support services because they can make rapid and highly effective use of them, especially education and group services. They often resent not having access to such services. As one patient said, "I knew I could cope well with a cancer diagnosis and I did, but I might have coped better with some help and would have liked to have known about counselling that could have been available to me."

The recent findings of Spiegel and associates may support the validity of the resilient patients' concerns [2]. In a 1-year randomized prospective study of metastatic breast cancer patients randomly assigned to group therapy or no group therapy (control), the patients who had group therapy had lower mood-disturbance scores on the Profile of Mood State scale, had fewer maladaptive coping responses, and were less fearful than the control group. Spiegel recently reported on a 10-year followup of this group [3]. Most surprisingly, he found that those participating in the group therapy on average lived a year and a half longer than those in the control group. Further research may clarify how the intervention affected survival time.

There are four tasks that need to be confronted by the cancer patient during the stage of diagnosis:

1. Coping with the confrontation with one's own mortality
2. Coping with the emotional overwhelm that is a part of the diagnostic process
3. Moving from denial of the reality of the disease to constructive processing of disease and treatment information
4. Making decisions about the appropriate treatment

All patients report that the diagnostic process involves a confrontation with the reality of one's mortality, even if the biopsy proves to be negative. They are emotionally overwhelmed and often say that for them life will never be the same again because they will always have a heightened sense of their own personal vulnerability. Interventions need to be aimed at ways of quickly reducing patients' anxiety in order to enable them to integrate the information they need to make vital treatment decisions.

Critical interventions during diagnosis include education, the provision of information, and crisis intervention. In fact there are few programmatic interventions offered systematically to patients and their families during the diagnostic process.

One intervention at diagnosis is the Sunday admissions program at MSKCC [4]. Group sessions are conducted by social workers to orient family members to the hospital system and medical procedures, informing them about, for example, where to wait for the results of surgery, how to find out information about such things as visiting hours, housing and parking, and the availability of support services. This begins to restore their sense of control over their environment and helps to contain anxiety. Patient volunteers also attend these groups. These are recovered patients who have regained a good deal of their former level of functioning and who are trained to share their experiences effectively with other patients. Their very presence reduces family members' anxiety as they demonstrate the potential to survive and continue living effectively. The patient volunteers provide information about the illness and treatment experience, the usual thinking and feeling states of the patient, and make suggestions about useful ways of communicating about the distress caused by the experience. Both the information and the experience of talking with a recuperated patient are reassuring to families and therefore facilitate a better understanding of the issues.

A veteran patient visit with the newly diagnosed patient is also offered during this admissions process. Patients have described feeling reassured by a discussion with another patient at diagnosis. Veteran patients who have completed their treatment and returned to normal life can be especially helpful when appropriately trained and supervised. Their contact with the patient can rapidly instill a powerful feeling of optimism and hope. One patient, Mrs. L., left the hospital and returned to her office after receiving the diagnosis of breast cancer. She described herself as being in a state of disbelief that such a strong person as herself could be so vulnerable. She felt as though her life had ended. Because she had experience as a senior executive in her company, she was able to appear composed and in control until she closed her office door. When her secretary discovered her in tears, she offered to contact Mrs. L.'s husband. That night a friend who had had breast cancer learned of her plight and phoned to share her treatment experience and her return to normal living. Mrs. L. said that it was hard to describe the enormous relief she experienced after this conversation. "For the first time I believed I would live." We are planning to offer such veteran patient contact in a more systematic way in the new Off Site Breast Center planned at MSKCC.

Treatment Side Effects

There are four tasks patients need to confront during the stage we call "treatment side effects." These are:

1. Rebuilding self-esteem in the face of effects such as the loss of a body part, hair loss, weight loss, and fatigue
2. Coping with the ambivalence about treatment caused by such negative effects of treatment
3. Developing ways to have some control of side effects
4. Incorporating the physical demands of treatment into ongoing personal and family life

Patients often need to learn specific strategies for coping with the impact of negative treatment effects on their physical and psychological functioning. These symptoms may cause people to become ambivalent about continuing treatment and hence they may fail to comply with treatment requirements or terminate treatment altogether. Interventions used at this stage include group and individual emotional support of the patient, visits from veteran patients, obtaining financial and other practical assistance, and learning relaxation and other behavioral techniques.

The Breast Surgery Rehabilitation Group [5] developed by social work at MSKCC is an example of a group intervention aimed at helping patients cope with the effects of treatment. Ninety-five percent of all patients undergoing breast surgery attend this group which is co-led by a nurse, physical therapist, and a patient-to-patient volunteer three times a week. The goal of the group is to inform patients of the physical and psychological tasks of recovery from their surgery and to normalize many of their reactions and concerns. In addition to information about physical recovery, patients learn about universal reactions such as fears of recurrence, changes in body image, reluctance to communicate with others about the surgery, and problems with depression and emotional control. In this way they are encouraged to become active participants in their physical and psychological rehabilitation.

Recent medical findings have led to a dramatic increase in the number of women receiving adjuvant chemotherapy for breast cancer. These women face the crisis of chemotherapy before the crisis of a breast cancer diagnosis has been resolved. They need reassurance that they are not being treated with chemotherapy because of documented cancer metastasis, but because they are at increased statistical risk of metastases. In fact, as adjuvant therapy is recommended to increasing numbers of women who are node-negative, it is viewed by them less as a statement of a poor prognosis and more as a routine treatment for the disease.

In addition to hair loss, women face a series of physically debilitating side effects, ranging from mouth sores and fatigue to decreased resistance to infection, and sometimes severe nausea and vomiting. Furthermore, women must cope with the ambiguity surrounding the need for this treatment, the persistent reminder of disease caused by ongoing treatment, financial expense, and the difficulty of managing ongoing family and work responsibilities.

We have found that patients benefit enormously from frank discussions of treatments effects and advance preparation for how they will cope with them. For example, they can plan dietary changes, organize time for exercise, purchase a wig, and learn ways of using make-up to improve their appearance. The Look Good, Feel Better program, sponsored by the American Cancer Society, offers free make-up consultation to these patients. Patients also benefit from learning relaxation and other stress reduction techniques in advance of treatment so they have an additional means of coping with nausea, vomiting, and symptoms of anxiety. Their experience of adjuvant chemotherapy can be dramatically altered by such advance preparation and development of specific coping skills for managing symptoms and side effects.

Normalization and Survivorship

Because of the large increase in cancer survivors, we have been concentrating our attention in the last 3 years on the special needs of the cancer patient who may be cured of the disease or living with it in remission. The general processes involved in the development of any new program in our center include

1. Identification of the problem
2. Assessment of extent and pervasiveness of the need
3. Piloting interventions
4. Implementing a program of interventions. These include finding funding, space, etc.
5. Evaluation of the effectiveness of the program

We encountered an unusual problem in identifying the problems for which psychosocial intervention is indicated among cancer survivors. Initially, research focused on the physical late effects of cancer treatment. Gradually, more research looked at the psychosocial consequences of these late effects. This research, however, was limited because it relied on the more traditional markers of patient emotional disorders such as clinical depression and clinical anxiety. Such symptoms were not generally found in these patients who were now off treatment. The whole framework that we had used for identifying needs for patients who were still on treatment was less germane to patients in the post-treatment period. We had used the framework of severe emotional distress as a flag for the need to develop a new intervention. We were looking for acute stress, severe depression, acute disorganization of family or planning ability etc.

These findings, however, did not fit with our clinical experiences with survivors and with our gut feelings based on contact with patients who were now off treatment. Survivor patients told us something different. The survivors, some of whom volunteered at the center, served on our boards, wrote books about their cancer experience, and others, all shared a quieter but still powerfully felt chronic disfunction: a general anomie, malaise, a tendency to frequent rumination; i.e., a more subtle but quite possibly important psychological barrier to optimal function.

For example, while most breast cancer patients resume their prediagnosis life style in a physical and mechanical way, they often say that while they may appear well and behave "normally," emotionally they do not feel the same as they did before the diagnosis. Indeed, patients often say they felt frustrated and distressed by the general lack of awareness and understanding among the public of the types of residual psychosocial difficulties the cancer survivor may experience. They feel they are often reminded they are "lucky" to have survived a potentially fatal illness. They consequently feel unable to assert their needs or express their resentment and anger over the social, psychological, and physical sequelae of their illness and its treatment.

Patients may also be reluctant to discuss their dissatisfactions or concerns about their lives following successful treatment with their physicians [6, 7]. They worry that they will be regarded as being ungrateful for having their lives saved, or as neurotic. They may also think it is inappropriate to burden their physician with psychosocial problems of adjustment.

Patients are further stressed by the notion commonly held in our culture that individuals should be able to emerge from a crisis "without missing a beat." This suggests that once treatment is over, patients should be able to pick up from where they left off before the diagnosis. However, most patients find that cancer constitutes a major discontinuity in their lives, bringing about lasting changes in the way they view themselves and their future possibilities. They feel their experience has made major changes in their self-concept, values, roles, and time perspective, and they cannot return to their former sense of self.

In our own center we worked closely with our veteran patient group, who were comfortable enough with us to share some of these experiences. These patients were often helpful in fund raising for the center as they became articulate in sharing their often very poignant experiences. From the more recent research [1], our own research on Hodgkin's disease survivors [7], and our own experiences with patients we identified the following tasks of normalization and survivorship:

1. Leaving the patient role
2. Resumption of normal activities with a change of time frame
3. Accepting remaining physical impairment
4. Coping with fear of recurrence
5. Rebuilding self-esteem with a new sense of self
6. Regaining a sense of competence, mastery, and control
7. Integrating changes in values, goals, and priorities

Three years ago, our chief physician became more aware of survivors' concerns and asked for the identification of programs that might address their needs. I developed the concept of a kind of clinic for cancer survivors that would offer a range of services to meet their psychosocial needs and that would foster the formation of a network of patients off treatment, through which they could find and relate to each other. Together with the Department of Psychiatry we developed what is now called the Post Treatment Resource Program to assist patients in accommodating these changes. Dr. Vincent DeVita, our new chief physician, has contributed enormously to the support and direction of this program.

Initially the program focused on individual counselling for patients, using a kind of mental health clinic model with some educational workshops. We soon learned from patients that while individual counselling is an essential component of such a program, they were more generally responsive to the education programs. We found that meeting with each other at workshops was a powerful motivation for patients' participation. Therefore we revised the programs offered to include the following:

1. A seminar series that provides updated information on current treatments, health promotion, and innovative strategies for improving the fabric of life after cancer
2. Open house meetings which offer informal meetings with other patients for sharing experiences and for socializing with others who had had similar life experiences. These are run by a professional staff member and a patient volunteer and organized around a specific topic. Once a month they function to orientate patients newly leaving treatment to the services of the program.
3. Ongoing group sessions that provide a forum for working on problems participants are experiencing in adapting to physical and psychosocial changes following treatment
4. Individual consultation for help with specific adjustment problems
5. Employment and insurance consultation to advocate for patients who encounter obstacles and discrimination in these areas. This can represent a special problem in our system where patients may lose their insurance after having cancer or may not be eligible for insurance if they change jobs. They may be unable to find jobs as employers are reluctant to insure them. These are some of the unfortunate consequences of our health care system.

In its 1st full year of operation over 1500 patients participated in these programs. The breast cancer groups that meet in the Post Treatment Program generally address a range of issues including a sense of vulnerability, fear of recurrence, and uncertainty about the future; a loss of a sense of control and mastery over the exigencies of life; and changed relationships with family, friends, and colleagues. The central theme of the group is often the fear of recurrence and all the images and fantasies associated with recurrent disease; pain, debilitation, dependency, and death. This fear affects patients' sense of self and lowers self-esteem. They may describe themselves as "in the community of people with the dreaded disease," "on the other side of the line," "different and less than others." While they are now physically strong enough to return to work and participate in family life, they may feel they are going through the motions of life without full participation.

The group members search for the meaning in their experience as they work to regain a sense of mastery and control over their lives. Through sharing of emotions and assisting in problem solving, the women are able to integrate their experience in a more positive way. Regularly patients report increased assertiveness in daily activities. They share newfound strengths and coping techniques. One patient was able to pursue legal advice for a problem she had been fearful of for several years: "If I could get through a mastectomy and chemotherapy I can face anything." Another patient who had been hurt by her family's perceived lack of support was able to contact them and discuss her disappointments. As the group progresses, patients are able to reframe their experience and find meaning in their struggle. By the end of the group sessions they generally feel they have achieved significant emotional growth and strength as a result of their cancer experience. While the threat of recurrence still exists, it no longer pervades their lives. They are able to see this "threat" in a positive way. As one patient explained, "The difference between us and others is a matter of delusion. Others believe they can control their futures; cancer patients no longer have that delusion. I know I must make the most of each day."

Funding for the Post Treatment Program staff includes patient insurance reimbursement and fees for group and individual therapy, and a major donation that served to provide the support of the basic staff. The staff now includes one full-time coordinator, one half-time insurance and employment specialist, and one secretary. A number of psychiatry and social work staff work as group leaders in the evenings, paid on a consultant basis. Other center staff also contribute their time. Dr. Jimmie Holland is the medical director, I am the program director, and an administrator from the hospital assists with budgets, personnel etc. Medical staff function as the major faculty for the seminar series.

Conclusion

In the development of a new program to address specific needs, given our market economy, we are most successful if we follow the sequence of determining the presence of an unmet need, defining the extent or pervasiveness of that need within the subpopulation, and identifying practical ways of meeting that need. We then pilot interventions. We then concern ourselves with the financial feasibility of implementing these wonderful ideas. In the US, the rocks on which the boat of good ideas primarily founders is the latter – the financial feasibility. Although I have presented the way in which new programs can be developed within the context of a capitalist market system, my hope is that some of these ideas may have a practical utility to those of you working within a government-sponsored and-controlled, tax-based health system.

References

1. Christ G, Adams-Greenly M (1984) Therapeutic strategies at psychosocial crisis points in the treatment of childhood cancer. In: Christ AE, Flomenhaft K (eds) Childhood cancer: impact on the family. Plenum NY, pp 109–128
2. Spiegel D, Bloom J, Yalom ID (1981) Group support for patients with metastatic breast cancer. Arch Gen Psychiatry 38: 527
3. Spiegel D, Bloom JR, Kraemer HC, Gottheil E (1989) Effect of psychosocial treatment on survival of patients with metastatic breast cancer. Lancet: 888–891
4. Mastrovito R, Moynihan R, Parsonnet L (1989) Self help and mutual support programs. In: Holland JC, Rowland JH (eds) Handbook of psychooncology. Oxford University Press, Oxford, pp 502–515
5. Christ GH, Bowles ME, Bauman TG, (1987) Educational and support groups for breast cancer patients and their families. In: Harris G, Hellman S, Henderson IG, Kinne DW (eds) Breast diseases. Lippincott, Philadelphia, pp 648–656

6. Christ GH (1987) Social consequences of the cancer experience. Am J Pediatr Hematol Oncol 9: 84–88
7. Siegel K, Christ GH (1990) Psychosocial consequences of long term survival of Hodgkin's disease. In: Lacher MJ, Redman JR (eds) Hodgkin's disease: the consequences of survival. Lea and Febiger, Philadelphia, pp 383–399

Aspects of Nonverbal Communication

S. Porchet-Munro

Medizinische Klinik C, Kantonsspital, 9007 St. Gallen, Switzerland

It is within the interventions and exchanges directly concerned with psychosocial support that patients often dare to reveal the many issues of nonverbal communication which increase their difficulties in dealing with cancer and the various treatment situations. For, rightly or wrongly, some cringe at the infringements on their personal space or the sterility of the clinical environment; some feel intimidated and/or baffled by the double messages of body language; some fear and mistrust the eye expressions of care givers; but most of these patients argue within themselves that they should be able to cope with such adversities and not let them have such impact, while, on the other hand, care givers often tend to think of themselves as experts at interpreting nonverbal messages from their patients and family but frequently are oblivious of their own.

Patients receive potent messages through these nonverbal channels – messages which at times seem to undermine the best intended supportive care, the most carefully chosen words, or the most skilfully administered treatment. Let us therefore consider some of the dimensions of what happens at a nonverbal level in patient care.

Environment

One may consider the nonverbal impact of the clinical environment of little importance, but this dimension can enhance or counteract the multiple efforts to treat and support the patient. An individual who is confronted with a lifethreatening disease and is facing the unknown impact of various treatments often finds it very difficult to cope with the environment in which s/he is placed.

The view from a hospital bed, of hospital hallways or hospital equipment may become the only views to see for weeks. Depending on whatever else happens in those weeks, this will be of greater or lesser consequence. If we remember how much a person is influenced, motivated, renewed, touched or moved by the impressions which s/he takes in, and how we seek out views to recharge our spirit, we may begin to grasp the impact of a drab environment on an ill person. Emptily staring at a bare ceiling or wall or at a picture which does not speak to the individual reflects for some patients the emptiness they feel within themselves. Sensitive care givers, on the other hand, can add immeasurable support if they are aware of the potent messages of the individual person's need to see meaningful things, and take the initiative to creatively change a drab environment. The patient who spontaneously creates his/her own environment with personal things, even in the hospital, and thus consciously keeps a healthy perspective close at hand is rather rare and often younger. Staff see such a patient far more as the individual s/he was before becoming ill and themselves relate to the person accordingly.

For many patients, the evidence of failing strength and loss of independence is almost unbearable and again often outweighs the efforts of staff to provide psychosocial support. Little things, such as an overhead light left on which can't be turned off because one is too weak to move or in pain, a commode advertising to every visitor the extent of one's helplessness, or the sight of a cane, symbolizing growing dependence – all these are nonverbal messages we often don't notice.

On the other hand, attention to a detail – a flower moved into the field of vision, a decoration on a meal tray or the occasional use of pretty china to contrast with everyday hospital ware – may break through sadness or lift a depressed spirit where words fail to have effect.

Body Language

Body language is inescapably tied to all interactions but rarely receives close attention. Of course, when one is confronted with explicit examples of body language, such as in mime or the silent movies of Charlie Chaplin, and watches the hundred and one ways in which the body talks, one is amused and things seem very obvious. Few of us, however, have sharpened our awareness about our own personal body language, despite the reality that a major part of all communication happens through body signals, gestures, mimicry and actions (Morris 1978). Molcho (1988) suggests that up to 80% of our decisions are influenced by such nonverbal communication.

Our posture, our particular way of moving, with its speed and rhythm;our gestures, some of them acquired in childhood, influenced by culture and reflecting our upbringing: all these speak – not infrequently more strongly than or contrary to our words – and influence the way we are perceived by others. It is body language which we use consciously or unconsciously to assert a particular position or rank, to reflect attitudes or emphasize our words: "One could – on the one hand – wait and re-examine your status in 3 months, or one could try – on the other hand (*with a higher hand gesture, indicating a preference*) – giving you another cycle of chemotherapy."

Our body language influences the body language of others – we mirror or complement the body of others. Body language also gives away our uncertainties, our tensions, our ambivalent feelings when we would least like them to show. It unmasks words. While we may pretend to be giving a patient our attention facially, our body may be indicating that we are only half present or anxious to leave, with a foot already pointing to the door. This may be a posture chosen on purpose to indicate to the patient that we need to leave, but it may also be taken up unconsciously when the subject of conversation is difficult or emotionally charged.

When a delicate issue is discussed with a patient, tension behaviours or compulsive gestures in the care giver, such as lip biting, head scratching or fiddling with the stethoscope may betray the carefully chosen words intended to reassure the patient.

On the other hand, the patient's nonverbal body messages are often skilfully overlooked if they speak of defence or withdrawal when treatment options are under discussion.

In a crisis situation, the eyes of patients read signals from the movement of care givers. Consciously measured movements will project calm, and transmit reassurance and an impression of competence, while hurried rushing around may not necessarily get a task accomplished more quickly but will certainly add to the impression of tension and danger the patient receives. At the same time, the pace of rushing about also builds up unnecessary tension within the care giver.

Patients also observe carefully the body language of and between the different members of the care team, and watch for signs of agreement, indifference, disagreement or uncertainty.

Personal Space

Body language is closely related to personal space. "We don't know how much space is necessary to any individual man, but what is important in our study of body language is what happens to an individual man when his shell of space or territory is threatened" (Fast 1970). In everyday life situations, healthy individuals manoeuvre their movements and actions in order to have the space to suit their needs and liking, and if circumstances cramp their style for a time, they usually adjust easily. In general, one simply expects the same adjustment from patients to the given situation of a day clinic or an in-patient unit. Too frequently however, these settings exacerbate the suffering of someone who is having to cope with a lifethreatening illness, the uncertainties about the outcome of investigations, and or unpleasant treatments. Patients feel invaded, humiliated, manipulated or even outcast by what they experience.

Gerdes (1986), in pointing out that life of a patient diagnosed with cancer is simply never as before again, compares the experience of living with this disease to that of people sentenced to death without just cause and without knowing whether the sentence will be carried out or not. They have to wait . . . and wait . . . and watch as others come and go . . . and some don't come back. The dread of waiting for investigations, for answers, for treatments is difficult enough in itself, and the waiting areas, sometimes with closely arranged chairs in a hallway or some other waiting space, add to the tension and frustration.

Hospital situations often force the patient into an environment where comfortable personal space is neither considered nor respected but rather threatened. To have a stranger's bed only an arm's length away when one is having to cope with nausea, vomiting or diarrhoea is rarely what any person would choose. In the same way, the sharing of toilets adds to feelings of frustration or even humiliation.

The frequent lack of space makes for nightmares for patients and staff alike. Occasionally, taking a patient out of a room for an investigation can be reminiscent of moving day, and manoeuvring a chair to the bedside may be equally trying; thus, in such an environment, infringement of personal space is unavoidable. The patients know as well as the care givers and administrators that such circumstances cannot always readily be remedied, but this kind of rational reasoning cannot regenerate the cancer patient's battered self-esteem or compensate feelings of desolation, which thus are exasperated by circumstances.

Knowingly or unknowingly, care givers too invade the personal space of patients, whether while carrying out routine procedures or during other interactions. We bend over patients to inspect a symptom or a catheter, or bend down close in order to better understand the person. This is considered routine by the care giver, but in an "unreasonable" way makes the patient uneasy and uncomfortable. If s/he in turn manifests this uneasiness and withdraws however, the care giver may be baffled and become self-conscious.

Eye Expression/Eye Contact

All interpersonal interactions are accompanied and influenced by eye contact and eye expression, which to some degrees cannot be controlled. In cancer care, the topic of the nonverbal impact of eye expression and contact is rarely raised, yet patients always anxiously search the eyes of care givers for messages, and care givers interpret the patient's eye signals. What happens in these exchanges?

The dozens of possible movements of the skin around the eyes allow the signalling of almost any message. Not only are thoughts and emotions mirrored in the eyes, but emotional changes even affect the size of the pupils. Studies have indicated that the pupils expand when something excites us, whether in pleasurable or fearful anticipation (Morris 1978; Bonnafont 1979). These changes normally occur without our knowledge and are also largely beyond our control. Pupil signals are not only unconsciously transmitted, they are also unconsciously received. They constitute a secret exchange of signs operating below the level of contrived manners and posed expression, and are part of the phenomenon of visual communication. Eye expressions speak strongly and can leave us guessing, amused or perplexed at their messages. Eye contact feeds subjective projection and incites the transfer of feelings. Messages are sent and received at a speed which is often too fast for reason to intervene.

Eye contact is to some degree maintained or shifted by one's choosing, and in some cases partly dictated by culture, but again, a significant amount of eye manoeuvre escapes control. Eye movement is intimately tied to emotions and thoughts and can easily betray words and gestures. It is much easier to intend to "look someone straight in the eye" than to actually do so. When one looks into eyes, one sees beyond them, behind them; when others look into one's own eyes, one becomes vulnerable and exposed. If we do not look at a person, s/he becomes a "nonperson". Care givers or relatives and friends often exclude patients from conversations in this way: they talk "over their head", and this signals to the patient, "I shouldn't hear, I don't exist or matter, I'm excluded." Not to receive eye contact for an extended time span leaves one feeling uncomfortable, irritated or rejected, and it becomes very difficult to counteract the communication of such nonverbal exclusion. Not to make eye contact, on the other hand, may be precisely a manoeuvre to avoid being questioned.

Eyes reflect, mirror, speak – not infrequently more strongly than words and body language combined. While chart entries may document a patient's visual expression or lack of eye contact, care givers rarely observe their own "eye language". In the care of cancer patients, there are many occasions when questions asked and subjects raised do not have a definite answer or an answer at all, and eye expressions reflect the care givers' dilemmas, which patients sense. Rosenthal (1973) writes, "I never really saw what fear was until I looked at everybody else looking at me." Most certainly, fear was the last thing those care givers or the loved ones wanted to transmit.

True supportive care in this way may mean care givers' choosing to look a patient consciously in the eye while giving an honest, also often difficult answer. "I don't know" or "Yes, you are going to die," if the eyes of the care giver remain focused and reflect his/her difficulty, pain and uncertainty about the patient's plight, may be easier to hear than a pretence answer with shifting eye contact which still tells the patient the truth.

One further potent nonverbal impact which leaves its mark on care givers, and which is rarely acknowledged, is the many impressions their eyes absorb of wasting or mutilated bodies, or of faces which change in the course of the disease or mirror suffering, loss or grief. Eyes can't be shut to these.

Touch

Health care techniques invariably involve touching the patient, yet the issue of touch is deliberately rarely addressed. As a matter of fact, when it is brought up, it often elicits uneasiness or ridicule.

Touch is defined as "the act of feeling something with the hand or another bodily part" (Webster 1982). The operative word is *feeling*. Although touch is not in itself an emotion, its sensory elements include those neural, glandular, muscular and mental changes which in combination we call an emotion. Hence, touch is not experienced only as a simple physical modality, as sensation, but also affectively, as an emotion. Tactile function is frequently alluded to in expressions with subtle connotations: rubbing someone the wrong way, getting in touch, handling people, reaching out to people, having a soft touch.

In just this way, patients receive messages each time they are "handled" in the many care situations. They sense and feel uneasiness, nervousness, tension, anxiety and also carelessness being transmitted, through the interpretation of the body language of care givers and close ones, as described earlier, but also in the way they are touched while being cared for. While the words accompanying the manual interventions may be chosen to conceal any difficulty or impatience on the part of the care giver, the sensory input through the hands often speaks another truth which frequently increases the patient's feeling of dependency.

Touch may be the best or only way to transmit empathy, understanding or reassurance, and will often outweigh words. In the complexity of the care of cancer patients, an astute awareness of these matters makes for competent care giving. The nonverbal communication of conscious comfort care – for example, as in an especially carefully given bedbath or back rub – may be the most meaningful or the only possible communication. But for this, the care giver has to decide *knowingly* what message s/he wants to or can transmit through touch and concentrate her/his effort accordingly. An arm can be scrubbed or it can be washed carefully; a hand or a leg can be grabbed or gently and securely lifted – each time the communication comes directly through the hands. Touch in this modality has the potential of being received as effective and affective stimulation. This important duality may make a significant difference for patients whose pain is difficult to control, just as for someone who can't fall asleep. It is in the attention to such detail, also, that the self-esteem of patients regains some strength, because they sense respect for their personhood. Such care does not necessarily involve a bigger time commitment, but it requires conscious attention in its execution to be perceived by the patient as psychosocial, supportive care.

The importance of the patient's own sense of touch is often forgotten. In touching numberless items and surfaces in the course of a day, one experiences, mostly unconsciously, orientation in the reality of one's environment. Bedridden patients invariably miss out on much of this sensory input at a time when they need it, for "memory exists in the nostrils and the hands, not only in the mind" (Cassell 1982). While children will stubbornly cling to a toy or a cloth which symbolizes comfort for them, adults, particularly within the hospital environment, are often embarrassed to spell out their need for such nonverbal comfort, be it the longing to feel the fur of a treasured pet or to hold a precious sign of friendship in their hand. Sensitive staff will reassure the individual that they understand the importance of such things.

The palliative care philosophy has done much to stress the importance of such nonverbal gestures as holding a hand, or stroking a forehead when verbal communication is no longer possible or inappropriate. Such contact, however, can be the best psychosocial support at any time during the illness, and certainly occasionally outweighs the most carefully chosen words or some other form of treatment.

All these issues require awareness and sensitivity from all health care professionals, be they nurses, doctors or others. They demand a being in touch and a philosophy of care which values these subtle details as much as various other treatment modalities. Invariably, patients also search farther beyond the actions of care givers in the hope of finding a communication through being. It is that way of being which helps the competent professional to do ordinary things in extraordinary ways.

Conclusion

In the midst of ever-increasing knowledge about cancer and cancer treatment, it may seem exaggerated to highlight these nonverbal factors. Considered in the light of psychosocial support, however, they have a role to play in terms of the patient's quality of life or ability to cope.

The difficulty with these issues is that they cannot easily be packaged as a programme to be instituted or offered, but that, for a start, they demand a certain kind of view or attitude on the part of care givers. Sensitivity and skill in nonverbal communication, for one, can be developed, taught and learned, yet such topics rarely receive major attention in health care curricula, for they are closely linked to individual perception and demand personal introspection. They require awareness, consciousness, observation and practice, which in this area would mean practice with our own bodies, our own hands and eyes, to become aware of the subtle nuances involved. Such experiential learning, however, is far less popular than a lesson about a new treatment technique. It is often perceived as threatening and therefore preferably left aside. While nursing programmes tend to include various experiential techniques and role play, the same is rarely true of medical training. In the daily routine, therefore, a lack of openness to various priorities or to the subtle perspective of nonverbal dimensions often prevails.

Cancer care is complex, and the relief of suffering rather than just the treatment of disease will continue to be a demanding challenge. Medical and pharmacological treatments are vital and will continue to absorb a large portion of time from the various care givers. While psychosocial support and care receives some attention, technical and medical matters still frequently demand priority and outweigh the efforts towards genuine whole-person care. Patients are certainly grateful for the many available treatments; the ambivalences of the nonverbal messages and communication, however, still play a larger role for them than one generally likes to acknowledge.

It will never be easy to balance all aspects of care appropriately for each patient, but it will remain important to consider and weigh up the importance of different treatment approaches and aspects as significant contributing factors to competent care.

References

Bonnafont C (1979) Die Botschaft der Körpersprache. Ariston, Genf, p 21

Cassell E (1982) The nature of suffering and the goals of medicine. N Engl J Med 306: 642

Fast J (1970) Body Language. Simon and Schuster, New York, p 16

Gerdes N (1986) Zurück zur "Normalität"? Onkol Forum Chemotherapie 3: 12–17

Molcho S (1988) Körpersprache als Dialog. Mosaik, München, p 49

Morris D (1978) Der Mensch mit dem wir leben. Droemersche Verlagsanstalt, München, p 169

Rosenthal T (1973) How could I not be among you. Avon, New York, p 28

Webster's New World Dictionary (1980) 3rd college edn. Simon and Schuster, New York

Alterations of Host Defenses: The Key to the Multifaceted Spectrum of Infections in Immunocompromised Patients

M.P. Glauser

Division of Infections Diseases, Département of Internal Medicine,
Centre Hospitalier Universitaire Vaudois, 1011 Lausanne, Switzerland

Since bacterial infection remains a frequent cause of death in patients with cancer, especially those with hematological malignancies, it is important to understand fully the mechanisms responsible for increased infection in these patients. Patients with cancer have a heightened risk for infection, either because of their underlying disease, or from the treatment directed against their underlying disease, or, additionally, from factors resulting from prolonged hospitalization and exposure to nosocomial foci of infection. Since the underlying disease itself dictates the type of therapy used, the length of time for which the risk of infection is increased varies considerably with the type of malignancy. In addition, the range of infecting organisms varies with the type of malignancy and the degree of depression of host defenses.

Defects Inherent in the Underlying Malignant Disease

There are several routes of acquisition of infections that relate directly to the particular type of malignancy affecting the patient.

Anatomical Defects

Rupture of Anatomical Barriers

Primary tumors of the skin or metastatic lesions to the skin from many other tumors may result in ulcerations or erosion and consequent rupture of this important anatomical barrier. Although infection is not a major occurrence in these patients unless there are other predisposing factors, serious bacteremia due to *Staphylococcus aureus* or Group A ß-hemolytic *Streptococcus* may be seen.

Mucous membranes or mucosal surfaces in the oral cavity and nasopharynx may be affected by ulcerating carcinoma, and local infection in the mouth, nose, throat, or sinuses may occur secondary to mucous membrane rupture. In these conditions, mixed anaerobic necrotizing infections or infections due to strepto-cocci, including *Streptococcus pneumoniae*, and *Haemophilus influenzae* may occur. Spread of infection from these sites, with or without direct invasion or erosion by the tumor, may reach the meninges, and meningitis or severe osteomyelitis of the sinuses with subsequent cerebral abscess may occur.

Mucous membrane ulceration in the gastrointestinal tract, such as is seen with ulcerating carcinoma or in patients with acute leukemia, may result in local abscess formation, actinomycotic infection, and bacteremia due to gram-negative rods, which may enter the general circulation from this site. The possibility of fungal infection increases further if the patient has been on broad-spectrum antibiotic therapy.

Rupture of anatomical barriers in the female genital tract can occur in association with ulcerating gynecological malignancies, but systemic infection is not a routine occurrence. When bacterial invasion of these sites does occur, it is usually due to anaerobic gram-negative rods, enteric gram-negative rods, *Clostridia* spp., or enterococci. The skin and mucous membrane sites also may be damaged by radiation therapy for adjacent tumors, and occasionally this may be the portal of entry for invasive bacteria.

Obstruction

The expansion of malignant lesions frequently leads to partial or complete obstruction of various passages and cavities. Among the secondary effects of such obstruction is infection, due usually to local resident flora. For example, obstruction of a major bronchus secondary to an expanding tumor may result in retained secretions which become infected with mouth and upper respiratory flora, and pneumonia with or without abscess formation may then occur. *Streptococcus pneumoniae* and anaerobes are frequently the causative agents of pneumonia in patients who acquire their infection outside of the hospital. Pathogenic aerobic gram-negative rods including *Klebsiella*, *Enterobacter*, *Acinetobacter* spp., *Pseudomonas*, etc., must be considered likely pathogens in patients who acquire their infections while hospitalized. These nosocomial organisms are often more antibiotic-resistant than are community-acquired strains.

Obstructive tumors of the genitourinary tract may result in hydronephrosis or pyonephrosis. Lower urinary tract and bladder tumors may favor incomplete emptying of the bladder, allowing repeated episodes of bacteremia secondary to urinary tract infection (by loss of the normally protective voiding mechanisms).

Tumors that obstruct vascular sites, especially those relating to the oropharynx, the gastrointestinal tract including the anus and rectum, or the female pelvic organs, may result in the development of septic thrombophlebitis, which may or may not be secondarily infected.

Dysfunction Secondary to Invasion

Depending on the type of malignancy, various organ functions may be impaired due to invasion by the malignant process. Since the spleen is able to clear bacteria from the blood even in the relative absence of specific antibody, normal splenic function is essential for recovery from bacteremia. In the absence of the spleen, the Kupffer's cells and reticular structures of the liver facilitate the clearing of organisms, but this process is more efficient when preexisting antibody is present. Serious invasion of the liver and spleen with extensive tumor involvement could increase the mortality associated with bacteremia by virtue of the decreased efficiency of this clearance mechanism. In the absence of the spleen, and presumably if splenic function is severely reduced by malignancy, encapsulated bacteria such *Streptococcus pneumoniae* and *Haemophilus influenzae* cause the greatest problems.

Humoral Defects

B-cell function and the production of humoral antibodies may be impaired in patients with chronic lymphocytic leukemia, Hodgkin's or other lymphomas, multiple myeloma or other plasma cell dyscrasias, Waldenström's macroglobulinemia, or overwhelming metastatic carcinoma. This occurs especially in patients undergoing treatment for these malignancies. Although any bacterial pathogen may overwhelm the host's defective humoral immunity, infections due to encapsulated bacteria, especially *Streptococcus pneumoniae*, *Haemophilus influenzae*, and *Neisseria meningitidis*, are common. Enteric gram-negative bacilli and *Pseudomonas aeruginosa* may also cause infection in patients with defective humoral immunity.

The human complement system is critically involved in the defense against infection. Complement activation plays an important role in the chemotaxis of polymorphonuclear lymphocytes, immune adherence, neutralization of viruses, phagocytosis, and the antibody-mediated, complement-dependent bactericidal activity of normal serum. In some patients who have undergone splenectomy the production of complement components may be deficient, and this may contribute to their increased susceptibility to and mortality from a variety of bacterial infections.

Cellular Defects

Granulocytopenia

Cellular defects may be extremely serious abnormalities inherent in the underlying malignancy; for example, patients with leukemia may have a reduced absolute number of circulating granulocytes secondary to invasion of the bone marrow or due to proliferation of nonfunctional lymphoid or myeloid precursor cells. Marrow infiltration with other tumor cells may also occur. In addition, diminished chemotactic responses and bactericidal activity of monocytes may occur in patients suffering from Hodgkin's disease and hairy cell leukemia.

The ultimate net effect of granulocytopenia or impaired neutrophil function is bacteremia. It has been shown that patients who remain severely neutropenic (less than 100 circulating neutrophils/mm^3) ultimately become infected within 3 weeks of the onset of severe neutropenia. Patients with lesser degrees of neutropenia (that is, 500–1 000 granulocytes/mm^3) have a lower frequency of bacterial infections, but the risk of bacterial infection rises with the duration of granulocytopenia.

Several studies have examined the types of infection that occur in neutropenic patients. The distribution of organisms may be dependent on the colonization of the gastrointestinal tract and other body sites prior to the onset of neutropenia. Clusters of particular pathogenic bacteria have been reported from cancer services, suggesting that local hospital flora may play an important role in determining which organisms are the predominant offenders. In most series, however, three gram-negative rods, *Escherichia Coli*, *Klebsiella pneumoniae*, and *Pseudomonas aeruginosa*, plus *Staphylococcus aureus*, were the organisms most frequently isolated from infected neutropenic patients. Over the last 10 years, new organisms have emerged as pathogens in many centers caring for neutropenic adult and pediatric patients, e.g., viridans group streptococci and coagulase-negative staphylococci (mostly *Staphylococcus epidermidis*). The observed shift from 2/3 gram-negative rod bacteremia in the 1960s and 1970s to 2/3 gram-positive coccal bacteremias by the end of the 1980s is not well understood; it may possibly be related to the wider use of quinolone antibiotics for oral prophylaxis of infection and/or to the more severe mucositis observed in the patients following the development of new anti-cancer regimens. Bacteremia due to *Bacteroides fragilis* is relatively uncommon in neutropenic leukemia patients unless there is associated gastrointestinal or gynecological invasive disease.

Fungi, notably *Candida albicans* and *Aspergillus fumigatus*, are also pathogens in severely neutropenic patients. These infections may occur concomitantly with bacterial invasion or may become manifest during treatment with broad-spectrum antibiotics for primary bacterial infection. The occurrence of *Aspergillus* infections is directly related to the duration of neutropenia.

Another clinical manifestation of severe neutropenia is difficulty in the mobilization of white blood cells to the site of inflammation. Since most local bacterial infections incite an acute pyogenic response, with migration of polymorphonuclear leukocytes to the affected site, it follows that a drop in the number of available neutrophils will hamper the usually brisk neutrophil response. Thus, patients with prolonged neutropenia may not be able to locally limit the spread of bacteria. The clinical ramifications of this failure include a relative decrease in the usual signs of inflammation, i.e., swelling, tenderness, heat over the affected area, and the ability to form abscesses. Thus, the appearance of local infections in severely neutropenic patients may be more subtle and they may be more easily overlooked than in normal hosts. Similarly, the radiologic signs in pneumonia, for example, may be delayed, and infiltrates may not appear for several days after the onset of pneumonitis. For this reason, frequent chest X-rays should be taken in neutropenic patients who develop fever, to help identify its source. Frequent intensive physical examinations, especially over the lungs and the perirectal area, should be performed to detect early inflammatory responses in potential spaces, especially in association with anal fissures.

Defects in Cell-Mediated Immunity

Hodgkin's disease and other lymphoproliferative disorders, as well as advanced metastatic cancer of any source, may be associated with defects in cell-mediated immunity. Defects in T-cell function may present with a failure to respond to skin tests, and profound lymphopenia may be present. Although the classical T-cell defects are associated with viral (varicella-zoster, cytomegalovirus, etc.) infections, fungal (*Candida* spp. *Aspergillus*) and protozoal (*Toxoplasma gondii*, *Pneumocystis carinii*) infections may occur in these patients. Notably, *Listeria monocytogenes* and intracellular gram-positive rod may cause meningitis or other systemic infections in these patients. Tuberculosis or infections due to atypical mycobacteria may occur with increased frequency in cancer patients with defective T-cell immunity, especially in those with Hodgkin's disease and hairy cell leukemia. *Salmonella* infections, which may involve lymphoid tissue in the gastrointestinal tract, also occur in association with these immune defects.

Defects Resulting from the Treatment of the Underlying Malignancy

Chemotherapy

With the introduction of potent new chemotherapeutic agents active against many tumor cell types, the clinician must face the unwanted results of some of the side effects of these agents, many of which increase the patient's risk of infection.

Bone marrow suppression and neutropenia can be consequences of the action of most cancer chemotherapeutic agents. The effects are often dose-related, but the lag period from administration to the nadir of the depression is quite variable and the latter may appear as late as 6 weeks after drug administration. Some cytotoxic drugs also inhibit certain functions of neutrophils, including migration and chemotaxis. Large doses of corticosteroids may also inhibit the bactericidal activity of polymorphonuclear leukocytes. The effects of these drugs are usually reversible, and the recovery time is usually predictable on the basis of the administered dose.

Many cancer chemotherapeutic agents may produce severe mucosal ulcerations in the mouth, esophagus, small and large intestines, and rectum. These ulcers may allow the invasion and erosion by bacteria resident at the site of ulceration. These may be the sources of bacteremia due to gram-negative rods and gram-positive cocci (notably streptococci and coagulase-negative staphylococci), or the cause of fever possibly due to the absorption of endotoxins from the bacteria in the gut. These lesions may also provoke the development of anorectal abscesses secondary to mucosal ulceration. Bleomycin and methotrexate cause skin lesions which may ulcerate and provide a ready means of access to staphylococci and other skin bacteria. Some cancer chemotherapeutic agents may be particularly irritating to the veins, producing phlebitis and increasing the risk of bacteremia via this route.

Some agents, notably methotrexate, cyclophosphamide, and 6-mercaptopurine, may result in a reduction in humoral antibodies, and the same agents, along with high doses of corticosteroids, may produce cellular immune defects by their lympholytic actions.

Radiation Therapy

Radiation therapy may also result in marrow depression with neutropenia, but these adverse effects are not common in cases with local irradiation of small areas. Neutropenia may occur following total body irradiation, but this is reversible. High doses of radiation may also depress cell-mediated immunity and antibody production, presumably by means of the suppression of precursor cells and by their lympholytic effect. Secondary infection may occur after radiation therapy if, for example, stenosing lesions develop in the respiratory, gastrointestinal, or urinary tracts. These defects would be similar to those due to the tumor itself, as described above.

Surgery

Extensive surgery, sometimes necessary for an advanced invasive tumor, may increase the risk of infection by removing large areas of otherwise protective tissue; this may occur in extensive pelvic, gastrointestinal, or maxillofacial surgery. Furthermore, surgery breaks the anatomical barriers, with the infectious danger such leakages carry with them, especially in patients with compromised host defenses. Recurrence of tumor at suture sites may result in further leaks across anatomical barriers and extravasation of material containing bacterial flora. The removal of critical organs such as the spleen produces immunological and other defects as outlined above.

Iatrogenic and Nosocomial Factors

All hospitalized patients are subject to colonization of skin and mucous membranes with potential pathogens resident in the hospital flora. Studies have correlated the increasing presence of potential pathogenic organisms at naso-pharyngeal and other body sites with increasing degrees of illness. Schimpff et al. [14–16] have demonstrated that neutropenic patients undergoing treatment for leukemia may be colonized at various body sites, including nasal and orophar-yngeal mucosa, axilla, groin, rectum, and perirectal areas, with pathogenic gram-negative rods including *Pseudomonas aeruginosa*. This colonization may precede subsequent bacteremia involving these organisms. The use of broad-spectrum antibiotics, especially for extended prophylactic use, results in the selection and overgrowth of multiple-antibiotic-resistant bacteria. Given the compromised nature of the patients, either because of their disease or because of therapy, as outlined above, secondary infection with these colonizing organisms may occur.

The intravenous catheter, introduced originally as a convenience device, now has a well-known role in the etiology of hospital-acquired infections. Plastic intravenous catheters have been implicated as a source of nosocomial bacte-remia, and the risk of sepsis increases with the duration of catheterization. Similar risks are associated with the long-term use of parenteral accesses, such as with the Hickman, Broviak, Portacath and other devices. Certain nonbacterial infections can be spread by blood and blood products, notably cytomegalovirus, hepatitis viruses, and HIV infection. Postoperative complications of infection and infections associated with tracheostomy and with the use of respiratory ventilators are also increased in this patient population, and careful attention must be paid to the care and maintenance of these instrument sites.

It is unusual for any of the above factors to operate alone. Rather, patients with cancer may develop bacterial infection via a combination of the above defects; and, depending on the clinical situation, fairly typical infections can be predicted. For example, patients undergoing chemotherapy for acute lymphocy-tic leukemia will become neutropenic for several days, and these patients are at increased risk of developing gram-negative rod bacteremia and bacteremia due to *Staphylococcus aureus*, especially after prolonged granulocytopenia with less than 100 neutrophils/mm^3. After prolonged antibiotic therapy for this bacterial infection, patients are likely to develop oral and possibly gastrointestinal fungal colonization and infection. It is not clear what additional role mucosal ulceration due to the cancer chemotherapeutic agent plays in this process. Often after successful treatment of a bacteremic episode, severely neutropenic patients treated with a variety of chemotherapeutic agents will develop invasive fungal infections such as those due to *Aspergillus*.

Summary

Patients with cancer are subject to bacterial infections because of a variety of specific defects. Patients may suffer increased susceptibility to infection by virtue of the invasiveness and obstructiveness of their basic malignancy as well as because of malignant processes directly involved in the hematopoietic and lymphoid systems. Also, the potent therapeutic modalities useful in treating

Spectrum and Treatment of Bacterial Infections in Cancer Patients with Granulocytopenia

T. Calandra

Division of Infectious Diseases, Department of Internal Medicine,
Centre Universitaire Vaudois, Lausanne, Switzerland

In cancer patients with myelosuppression induced by chemotherapy, bacterial infections remain a frequent clinical problem associated with significant morbidity and mortality [1, 2]. In these patients, the incidence of infections begin to rise when the granulocyte count drops below $500/\mu l$. Most of the severe infections and almost all bacteremias occur in patients with less than 100 granulocytes/μl [3]. In granulocytopenic patients the classical signs of infection such as pain, heat, redness and swelling are often absent. Fever remains the first and most frequently the only sign of infection in these patients [4]. However, not all febrile episodes are due to microbiologically documented infections, as was shown by the results of a recently published multicenter study of empirical therapy of fever in granulocytopenic cancer patients [5]. Of 887 episodes of fever, 320 (36%) were caused by a microbiologically documented infection (252 were bacteremias, 53 were focal bacterial infections with negative blood cultures and 15 were viral or fungal infections), 225 (25%) were associated with a clinically documented infection, but without microbiological proof of its etiology, and 342 (39%) were classified as a fever of unknown origin (i.e., possible infection). Thus, only 34% of the total number of primary febrile episodes were due to a documented bacterial infection. Since 30%–35% of the clinically documented and possible infections respond rapidly to empirical antibiotic therapy, it is likely that an overall 65%–70% of the febrile episodes are due to bacterial infections, half of those being microbiologically documented. The ratio of bacterial to fungal and viral infections is highest when the infection develops in the early phase of granulocytopenia. When secondary infections develop in patients with granulocytopenia of prolonged duration (>2 weeks), the proportion of bacterial infections decreases, owing to a rise in the incidence of viral and fungal infections.

Microbiology and Sites of Infection

In the past decade, most cancer centers have experienced a major change in the etiology of bacterial infections occurring in cancer patients with granulocytopenia. While gram-negative bacteria predominated in the previous two decades, gram-positive bacteria have recently increased in frequency [6–11] and are now the prevalent pathogens in many institutions. As an example of this change, the percentage of single-agent gram-positive bacteremia increased from 29% in the first trial (1973–1976) conducted by the International Antimicrobial Therapy Project Group of the European Organization for Research on Treatment of Cancer (EORTC) to 63% in the fifth trial (1986–1988) of this group [12, 13]. Similarly, in a recent study carried out at the National Cancer Institute in the United States, gram-positive aerobes accounted for 55% of the primary bloodstream infections [14]. In 1988, 123 febrile episodes were recorded in neutropenic cancer patients at the Centre Hospitalier Universitaire Vaudois (Lausanne, Switzerland). Of those, 42 were associated with bloodstream infections, which were due to gram-positive bacteria in 59% of the cases, gram-negative bacteria in 29%, anaerobes in 7%, and yeasts in 5%. In 1989, the proportion of gram-positive bacteremia increased to 66%.

Although the relative prevalences of the various bacterial pathogens causing infections in cancer patients with neutropenia may vary from center to center, some general statements can be made that apply for most institutions. With respect to gram-positive infections, about 80%–85% of all these infections are caused by coagulase-negative staphylococci, *Staphylococcus aureus* or viridans and α-hemolytic streptococci. *Streptococcus pneumoniae*, *Streptococcus pyogenes*, enterococci, *Corynebacterium* spp. and a few species of anaerobes account for most of the remaining 15%–20% of gram-positive infections.

Among gram-negative bacteria *Escherichia coli*, *Pseudomonas* spp. and *Klebsiella* spp. are responsible in most studies for approximately 80% of all gram-negative infections.

According to the results obtained in the most recent multicenter study of the EORTC, which included 278 patients with bacterial infections, the primary site of these bacterial infections could be determined in only 52% of the cases [13]. The site of infection was the oral cavity and the pharynx in 17% of the patients, the skin and soft tissue in 16% and the respiratory tract in 10%. The gastrointestinal tract (4%), the urinary tract (3%) or other sites (2%) were infrequently recognized as foci of infection.

Epidemiological Data

The reason or reasons for the increased incidence of gram-positive infections in cancer patients have not yet been fully clarified. The striking increase is coagulase-negative staphylococcal infections is probably related, at least partly, to the extensive use of intravenous catheters, particularly those inserted for long periods of time. However, a number of these infections may also originate from other sites. The gastrointestinal tract, particularly in patients not receiving oral prophylactic antibiotics active against coagulase-negative staphylococci, has recently been identified as a portal of entry of these infections [9]. Indeed, studies conducted by investigators of the University of Maryland Cancer Center

(Baltimore, USA) have recently shown that in some patients the plasmid profile of coagulase-negative staphylococci isolated from blood was similar to that of strains of coagulase-negative staphylococci isolated from surveillance cultures of nose, gum or rectum [15]. These results suggest that coagulase-negative staphylococcal infections may not all be catheter-related, and also indicate that preventing the colonization of the gastrointestinal tract might help to reduce the incidence of these bacteremias.

Recent reports have shown that viridans and α-hemolytic streptococci (designated "viridans streptococci" in the remainder of this article) are frequent pathogens in febrile neutropenic patients with acute leukemia, lymphoma, or solid tumors [7, 10, 16–18]. In some institutions today, these organisms comprise the second most common cause of bacteremia and are outnumbered only by coagulase-negative staphylococci [13, 19]. These streptococcal infections may be severe and present with septic shock [10, 16, 17] or acute respiratory distress syndrome [16, 17, 20]. Since viridans streptococci are normal inhabitants of the mouth and pharynx, it has been hypothesized, but so far not proven, that these infections arise from the oral cavity. These streptococcal infections may be secondary to the development of severe mucositis following radiation therapy or chemotherapy, particularly in patients treated with high-dose cytosine arabinoside [17, 19], but may also be secondary to oral ulcerations due to herpesvirus infections. Another factor predisposing patients to these streptococcal infections may be the use of quinolone antibiotics for the prevention of bacterial infection. These antibiotics are highly active against gram-negative bacteria but have limited anti-gram-positive activity, and therefore may not prevent the development of streptococcal infections, particularly in the oral cavity, where the concentration of antibiotic is likely to be low. However, the frequency of viridans streptococcal infections seems to be also increasing in cancer centers not using quinolone prophylaxis, indicating that the causes for these infections are probably multifactorial.

It is likely that the cause of the sharp decline in the frequency of gram-negative infections, as observed in most European countries, is the use of quinolone antibiotics for the prophylaxis of infection in these patients. However, it has been argued that quinolone prophylaxis might convert documented infections, particularly those caused by gram-negative bacteria, into fever of undetermined origin and therefore does not decrease the need for parenteral antibiotics [21].

Treatment

The concept of empirical therapy [22] of suspected infection in cancer patients with granulocytopenia is founded on the following considerations: (a) in these patients the classical signs of infection are often absent and in most circumstances fever is the only sign of infection (4); (b) the results of microbiological cultures take days to arrive; and (c) a delay in the initiation of antibiotic therapy may be disastrous in the immunocompromised host. Although this concept has never been proven in a prospective, randomized study, its use has been shown to markedly improve the outcome for patients with bacteremia due to *Pseudomonas aeruginosa* [23].

Until the early 1980s the standard empirical therapy for suspected infection in a granulocytopenic patient consisted of the combination of an extended-spectrum penicillin or a third-generation cephalosporin and an aminoglycoside [24]. Three arguments constituted the rationale for using such antibiotic combinations. First, these combinations offer a broad-spectrum antibacterial coverage. Second, they usually induce high bactericidal activity with synergistic antibacterial effects, which are important factors in the outcome of gram-negative bacteremia in patients with profound and persistent granulocytopenia [25–26]. Third, they may limit the emergence of resistance [5, 27].

However, with the advent in the therapeutic armamentarium of new antibiotics with an extended spectrum of activity, such as the third-generation cephalosporins and the carbapenems, empirical monotherapy has become a possible alternative to combination therapy in febrile neutropenic cancer patients [28]. In a randomized study of 550 episodes of fever and neutropenia, Pizzo et al. compared ceftazidime monotherapy with a combination of cephalothin, gentamicin and carbenicillin (KGC) (14). In the 394 episodes of unexplained fever, representing 72% of the total number of evaluable febrile courses, 78% of the patients treated with ceftazidime and 77% of those treated with KGC responded without modification of empirical therapy, 20% and 21% respectively responded with modification of empirical therapy, and 2% failed in each treatment group. In this study failure meant death of the patient. In the 156 episodes of documented infections (28% of the total), only 30% of the patients treated with ceftazidime and 31% of those treated with KGC responded without modification of empirical therapy, 59% and 60% respectively responded with modification of therapy, and the remaining 11% and 9% died of infection. These results should be compared with those obtained by the EORTC (5). In this large multicenter study of empirical therapy, ceftazidime was combined with a short (3 days) or long (at least 9 days) course of amikacin. Failure was defined as death of the patient within 9 days of the initiation of therapy or as a change in empirical therapy to improve the patient's response. Patients with gram-negative bacteremia fared significantly better when on ceftazidime and long amikacin than on ceftazidime and short amikacin (response rates: 81% versus 48%, $p = 0.002$). Ceftazidime and long amikacin were particularly efficacious in patients with profound (< 100 granulocytes/μl) and persistent (i.e., throughout therapy) granulocytopenia and in those with *Pseudomonas aeruginosa* bacteremia. In the other categories of infections the response rates of the two ceftazidime treatment groups were similar. Thus, although not absolutely comparable, these two studies seem to suggest that ceftazidime monotherapy is an alternative to combination therapy for patients with non microbiologically documented infections. However, for patients with gram-negative bacteremia, ceftazidime should be combined with an aminoglycoside. A report on a recently completed but not yet published study seems to suggest that imipenem–cilastatin monotherapy is as efficacious as the combination of piperacillin and amikacin for the empirical therapy of fever in granulocytopenic cancer patients [29].

Until recently, antibiotic regimens of empirical therapy in neutropenic patients have been designed for optimal coverage of gram-negative infections, which were associated with the highest mortality. As a consequence, the response rate of gram-positive infections to these empirical regimen was generally low, i.e., in the range of 40%–50%, but the mortality associated with these infections was lower than 5%. In the past 5 years considerable controversy has been generated as to the need for empirical specific anti-gram-positive therapy at the onset of the treatment of fever in granulocytopenic patients. Although some authors have suggested that the addition of vancomycin at the initiation of empirical therapy is preferable, others have not supported this concept. It is obviously beyond the scope of this article to review all these studies, so only the results of four recent studies that have addressed the issue of the empirical use of vancomycin in neutropenic cancer patients will be presented here. In a double-blind, randomized, placebo-controlled trial in 60 adult patients with acute leukemia and prolonged granulocytopenia, Karp et al. showed that treatment with vancomycin resulted in a more rapid resolution of fever related to primary infections, fewer total febrile days during the granulocytopenic course, and a significant reduction of subsequent gram-positive infections [30]. No increase in toxicity was noted in patients treated with vancomycin. Rubin et al. retrospectively reviewed the use of vancomycin in 75 patients with either primary or secondary gram-positive infections [31]. Vancomycin was used in only 43 (57%) of these patients, of whom 39 had vancomycin therapy initiated after documentation of the gram-positive infection. Only one failure to cure infection was documented, and therefore it was concluded that vancomycin should not be routinely used as empirical therapy of fever in neutropenic patients, but should be added when clinical or microbiological data suggest the need. In a double-blind study in 101 neutropenic children with cancer, Shenep et al. showed that a combination of vancomycin, ticarcillin, and amikacin was more effective than a combination of ticarcillin-clavulanate and amikacin for the empirical treatment of fever (response rates: 85% versus 62%, $p = 0.01$) [19]. The difference in response rates was due to a higher proportion of breakthrough gram-positive bacteremias (one of which was fatal) in patients not receiving vancomycin (9/48 versus 1/53, $p = 0.006$). In the most recent trial of the EORTC, 747 evaluable patients with fever and granulocytopenia were randomly assigned to receive ceftazidime and amikacin, with or without vancomycin [13]. In both the 135 patients presenting with primary single gram-positive bacteremias and the 612 patients who did not have such infections, the empirical use of vancomycin did not reduce the mortality or the morbidity associated with these infections. Moreover, the use of vancomycin in combination with amikacin caused increased nephrotoxicity.

The results of these four studies do not support the empirical use of vancomycin in all febrile neutropenic cancer patients. Indeed, in none of these studies did vancomycin reduce the overall mortality or the mortality due to gram-positive infection, and in only two did it to some extent reduce morbidity in a limited number of patients. Furthermore, the clinical benefit of this reduction in morbidity should be weighed up against the problem of costs and toxicity when vancomycin is given empirically to all febrile granulocytopenic cancer patients.

Lastly, it appears that in patients with documented gram-positive infections not responding to empirical therapy, successful treatment can be easily obtained after the identification of the pathogen.

Summary

Bacterial infections remain a frequent cause of morbidity and mortality in cancer patients with granulocytopenia. In recent years the proportion of patients with gram-positive infections, caused mainly by coagulase-negative staphylococci and viridans streptococci, has increased markedly in many institutions. The precise reasons for this recent change in the epidemiology of infection in cancer patients are as yet not fully ascertained. Although less prevalent, gram-negative infections are still the major threat, since they are associated with higher mortality. What constitutes the optimal empirical antibiotic therapy remains a controversial issue. One should however recognize that the results of one particular study may not be relevant to other institutions where the predominant pathogens and the pattern of antibiotic resistance may be different. In addition, the results of studies using various antibiotic regimens should be compared with caution. However, with these limitations in mind, the results of the most recently published studies support the following recommendations: in patients with nonmicrobiologically documented infections, monotherapy with a third-generation cephalosporin or a carbapenem is a safe alternative to combination therapy. For gram-negative bacteremia, combined therapy with an extended-spectrum β-lactam antibiotic and an aminoglycoside appears preferable. For gram-positive infections, a specific anti-gram-positive antibiotic is not needed in every patient and can safely be added upon identification of the pathogen in those patients not responding to empirical therapy.

References

1. Schimpff SC (1990) Infections in the compromised host: an overview. In: Mandell GL, Douglas RG, Bennett E (eds) Principles and practice of infectious diseases. Churchill Livingstone, New York, pp 2258–2265
2. Brown AE (1984) Neutropenia, fever, and infection. Am J Med 76: 421–428
3. Bodey GP, Buckley M, Sathe YS, Freireich EJ (1966) Quantitative relationships between circulating leukocytes and infection in patients with acute leukemia. Ann Intern Med 64: 328–340
4. Sickles EA, Greene WH, Wiernik PH (1975) Clinical presentation of infection in granulocytopenic patients. Arch Intern Med 135: 715–719

5. The EORTC International Antimicrobial Therapy Cooperative Group (1987) Ceftazidime combined with a short or long course of amikacin for empirical therapy of gram-negative bacteremia in cancer patients with granulocytopenia. N Engl J Med 317: 1692–1698
6. Ladisch S, Pizzo PA (1978) Staphylococcus aureus sepsis in children with cancer. Pediatrics 61: 231–234
7. Pizzo PA, Ladisch S, Witebsky FG (1978) α-Hemolytic streptococci: clinical signtficance in the cancer patient. Med Pediatr Oncol 4: 367–370
8. Sotman SB, Schimpff SC, Young VM (1980) Staphylococcus aureus bacteremia in patients with acute leukemia. Am J Med 69: 814–818
9. Wade JC, Schimpff SC, Newman KA, Wiernik PH (1982) Staphylococcus epidermidis: an increasing cause of infection in patients with granulocytopenia. Ann Intern Med 97: 503–508
10. Cohen J, Donnelly JP, Worsley AM, Catovsky D, Goldman JM, Galton DAG (1983) Septicemia caused by viridans streptococci in neutropenic patients with leukemia. Lancet II: 1452–1454
11. Winston DJ, Dudnick DV, Chapin M, Ho WG, Gale RP, Martin WJ (1983) Coagulase-negative staphylococcal bacteremia in patients receiving immunosuppressive therapy. Arch Intern Med 143: 32–36
12. The EORTC International Antimicrobial Therapy Project Group (1978) Three antibiotic regimens in the treatment of infection in febrile granulocytopenic patients with cancer. J Infect Dis 137: 14–29
13. The EORTC International Antimicrobial Therapy Cooperative Group. Vancomycin added to empirical combination therapy for fever in granulocytopenic cancer patients. (submitted)
14. Pizzo PA, Hathorn JW, Hiemenz J, Browne M, Commers J, Cotton D, Gress J, Longo D, Marshall D, McKnight J, Rubin M, Skelton J, Thaler M, Wesley R (1986) A randomized trial comparing ceftazidime alone with combination antibiotic therapy in cancer patients with fever and neutropenia. N Engl J Med 315: 552–558
15. Khabbaz RF, Cooksey RC, Saba G, Wade JC (1987) The alimentary tract as a source of S. epidermidis bacteremia in patients with cancer: clues from molecular epidemiology In: Program and Abstracts of the 27th Interscience Conference on Antimicrobial Agents and Chemotherapy (abstract 1036). New York
16. Henslee J, Bostrom B, Weisdorf D, Ramsay N, McGlave P, Kersey J (1984) Streptococcal sepsis in bone marrow transplant patients. Lancet I: 393
17. Kern W, Kurrle E, Vanek E (1987) High risk of streptococcal septicemia after high dose cytosine arabinoside treatment for acute myelogenous leukemia. Klin Wochenschr 65: 773–780
18. Sotiropoulos SV, Jackson MA, Woods GM, Hicks RA, Cullen J, Freeman AI (1989) α-Streptococcal septicemia in leukemic children treated with continuous or large dosage intermittent cytosine arabinoside. Pediatr Infect Dis 8: 755–758
19. Shenep J, Hughes WT, Roberson PK, Blankenship KR, Baker DK, Meyer WH, Gigliotti F, Sixbey JW, Santana VM, Feldman S, Lott L (1988) Vancomycin, ticarcillin, and amikacin compared with ticarcillin-clavulanate and amikacin in the empirical treatment of febrile, neutropenic children with cancer. J Engl J Med 319: 1053–1058
20. Ognibene FP, Martin SE, Parker MM, Schlesinger T, Roach P, Burch C, Shelhamer JH, Parillo JE (1986) Adult respiratory distress syndrome in patients with severe neutropenia. N Engl J Med 315: 547–551

21. Young LS (1987) The new fluorinated quinolones for infection prevention in acute leukemia. Ann Intern Med 106: 144–146
22. Klastersky J (1986) Concept of empiric therapy with antibiotic combinations: indications and limits. Am J Med 80 (suppl 5C): 2–12
23. Schimpff S, Satterlee W, Young VM, Serpick A (1971) Empiric therapy with carbenicillin and gentamicin for febrile patients with cancer and granulocytopenia. N Engl J Med 284: 1061–1065
24. Klastersky J (1983) Empiric treatment of infections in neutropenic patients with cancer. Rev Infect Dis 5 [Suppl]: S21–S31
25. Klastersky J, Meunier-Carpentier F, Prevost JM (1977) Significance of antimicrobial synergism for the outcome of gram-negative sepsis. Am J Med Sci 273: 157–167
26. de Jongh CA, Joshi JH, Newman KA, Moody MR, Wharton R, Standiford HC, Schimpff SC (1986) Antibiotic synergism and response in gram-negative bacteremia in granulocytopenic cancer patients. Am J Med 80 (suppl 5C): 96–100
27. Gribble MJ, Chow AW, Naiman SC, Smith JA, Bowie WR, Sacks SL, Grossman L, Buskard N, Growe GH, Plenderleith LH (1983) Prospective randomized trial of piperacillin monotherapy versus carboxypenicillin-aminoglycoside combination regimens in the empirical treatment of serious bacterial infections. Antimicrob Agents Chemother 24: 388–393
28. Hathorn JW, Rubin M, Pizzo PA (1987) Empirical antibiotic therapy in the febrile neutropenic cancer patient: clinical efficacy and impact of monotherapy. Antimicrob Agents Chemother 31: 971–977
29. Wade J, Bustamante C, Devlin A, Finley R, Drusano G, Thompson B (1987) Imipenem vs. piperacillin plus amikacin, empiric therapy for febrile neutropenic patients: a double-blind trial. In: Program and Abstracts of the 27th Interscience Conference on Antimicrobial Agents and Chemotherapy (abstract 1251), New York
30. Karp JE, Dick JD, Angelopulos C, Charache P, Green L, Burke PJ, Saral R (1986) Empiric use of vancomycin during prolonged treatment-induced granulocytpenia. Randomized, double-blind, placebo-controlled clinical trial in patients with acute leukemia. Am J Med 281: 237–242
31. Rubin M, Hathorn JW, Marshall D, Gress J, Steinberg SM, Pizzo PA (1988) Gram-positive infections and the use of vancomycin in 550 episodes of fever and neutropenia. Ann Intern Med 108: 30–35

Prevention of Infections in Granulocytopenic Patients by Fluorinated Quinolones

M. Rozenberg-Arska[1], A.W. Dekker[2], and J. Verhoef[1]

[1]Department of Clinical Microbiology and Laboratory of Infectious Diseases,
University Hospital Utrecht, P.O. Box 85500, 3508 GA Utrecht, The Netherlands
[2]Department of Hematology, University Hospital Utrecht, P.O. Box 85500,
3508 GA Utrecht, The Netherlands

Infections remain a major cause of morbidity and mortality in patients with hemotological malignancies (Young 1983; Bodey et al. 1978). Several factors predispose these patients to infections. The most important factor is profound and prolonged granulocytopenia due to the underlying disease or its treatment. Besides the myelosuppression, lesions in the skin and mucosal membranes caused by the cytotoxic agents also make the patient highly susceptible to infections. Medical procedures such as intravenous infusions and indwelling urinary and central venous catheters, which break the skin and/or the mucosal barrier, contribute to the susceptibility of the patient to infection. Immunosuppression as a consequence of corticosteroids is a further predisposing factor.

Most of the infections occur during the period when the granulocyte counts are below $500/\mu l$; the majority of severe and sometimes lethal infections are observed when the granulocyte count is below $100/\mu l$ (Bodey et al. 1966; Bodey et al. 1978). The commonest infections in granulocytopenic patients are pneumonia, oropharyngeal infections, and septicemia (Gurwith et al. 1978). Because of the impaired inflammatory response, patients with granulocytopenia often show fewer of the classical signs of localized infection; minor infections may become life-threatening in these patients and are often associated with positive blood cultures.

Although advances in antimicrobial therapy, extensive diagnostic procedures and better supportive care, have brought a dramatic decline in the death rate associated with infections, morbidity from infectious disease in granulocytopenic patients still remains a problem. Most of the infections develop from microorganisms colonizing the alimentary tract and the upper respiratory passages (*Escherichia coli, Pseudomonas aeruginosa, Klebsiella pneumoniae*, staphylococci, viridans streptococci, *Candida albicans* etc.). About half of the bacteria causing infections belong to the patient's endogenous flora; the rest are organisms acquired from the hospital environment which have colonized the gastrointestinal tract during the patient's stay in hospital (Schimpff et al. 1972).

These latter organisms are frequently more virulent and likely to be more resistant than are the endogenous flora. Logical approaches for infection prevention, therefore, are cutting down the acquisition of new organisms and suppressing those potentially pathogenic microorganisms already colonizing the patient.

In attempts to reduce acquisition, patients have been nursed in wards in strict isolation, such as laminar air flow rooms and plastic isolators. Often these patients are also treated prophylactically with oral nonabsorbable antimicrobial agents, to eliminate the potential pathogenic organisms from the skin and the mucosal surfaces. The effectiveness of simple protective isolation (single room treatment) or complete reverse isolation with laminar air flow equipment is not convincing (Pizzo and Schimpff 1983; Yates and Holland 1973; Dietrich et al. 1977; Levine et al. 1973; Schimpff et al. 1975; Buckner et al. 1978; Rodriguez et al. 1978; Lohner et al. 1979; Bodey et al. 1979). Despite several comparative studies, the question "Are protected environments effective in prolonging the life of selected neutropenic patients?" still cannot be answered. Because protective environments are difficult to maintain, require expensive equipment, a sterile food supply, and skilled nursing staff and are often a psychological burden to the patient, reverse isolation treatment cannot be recommended routinely.

Since the alimentary tract has been recognized as an important reservoir of potential pathogens, total decontamination of the alimentary tract without protective environment has also been tested.

Poor compliance, usually due to the unpleasant taste of the oral non-absorbable antibiotics, can be the cause of significant rebound overgrowth of potential pathogens and acquisition of resistant strains from the hospital environment (Schimpff 1980; Pizzo and Schimpff 1983). The combination of administration of oral nonabsorbable antibiotics with nursing under strict isolation conditions has improved these results. A substantial reduction (about 50%) in the incidence of infections was obtained with this combined approach in a number of studies (Yates and Holland 1973; Levine et al. 1973; Schimpff et al. 1975; Rodriguez et al. 1978; Buckner et al. 1978; Bodey et al. 1979). However, in other studies results were less convincing (Dietrich et al. 1977; Lohner et al. 1979).

In the light of these problems, another approach was developed by van der Waaÿ and coworkers (van der Waaij et al. 1971; van der Waaij et al. 1972; van der Waaij and Berghuis-de Vries 1974; van der Waaij and Berghuis 1974): selective decontamination of the alimentary tract. This procedure aims to eliminate potentially pathogenic aerobic gram-negative rods from the alimentary tract without affecting the anaerobic flora, and is based on the observation that most infections seen in neutropenic patients are caused by these potentially pathogenic aerobic gram-negative rods, and on the observation in mice that the anaerobic flora prevent the host from becoming colonized with bacteria from the environment (colonization resistance). If the anaerobic flora is left intact, the resistance to colonization by aerobic gram-negative bacilli is believed to be maintained and subsequent infection prevented.

Antimicrobial agents such as nalidixic acid, polymyxin B and trimethoprim-sulfamethoxazole have been used for selective decontamination. These agents selectively suppress the aerobic flora and do not change the anaerobic flora (van der Waaij 1979). They are also more palatable, leading to better compliance, and are cheaper than gentamicin and vancomycin. Another advantage of this approach could be that there is no need to nurse the patient in a laminar airflow room. The results of infection prevention based on selective decontamination that have been evaluated are encouraging (Guiot and van Furth 1977; Gurwith et al. 1979; Sleijfer et al. 1980; Guiot et al. 1983; Rozenberg-Arska and Dekker 1978).

Trimethoprim/sulfamethoxazole offers several potential advantages as a single oral prophylactic antimicrobial agent (Gurwith et al. 1979; Wade et al. 1981; Dekker et al. 1981; Watson et al. 1982; Starke et al. 1982; Kaufman et al. 1983; Gualtieri et al. 1983; Kurrle et al. 1986). This drug combination is not only effective in elimination of gram-negative bacilli from the gut but is in addition well absorbed and gives therapeutic levels in the blood and tissues. Several studies have shown the superiority of trimethoprim/sulfamethoxazole over nonabsorbable drugs (Wade et al. 1981; Watson et al. 1982; Starke et al. 1982; Kurrle et al. 1986).

One of the potential problems of using trimethoprim/sulfamethoxazole alone as a prophylactic agent is the emergence of resistant gram-negative bacilli which can colonize patients and can cause infections (Wade et al. 1981; Dekker et al. 1981; Kaufman et al. 1983; Gualtieri et al. 1983; Kurrle et al. 1986; Wilson and Guiney 1982; De Jongh et al. 1981; Jacoby 1982). That means that although trimethoprim sulfamethoxazole does not affect the anaerobic flora, it does affect colonization resistance, resulting in colonization by resistant microorganisms. The problem of emergence of resistant bacteria could be partially solved by adding colistin to the trimethoprim/sulfamethoxazole regimen (Rozenberg-Arska et al. 1983). Another potential disadvantage of the prophylactic use of trimethoprim/sulfamethoxazole could be an increased duration of the granulocytopenic period, which was shown in some studies (Dekker et al. 1981; Wade et al. 1983; Pizzo et al. 1983), and the development of hypersensitivity reactions, especially due to the sulfa component (Kurrle et al. 1986, Rozenberg-Arska et al. 1983; Young 1983).

These side effects and the lack of the activity against *Pseudomonas* associated with the use of trimethoprim/sulfamethoxazole encouraged the search for more efficacious and safer antimicrobial prophylaxis in patients with prolonged and profound granulocytopenia. The newly developed quinolone derivatives hold some attractive promises.

Rozenberg-Arska et al. (1985) studied the effect of ciprofloxacin, given 500 mg twice daily to 15 patients with acute leukemia, on flora of the alimentary tract. A rapid reduction in the number of Enterobacteriaceae in faeces was observed within 3–5 days and thereafter cultures remained negative for Enterobacteriaceae. In contrast to the rapid elimination of Enterobacteriaceae, no significant reduction in the number of anaerobic gram-negative bacilli and *Clostridium* occurred, although some effect was seen on anaerobic non-spore-forming gram-positive bacilli and anaerobic cocci. During the study period (mean duration of study 46 days) six resistant strains of *Pseudomonas* spp. were isolated from 186 fecal cultures, and one resistant *Pseudomonas* spp. and two *Acinetobacter* spp. were isolated from oropharyngeal samples, but none of these bacteria colonized patients or caused infections. Most of the patients became colonized with *Staphylococcus epidermidis*. The mean peak concentration of ciprofloxacin in serum 2 h after administration of the drug was 1.6 mg/l, with a range from 0.8 to 2.3 mg/l. All but one bacteriologically documented infections were caused by gram-positive cocci (*Staphylococcus epidermidis* and α-hemolytic streptococci); no infections caused by gram-negative bacilli were observed. Ciprofloxacin was very well tolerated, compliance was excellent, and no adverse reactions were seen. This study showed that ciprofloxacin was effective for selective decontamination of the the alimentary tract and prevented infections caused by gram-negative bacilli.

The results of a randomized study by Dekker et al. (1987) showed the superiority of ciprofloxacin administered 500 mg twice daily, especially for prevention of infection caused by gram-negative bacilli in adult patients treated for acute leukemia, over the combination of trimethoprim/sulfamethoxazole and colistin. In the group of patients receiving ciprofloxacin no infections caused by gram-negative bacilli occurred; most of the acquired infections were caused by gram-positive bacteria. Ciprofloxacin also prevented colonization of the alimentary tract with resistant gram-negative bacilli. Ciprofloxacin was very well tolerated, leading to excellent compliance, and no allergic skin reactions were seen. Although fewer bacteriologically documented infections occurred in the group of patients receiving ciprofloxacin, the need for parenteral antibiotics in both study groups was identical.

The increased number of infections caused by gram-positive bacteria (*Staphylococcus epidermidis* and viridans streptococci) led us to study the ability of an erythromycin derivative (roxithromycin) to prevent infections caused by these bacteria. Forty-five consecutive patients undergoing intensive cytotoxic treatment received a short course of roxithromycin (10 days 150 mg b.i.d. orally) in addition to ciprofloxacin. During the days on which roxithromycin was added, no infections caused by α-hemolytic streptococci occurred, while in the control group of 80 patients 16 bacteremias (20%) were seen (Rozenberg et al. 1989).

Other investigators (Karp et al. 1987; Winston et al. 1986) have shown the advantageousness of using norfloxacin prophylactically in patients with acute leukemia. Oral prophylaxis with norfloxacin suppressed infection caused by aerobic gram-negative bacilli during antileukemia therapy, without significant effect on the incidence of infections caused by gram-positive bacteria. In a prospective, double-blind, placebo-controlled trial Karp et al. (1987) studied the role of oral norfloxacin (400 mg b.i.d.) in preventing bacterial infections in adults with acute leukemia. In this study it was shown that norfloxacin reduced the incidence of infections by gram-negative bacteria. However, in 3 of 35 patients receiving norfloxacin, colonization of the oropharynx with gram-negative bacilli led to subsequent bacteremia. In those patients norfloxacin failed to prevent gram-negative infections originating outside the gastrointestinal tract. Norfloxacin was very well tolerated and did not predispose patients to the development of bacteria resistant either to norfloxacin or to other antibiotics. In this study all patients receiving either norfloxacin or placebo still received parenteral antimicrobial therapy after having a similar incidence of fever; ultimate survival was not affected.

Winston et al. (1986) evaluated the effect of norfloxacin (400 mg t.i.d.) for prevention of infections in granulocytopenic patients. The efficacy was compared with the efficacy of vancomycin-polymyxin. In patients receiving norfloxacin prophylactically no infections by gram-negative bacilli were seen. Non-*Pseudomonas aeruginosa* colonization occurred frequently, but none of the colonizing bacteria caused infection. There was no difference between the two groups in the use of parenteral antimicrobial therapy. Six of the 36 patients receiving norfloxacin and 2 of the 30 patients receiving vancomycin-polymyxin did not require intravenous antibiotics.

Kern et al. (1987) used ofloxacin (200 mg b.i.d.) prophylactically in granulocytopenic patients and demonstrated rapid elimination of gram-negative bacteria from the alimentary tract. However, 4 of 40 patients became colonized by gram-negative bacilli and two of three patients colonized with ofloxacin-resistant *Pseudomonas aeruginosa* strains developed *Pseudomonas* infections. Maschmeyer et al. (1988) concluded from the EORTC Gnotobiotic Project Group that ciprofloxacin and norfloxacin at a daily dosage of 1000 mg and 800 mg respectively can be used for infection prevention in severely granulocytopenic patients. Lower dosages of those antibiotics are not recommended because of persistent or de novo colonization by Enterobacteriaceae and non-fermenters.

Prophylactic use of antibiotics and especially new quinolone derivatives in granulocytopenic patients may lead to a change in the spectrum of infections seen in these patients, from infections caused by organisms such as Enterobacteriaceae or *Pseudomonas aeruginosa* to *Staphylococcus epidermidis*, α-hemolytic streptococci and other gram-positive bacteria (Rozenberg-Arska et al. 1983; Dekker et al. 1987; Karp et al. 1987; Winston et al. 1986; Kern et al. 1987; Maschmeyer et al. 1988). *Staphylococcus epidermidis* infections (mostly bacteremias) are often associated with the presence of long-term indwelling central venous catheters (Blacklock et al. 1980; Lowder et al. 1982). These infections are usually not life threatening and can be successfully treated with cephalotin or vancomycin without removal of the line.

In contrast to infections caused by *Staphylococcus epidermidis*, many infections caused by α-hemolytic streptococci, frequently related to intensive cytotoxic treatment, are severe. Intensive cytotoxic treatment leads not only to prolonged and profound granulocytopenia, but often also to ulcerations of the oropharynx and alimentary tract, which provide entry for streptococci with subsequent invasion of the bloodstream and deep tissues (Dekker et al. 1987;

Cohen et al. 1983; Peters et al. 1988; Henslee et al. 1984; Kern et al. 1987). The infections caused by α-hemolytic streptococci can be life threatening, often resembling adult respiratory distress syndrome and/or shock (Henslee et al. 1984; Kern et al. 1987; Steiner et al. 1988). In order to decrease the infections caused by α-hemolytic streptococci, Rozenberg-Arska et al. (1988) added roxithromycin (a new well-absorbed oral macrolide antibiotic) to a ciprofloxacin prophylactic regimen during the period of severe mucosal damage and bone marrow aplasia. Addition of roxithromycin prevented infections caused by α-hemolytic streptococci.

The authors concluded that patients receiving intensive cytotoxic treatment should receive for prophylaxis not only antimicrobial agents effective against gram-negative bacilli, but also gram-positive coverage until lesions are healed. The changing pattern of bacterial infection seen in patients receiving quinolones prophylactically suggests a need to include an antibiotic effective against gram-positive organisms in the initial therapeutic regimen. At present such a regimen can include cephalotin or vancomycin (depending on the incidence of methicillin resistance among staphylococci) or perhaps imipenem/cilastatin.

More studies are needed to ascertain the true efficacy of quinolone derivatives for prevention of infection. Careful monitoring for the emergence of resistant organisms remains mandatory. Moreover, it must be agreed with Young (1987) that the present therapeutic promise of the quinolones could undermine their ultimate prophylactic utility.

It still remains an open question why quinolones are able to prevent infections. It may be due to their effect on the gut flora or due to their systemic effect, or both. Studies comparing oral absorbable drugs with oral non-absorbable drugs (e.g., Kurrle et al. 1986) indicate that absorbable drugs are better able to prevent infections than nonabsorbable drugs, although both regimens are able to selectively decontaminate the gastrointestinal tract. This would be in line with findings published by Wells and other (Wells et al. 1987). This group showed that bacteria may translocate from the gastrointestinal tract to the mesenteric lymph nodes, where they can survive. These bacteria could then be an initial site of invasion into other tissues. Thus, the reason why oral nonabsorbable drugs are less effective than oral absorbable drugs (e.g., quinolones) is that they do not eliminate bacteria from the lymph nodes, allowing foci of infection to remain.

References

Bauernfeind A, Petermuller C (1983) In vitro activity of ciprofloxacin, norfloxacin and nalidixic acid. Eur J Clin Microbiol 2: 111–115
Blacklock HA, Hill RS, Clarke AG, Pillai MV, Matthews JRD, Wade JF (1980) Use of modified subcutaneous right-atrial catheter for venous access in leukemic patients. Lancet I: 993–994

Bodey GP, Buckley M, Sathe YS, Freireich EJ (1966) Quantitative relationships between circulating leukocytes and infection in patients with acute leukemia. Ann Intern Med 64: 328–340

Bodey GP, McCredie KB, Keating MJ, Freireich EJ (1979) Treatment of acute leukemia in protected environment units. Cancer 44: 431–436

Bodey GP, Rodriguez V, Chang H-Y, Narboni G (1978) Fever and infections in leukemic patients. A study of 494 consecutive patients. Cancer 41: 1610–1622

Buckner CD, Clift RA, Sanders JE, Meyers JD, Counts GW, Farewell VT, Thomas ED, Seattle Marrow Transplant team (1978) Protective environment for marrow transplant recipients. A prospective study. Ann Intern Med 89: 893–901

Cohen J, Donnelly JP, Worsley AM, Catovsky D, Goldman JM, Galton DAG (1983) Septicemia caused by viridans streptococci in neutropenic patients with leukemia. Lancet II: 1452–1454

Crump B, Wise R, and Dent J (1983) The pharmacokinetics and tissue penetration of ciprofloxacin. Antimicrob Agents. Chemother 24: 784–786

Dekker AW, Rozenberg-Arska M, Sixma JJ, Verhoef J (1981) Prevention of infection by trimethoprim-sulfamethoxazole plus amphotericin B in patients with acute non-lymphocytic leukemia. Ann Intern Med 95: 555–559

Dekker AW, Punt K, Verdonck LF (1987a) The use of amsacrine plus intermediate-dose cytosine arabinoside in relapsed and refractory acute nonlymphocytic leukemia. In: Büchner T, Schellong G, Hiddemann W, Urbanitz D, Ritter J (eds) Acute Leukemias. Springer, Berlin Heidelberg New York, pp 333–335 (Haematology and blood transfusion vol 30)

Dekker AW, Rozenberg-Arska M, Verhoef J (1987b) Infection prophylaxis in acute leukemia: a comparison of ciprofloxacin with trimethoprim/sulfamethoxazole and colistin. Ann Intern Med 106: 7–12

de Jongh CA, Schimpff SC, Wiernik PH (1981) Antibiotic prophylaxis in acute leukemia. Ann Intern Med 95: 783–784

Dietrich M, Gaus W, Vossen J, van der Waaij D, Wendt F (1977) Protective isolation and antimicrobial decontamination in patients with high susceptibility to infection. A prospective cooperative study of gnotobiotic care in leukemia patients. I. Clinical results. Infection 5: 107–114

Gualtieri RJ, Donovitz GR, Kaiser DL, Hess CE, Saride MA (1983) Double blind randomized study of prophylactic trimethoprim-sulfamethoxazole in granulocytopenic patients with haematologic malignancies. Am J Med 74: 934–40

Guiot HFL, van Furth R (1977) Partial decontamination. Br Med J 1: 800–802

Guiot HFL, van den Broeke JWM, van der Meer JWM, van Furth R (1983) Selective antimicrobial modulation of the intestinal flora of patients with acute non-lymphocytic leukemia: a double-blind placebo controlled study. J Infect Dis 47: 615–623

Gurwith MJ, Brunton JL, Lank BA, Ronald AR, Harding GKM (1978) Granulocytopenia in hospitalized patients. I. Prognostic factors and etiology of fever. Am J Med 64: 121–126

Gurwith MJ, Brunton JL, Lank BA, Harding GLM, Ronald AR (1979) A prospective controlled investigation of prophylactic trimethoprim/sulfamethoxazole in hospitalized granulocytopenic patients. Am J Med 66: 248–256

Henslee J, Bostrom B, Weidsdorf D, Ramsay N, McGlave P, Kersey J (1984) Streptococcal sepsis in bone marrow transplant patients. Lancet I: 393

Jacoby GA (1982) Perils of prophylaxis. N Engl J Med 306: 43–44

344   M. Rozenberg-Arska et al.

Karp JE, Merz WG, Hendricksen C, Laughon B, Redden T, Bamberger BJ, Bartlett JG, Saral L, Burke PJ (1987) Oral norfloxacin for prevention of gram-negative bacterial infections in patients with acute leukemia and granulocytopenia. A randomized, double-blind, placebo-controlled trial. Ann Intern Med 106: 1–7

Kaufman CA, Liepman MK, Bergman AG, Mioduszewski J (1983) Trimethoprim-sulfamethoxazole prophylaxis in neutropenic patients. Reduction of infections and effect on bacterial and fungal flora. Am J Med 74: 599–607

Kern W, Kurrle E, Vanek E (1987a) Ofloxacin for prevention of bacterial infections in granulocytopenic patients. Infection 15: 427–432

Kern W, Kurrle E, Vanek E (1987b) High risk of streptococcal septicemia after high dose cytosine arabinoside treatment for acute myelogenous leukemia. Klin Wochenschr 65: 773–780

Kurrle E, Dekker AW, Gaus W, Haralambie E, Krieger D, Rozenberg-Arska M, De Vries-Hospersd HG, van der Waaij D, Wendt F (1986) Prevention of infection in acute leukaemia: a prospective randomized study on the efficacy of two different drug regimens for antimicrobial prophylaxis. Infection 14: 226–232

Levine AS, Siegel SE, Schreiber AD, Hauser J, Preisler H, Goldstein IM, Seidler F, Simon R, Perry S, Bennett JE, Henderson ES (1973) Protected environments and prophylactic antibiotics. A prospective controlled study of their utility in the therapy of acute leukemia. N Engl J Med 288: 477–483

Lohner D, Debusscher L, Prevost JM, Klastersky J (1979) Comparative randomized study of protected environment plus oral antibiotics versus oral antibiotics alone in neutropenic patients. Cancer Treat Rep 63: 363–368

Lowder JN, Lazarus HM, Herzig RH (1982) Bacteremias and fungemias in oncologic patients with central venous catheters. Changing spectrum of infection. Arch Intern Med 142: 1456–1459

Maschmeyer G, Haralambie E, Gaus W, Kern W, Dekker AW, De Vries-Hospers HG, Sizoo W, König W, Gutzler F, Daenen S (1988) Ciprofloxacin and norfloxacin for selective decontamination in patients with severe granulocytopenia. Infection 16: 98–104

Peters WG, Willemze R, Colly LP (1988) Results of induction and consolidation treatment with intermediate and high-dose cytosine arabinoside and m-AMSA of patients with poor-risk acute myelogenous leukemia. Eur J Hematol 40: 198–204

Pizzo PA, Schimpff SC (1983) Strategies for the prevention of infection in the myelosuppressed or immunosuppressed cancer patient. Cancer Treat Rep 67: 223–34

Pizzo PA, Robichaud K, Edwards B (1983) Oral antibiotic prophylaxis in patients with cancer. A double blind randomized placebo controlled trial. J Pediatr 102: 125–133

Rodriguez V, Bodey GP, Freireich EJ, McCredie KB, Gutterman JU, Keating MJ, Smith TL, Gehan EA (1978) Randomized trial of protected environment–prophylactic antibiotics in 145 adults with acute leukemia. Medicine 57: 253–266

Rozenberg-Arska M, Dekker AW (1978) Prevention of bacterial and fungal infection in granulocytopenic patients. In: Peterson PK, Verhoef J (eds) Antimicrobial agents annual 2. Elsevier, Amsterdam, pp 471–481

Rozenberg-Arska M, Dekker AW, Verhoef J (1983) Colistin and trimethoprim sulfamethoxazole for the prevention of infection in patients with acute non-lymphocytic leukemia. Decrease in the emergence of resistant bacteria. Infection 11: 167–169

Rozenberg-Arska M, Dekker AW, Verhoef J (1985) Ciprofloxacin for selective decontamination of the alimentary tract in patients with acute leukemia during remission induction treatment: the effect on fecal flora. J Infect Dis 152: 104–107

Rozenberg-Arska M, Dekker AW, Verdonck LF, Verhoef J (1989) Prevention of gram-positive bacteremias by a short course of roxithromycin (RU) in granulocytopenic patients receiving ciprofloxacin (CF) prophylactically. Infection 17: 240–244

Schimpff SC (1980) Infection prevention during profound granulocytopenia. New approaches to alimentary canal microbial suppression. Ann Intern Med 93: 358–361

Schimpff SC, Young VM, Greene WH, Vermeulen GD, Moody MR, Wiernik PH (1972) Origin of infection in acute nonlymphocytic leukemia. Significance of hospital acquisition of potential pathogens. Ann Intern Med 77: 707–714

Schimpff SC, Greene WH, Young VM, Fortner CL, Jepsen L, Cusack N, Block JB, Wiernik PH (1975) Infection prevention in acute non-lymphocytic leukemia. Laminar air flow room reverse isolation with oral, non-absorbable antibiotic prophylaxis. Ann Intern Med 82: 351–358

Shannon KP, Phillips I (1985) The antimicrobial spectrum of the quinolones. Res Clin Forum 7: 29–36

Sleijfer DTh, Mulder NH, de Vries-Hospers HG, Fidler V, Nieweg HO, Van der Waaij D, Van Saene HKF (1980) Infection prevention in granulocytopenic patients by selective decontamination of the digestive tract. Eur J Cancer 16: 859–869

Starke JD, Catovsky D, Johnson SA, Donnelly P, Darrel J, Goldman JM, Galton DAG (1982) Cotrimoxazole alone for prevention of bacterial infection in patients with acute leukemia. Lancet I: 5–6

Steiner M, Villablanca J, Kersey J, Ramsay N, Ferrier M, Haake R, Weisdorf D (1988) α-streptococcal shock in bone marrow transplantation patients (abstract no. 1548). Blood 72 (suppl 1): 409A

van der Waaij D (1979) Colonization resistance of the digestive tract as a major lead in the selection of antibiotics for therapy. In: Van der Waaij D, Verhoef J (eds) New criteria for antimicrobial therapy: maintenance of digestive tract colonization resistance. Excerpta Medica, Amsterdam, pp 271–282

van der Waaij D, Berghuis JM (1974) Determination of the colonization resistance of the digestive tract of individual mice. J Hyg (Camb) 72: 379–387

van der Waaij D, Berghuis-de Vries JM (1974) Selective elimination of Enterobacteriaceae species from the digestive tract in mice and monkeys. J Hyg (Camb) 72: 205–211

van der Waaij D, Berghuis-de Vries JM, Lekkerkerk-van der Wees JEC (1971) Colonization resistance of the digestive tract in conventional and antibiotic-treated mice. J Hyg (Camb) 69: 405–411

van der Waaij D, Berghuis JM, Lekkerkerk JEC (1972) Colonization resistance of the digestive tract of mice during systemic antibiotic treatment. J Hyg (Camb) 70: 605–610

Wade JC, Schimpff SC, Hargadon MT, Fortner CL, Young VM, Wiernik PH (1981) A comparison of trimethoprim-sulfamethoxazole plus nystatin with gentamicin plus nystatin in the prevention of infections in acute leukemia. N Engl J Med 304: 1057–1062

Wade JC, de Jongh CA, Newman KA, Crowley J, Wiernik PH, Schimpff SC (1983) Selective antimicrobial modulation as prophylaxis against infection during granulocytopenia: trimethoprim-sulfamethoxazole vs. nalidixic acid. J Infect Dis 147: 624–634

Watson JG, Powles RL, Lawson DN, Morgenstern GR, Jameson B, McElwain TJ, Judson J, Lumley H, Kay HEM (1982) Contrimoxazole versus nonabsorbable antibiotics in acute leukemia. Lancet I: 6–9

Wells CL, Maddaus MA, Reynolds CM, Jechorek RP, Simmons RL (1987a) Role of anaerobic flora in the translocation of aerobic and facultatively anaerobic intestinal bacteria. Infect Immun 55: 2689–2694

346   M. Rozenberg-Arska et al.

Wells CL, Maddaus MA, Jechorek RP, Simmons RL (1987b) Ability of intestinal Escherichia coli to survive within mesenteric lymph nodes. Infect Immun 55: 2834–2837

Wilson JM, Guiney DG (1982) Failure of oral trimethoprim-sulfamethoxazole prophylaxis in acute leukemia: isolation of resistant plasmids from strains of Enterobacteriaceae causing bacteremia. N Engl J Med 306: 16–20

Winston DJ, Ho WG, Nakao SL, Gale RP, Champlin RE (1986) Norfloxacin versus vancomycin/polymyxin for prevention of infections in granulocytopenic patients. Am J Med 80: 884–890

Wise R, Lockley MR, Crump B, Adhami ZN (1985) The pharmacokinetics and tissue penetration of orally administered enoxacin, norfloxacin and ciprofloxacin. Res Clin Forum 7: 63–68

Yates JW, Holland JF (1973) A controlled study of isolation and endogenous microbial suppression in acute myelocytic leukemia patients. Cancer 32: 1490–1498

Young LS (1983) Antimicrobial prophylaxis against infection in neutropenic patients. J Infect Dis 147: 611–614

Young LS (1987) The new fluorinated quinolones for infection prevention in acute leukemia. Ann Int Med 106: 144–146

Influence of Infusion Time on the Acute Toxicity of Amphotericin B: Results of a Randomized Double-Blind Study

M. Arning, B. Dresen, C. Aul, and W. Schneider

Abteilung für Innere Medizin, Heinrich Heine-Universität Düsseldorf, Moorenstraße 5, W-4000 Düsseldorf, FRG

Despite the development of several new antifungal drugs, intravenous amphotericin B (amB) is still considered the drug of choice for the treatment of severe systemic fungal infections in immunocompromised patients. However, therapy is often limited by various side effects (Table 1). From the patients' point of view, the acute toxic reactions (fever, chills, nausea and vomiting) induced by the drug are particularly troublesome.

The package insert recommends that intravenous amB should be given over 4–6 h in an attempt to minimize the incidence and severity of toxic reactions, although it has not conclusively been shown that this is either necessary or effective. Administration of AmB over several hours often interferes with the scheduled administration of other intravenous drugs, blood products and hyperalimentation and leads to logistical problems in patients under intensive care. The standard infusion protocol also makes therapy on an outpatient basis difficult.

Several small studies have been performed evaluating the incidence and severity of amB-related toxicity after infusions lasting between 30 min and 2 h.

Table 1. Side effects induced by amphotericin B

Frequent	Rare
Chills	Anaphylactoid reactions
Fever	Hepatotoxicity
Nausea	Neurological symptoms
Vomiting	
Thrombophlebitis	
Anaemia	
Hypokalaemia	
Nephrotoxicity	

There are reports that no greater toxicity occurs after short-time infusions (Seabury and Dascomb 1958; Fields et al. 1971; Spitzer et al. 1989), and less toxicity has been reported with infusion of amB lasting 2–3 h (Utz et al. 1964; Campbell 1982) than with infusions over 4–6 h. However, most of the studies were retrospective, involved small patient groups, or used different premedications, which makes interpretation of the data difficult. We therefore performed a prospective, randomized, double-blind study to evaluate the incidence and severity of acute toxic reactions after a 2-h vs. a 4-h intravenous infusion of amB.

Patients and Method

25 adult patients (median age 48 years, range 21–72 years) suffering from acute non-lymphocytic or lymphocytic leukaemia gave their informed consent to participate in the study. Intravenous amB therapy was required because of suspected or microbiologically proven fungal infections occurring during chemotherapy-induced aplasia. Pregnant patients and those with known anaphylactoid reactions to amB or with renal failure were not eligible.

The study protocol is shown in Table 2. We used a cross-over design because of the fact that amB-related acute toxicity usually lessens with continuing treatment. Acute toxic reactions due to amB were studied during the first 8 days of treatment. On day 1, a test dose of 1 mg amB was given over 1 h to exclude severe anaphylactoid reactions. If no reaction occurred, the dosage was increased stepwise up to 1 mg/kg body weight on day 7. On day 2, patients were randomized to receive either a 2- or a 4-h infusion of amB. The infusion time then alternated every other day between 2 and 4 h. After each infusion, patients were asked to report symptoms probably related to the amB infusion. Toxicity was graded daily by one of us (DB) according to modified WHO criteria for adverse reactions (Tables 3, 4). On day 8, patients were asked whether they would prefer further antifungal treatment with the 2-h or the 4-h infusion regimen.

Table 2. Study protocol

Day 1	Test dose of 1 mg amphotericin B over 1 h i.v.; patients randomized		
	Drug dose	Infusion regimen 1	Infusion regimen 2
Day 2	5 mg	2 h	4 h
Day 3	15 mg	4 h	2 h
Day 4	30 mg	2 h	4 h
Day 5	45 mg	4 h	2 h
Day 6	60 mg	2 h	4 h
Day 7	1 mg/kg body weight	4 h	2 h
Day 8	Patients asked: further antifungal therapy with infusions over 2 or 4 h? Further treatment with dosage of 1 mg/kg body weight per day		

Table 3. Grading of amphotericin B-related acute toxicity: chills and fever. (Modified from WHO)

Grade 0:	No elevation of temperature
Grade 1:	Rise in temperature by up to 1°C over baseline temperature, shivering
Grade 2:	Minor chill, rise in temperature by up to 2°C over baseline, symptoms controlled by 1 g acetaminophen
Grade 3:	Major chills with dyspnoea and cyanosis, rise in temperature by up to 2°C over baseline, symptoms controlled by intravenous pethidine and/or corticosteroids
Grade 4:	Life-threatening reaction with elevation of temperature above 40°C with cyanosis, dyspnoea, bronchospasmus, and circulatory failure

Table 4. Grading of amphotericin B-related acute toxicity: nausea and vomiting. (Modified from WHO)

Grade 0:	No nausea or vomiting
Grade 1:	Nausea without vomiting
Grade 2:	Nausea with vomiting lasting <2 h after drug infusion
Grade 3:	Nausea with vomiting lasting >2 h, antiemetic therapy necessary
Grade 4:	Nausea with vomiting despite antiemetic therapy

No systematic premedication with corticosteroids, antihistamines or antipyretics was given. Precautions were taken to guarantee optimal supportive care when severe side effects occurred.

The double-blinding of the study was ensured as follows: the amB infusions were prepared by a nurse not involved in the care of the patients. The drug was infused in opaque Perfusor syringes and opaque lines using a central venous line. For infusions over 4-h the dose of amB was divided in two syringes each infused over 2 h. When given over 2 h, the drug was infused with the first syringe during the first 2 h, and a glucose 5% solution was then administered as placebo over the next 2 h.

Results

A total of 184 infusions was administered, 91 over 2 h and 93 over 4 h. There were no grade 4 reactions after administration of the drug and in no patient were side effects severe enough to lead to permanent discontinuation of amB therapy.

Chills

The incidence of amB-related chills is shown in Fig. 1. Shivering and overt chills occurred less often after the 2-h infusions, but the difference was not statistically

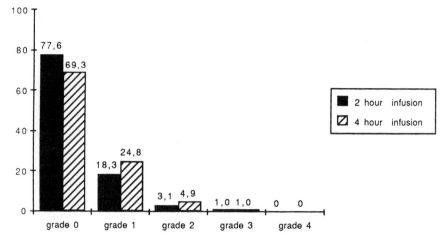

Fig. 1. Incidence of amphotericin B-related chills (% of infusions)

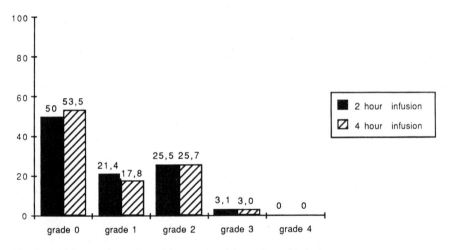

Fig. 2. Incidence of amphotericin B-related fever (% of infusions)

significant. Major chills with a subsequent rise of temperature to more than 40°C were rarely observed (after 1% of the infusions in both groups).

Fever

Fever occurred after 50% of amB infusions with approximately the same incidence after the 2- and 4-h infusions (Fig. 2). A rise in temperature by up to 2°C over baseline values without chills was observed after one quarter of the infusions in both groups. Temperature usually rose 2-h after the start of amB and peaked at 4 h. Acetaminophen at a dose of 1000 mg given orally was

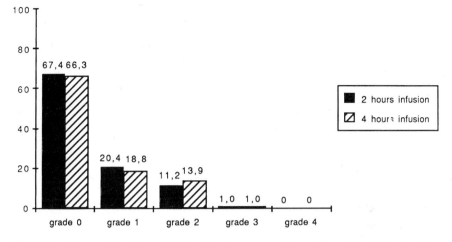

Fig. 3. Incidence of amphotericin B-related nausea and vomiting (% of infusions)

generally sufficient to return temperature to normal. When interpreting these data, one must remember that chills and temperature may not only be due to amB, but also due to the underlying suspected or documented fungal infection. Nearly all patients had at least low-grade fever due to infection at the time of randomization. Furthermore, it can not be excluded that other drugs administered in combination with amB may have caused fever and chills in these seriously ill patients. Although we tried to exclude fever not related to amB, the incidence of amB-induced febrile reactions may be overestimated. Nevertheless, in regard to amB-related acute toxicity there was no difference between the two infusion regimens, either in severity or incidence of fever or chills, suggesting that the two infusion schedules are equally pyrogenic.

Nausea and Vomiting

Nausea and vomiting accompanied amB infusions in approximately one third of all infusions studied, regardless of the infusion time (Fig. 3). Severe nausea despite antiemetic therapy was rarely observed. Again, there is a trend favouring the 2-h infusion as the better tolerated regimen, but there was no statistic difference. It may be argued that chemotherapy of the underlying disease has an influence on the incidence or severity of nausea and vomiting. However, as amB was given in therapy-induced aplasia usually 1–3 weeks after chemotherapy, it is unlikely that the latter had an influence. We also excluded drug-induced gastrointestinal disturbances caused by other, co-administered drugs.

Subjective Acceptance

As mentioned earlier, patients were asked on day 8 of amB therapy whether they would prefer further intravenous amB therapy performed with the long or short infusion time. Out of 25 patients, 24 wanted the 2-h infusion regimen. This was not because they actually had experienced less severe side effects when treated with the 2-h infusion, but because they appreciated the reduction of the infusion time by 2 h.

Conclusion

Based on these data we conclude that amB given over 2 h is as well – or poorly (!) – tolerated when given over 4 h. There were no more side effects using the 2-h infusion regimen. AmB given over 2 h reduces the demands on staff time and will facilitate treatment on an outpatient basis. Patients preferred the short infusion time because it shortened the overall infusion protocol and increased their mobility.

References

Campbell GD (1982) Using amphotericin B. Intern Med 3: 95–102

Fields BT, Bates JH, Abernathy RS (1971) Effect of rapid intravenous infusion on serum concentrations of amphotericin B. Appl Microbiol 22: 615–617

Loomer L, Cruz J, Powell B, Capizzi R, Peacock J (1988) Rapid intravenous (iv) infusion of amphotericin B (AmB) (abstract). Proc ASCO 7: 285

Seabury JH, Dascomb HE (1958) Experience with amphotericin B for the treatment of systemic mycoses. Arch Intern Med 102: 960–976

Spitzer TR, Creger RJ, Fox RM, Lazarus HM (1989) Rapid infusion amphotericin B: effective and well-tolerated therapy for neutropenic fever. Pharmatherapeutica 5: 305–311

Utz JP, Bennett JE, Brandriss MW, Butler T, Hill GJ (1964) Amphotericin B toxicity. Ann Intern Med 61: 334–354

New Antiviral Drugs for Treatment of Viral Infections in Immunocompromised Patients

U. Jehn

Medizinische Klinik III, Klinikum Großhadern, Ludwig-Maximilian-Universität, Marchioninistraße 15, W-8000 München 70, FRG

In non-immunocompromised individuals, herpes simplex virus (HSV) infections are among the most prevalent involving mucous membranes and the skin. HSV encephalitis is the most common cause of sporadic fatal encephalitis in the western world and is estimated to occur in approximately one in 250 000–500 000 persons per year [1]. Neutropenic cancer patients – particularly bone marrow transplant (BMT) recipients – are at very high risk for herpesvirus infections in addition to fungal infections. This is due to the defective cell-mediated immunity as well as to better control of serious bacterial infections which previously were lethal. It has been shown [2] that herpesviruses reactivate in these patients in a certain sequence and a high proportion of cases (Table 1). Cytomegalovirus (CMV) infections are clinically most relevant because they are one of the major causes of death. Over one half of the cases of interstitial pneumonitis in these patients are associated with CMV infection, and a high proportion of those in which no etiology is identified are probably undetected cases of CMV infection [3]. There is an increased incidence of CMV infections and interstitial pneumonitis in patients receiving granulocyte transfusions, particularly if the granulocytes were obtained from donors who show evidence of previous CMV infection [4]. CMV retinitis was seen relatively infrequently until the AIDS pandemic. Today it is diagnosed in 28% of AIDS patients. In AIDS, the immune defect is pronounced, and without therapy CMV retinitis – giving a "pizza-like" appearance to the retina – will lead to progressive retinal destruction [5].

The first antiviral drug for systemic use that was relatively effective and not too toxic was vidarabine. This drug has now been superseded by acyclovir due to both the efficacy and the safety of the latter [6]. As shown in Fig. 1, acyclovir, a nucleoside analogue, is phosphorylated to acyclovir monophosphate by a specific thymidine kinase provided by the target virus. The final activated triphosphate is then incorporated into the viral DNA, replacing deoxyguanosine triphosphate, thereby blocking viral replication. Acyclovir has a selective toxicity for HSV, varicella zoster virus (VZV), and to some extent, Epstein–Barr virus (EBV). CMV shows only limited susceptibility at high concentrations of

Table 1. Incidence and sequence of reactivation of viral infection after allogeneic bone marrow transplantation

HSV	42%	0–20 days (peak: 18).
EBV	60%	14–21 days (peak : 17)
CMV	70%	40–80 days (peak : 50)
VZV	35%	100–160 days (peak: 130)

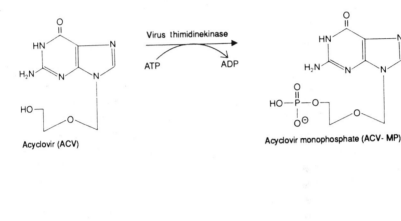

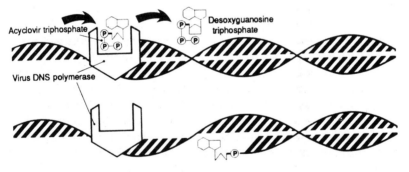

Fig. 1. *Above*: Phosphorylation and activation of acyclovir by the viral thymidine kinase. *Below*: Inhibition of viral DNA replication by activated acyclovir

the drug [7]. Acyclovir is the drug of choice for prevention of HSV infections in severely immunocompromised patients, as indicated by a placebo-controlled trial [8]. For the compromised host, in particular, the development of intravenous acyclovir has been a milestone and a major advance in the treatment of overt infections with HSV and VZV [9], for although usually self-limiting in the normal host, such infections may produce extensive and persistent ulcerative disease in the immunocompromised host [10].

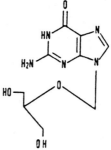

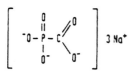

foscarnet (PFA)   dihydroxypropoxymethylguanine (DHPG)

Fig. 2   **Fig. 3**

Severe mucocutaneous infections due to acyclovir-resistant herpesvirus infections are now occurring with increasing frequency, pabticularly in AIDS
patients [11, 12]. Acyclovir resistance may arise from mutations in the genes for
thymidine kinase or DNA polymerase. The most common mechanism of
resistance in patients is the replication of mutants deficient in viral thymidine
kinase activity. Alternative therapies for HSV infections that fail to resolve with
acyclovir therapy include foscarnet [13], a pyrophosphate analogue (Fig. 2) that
inhibits HSV DNA polymerase without activation by viral thymidine kinase,
and, secondly, vidarabine, mentioned earlier. Vidarabine is activated to the
triphosphate form by cellular enzymes and also inhibits HSV DNA polymerase.
Furthermore, foscarnet is effective in diminishing the severity of generalized
CMV infections, as shown in preliminary clinical studies [14]. It is a trisodium
phosphonoformate hexahydrate. Toxicity studies in humans have shown only
mild adverse effects, including anemia and a rise in serum creatinine levels [15]. A
major disadvantage of the drug is related to the need for continuous infucion for
a 2- to 3-week period, due to its short half-life. The recomended dose is
2–8 g/day, reaching a steady state plasma level of 150 μg/ml.

Structurally related to acyclovir is dihydroxypropoxymethylguanine (DHPG)
or ganciclovir (Fig. 3). Compared to acyclovir it is 10-fold more potent in
inhibiting CMV and EBV viral replication in vitro [16]. It seems to be fairly
specific against CMV [17]. Because of this and the high clinical relevance of
CMV infections in immunocompromised cancer patients, several clinical trials,
mainly in BMT recipients, have been initiated to test its prophylactic and
therapeutic value in CMV-infected patients. In AIDS patients, ganciclovir has
been shown to stabilize CMV retinitis, but relapses occur in the vast majority of
patients shortly after therapy is discontinued [15, 18]. Furthermore, severe
neutropenia, the major adverse side effect of this drug, often limits its use in
patients with AIDS or after BMT because of its bone marrow toxicity. Finally,
the emergence of ganciclovir-resistant strains of CMV has been described

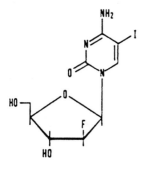

fluoroiodoaracytosine (FIAC)

Fig. 4

recently [19]. Foscarnet has been used in these three instances successfully and may be a reasonable alternative [15].

Fluoroiodoaracytosine (FIAC) (Fig. 4) is another new antiviral drug with potent in vitro activity against HSV, VZV, CMV, and EBV, but its in vivo therapeutic index is far from impressive. It is hampered by severe side effects, particularly myelotoxicity (dosage 400–600 mg/m² per day) [20].

Bromovinyldeoxyuridine (BVDU) (Fig. 5) is the most potent and the most selective of all anti-HSV and -VZV agents currently being investigated for therapeutic potential. Its potency to inhibit viral replication is superior to that of acyclovir [20]. As shown in a preliminary study by Tricot [21], the drug arrested progression of infection in the majority of patients suffering from HSV-1 or VZV infection within 1 day of treatment. BVDU has several advantages over acyclovir in the oral treatment of VZV infections and – most important – is still effective when treatment is initiated after prolonged infection, even if the latter is unresponsive to acyclovir.

Finally, emphasis must be placed on the development of newer drugs, which act against herpesviruses by different mechanisms or do not require thymidine-kinase for activation. One such agent is HPMPA (Fig. 6). This is an acyclic adenosine analogue and is phosphorylated intracellularly. The active form is probably its diphosphoryl derivative, targeting the viral DNA polymerase. This new compound has a potent and selective activity against a broad spectrum of DNA viruses in vitro and is also active against retroviruses (Table 2). It combines both good efficacy in animal models and apparent lack of toxicity at the active dosage schedules. It has not been tried in humans yet.

In summary (Table 3), there is a whole battery of new antiviral drugs both in clinical trials and under intensive investigation. With better understanding of their pharmacology and better knowledge of viral biochemistry, great progress has been made and more will come in the near future.

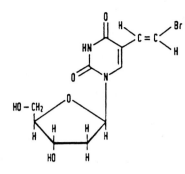

bromovinyldeoxyuridine (BVDU)

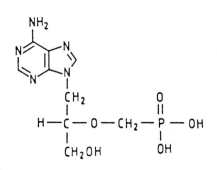

(S)-HPMPA

Fig. 5   **Fig. 6**

Table 2. Activity spectrum of (S)-HPMPA

HSV-1, HSV-2, HSV-TK⁻
VZV, VZV-TK⁻
CMV
Phocid (SeHV), simian (HVP), suid (SHV-1), bovid (BHV-1), and equid
herpesvirus (EHV-1)
African swine fever virus (ASF)
Human adenoviruses, vaccinia virus
Retrovirus: murine sarcoma virus (MSV)

Table 3. Antiviral drugs in use, undergoing clinical trial, or experimental

Drug	Target
Vidarabine (Ara A)	HSV, VZV, ACV-resistant HSV
Acyclovir (ACV)	HSV, VZV, (EBV)
Ganciclovir (DHPG)	CMV
Foscarnet (PFA)	ACV-resistant HSV, CMV, DHPG-resistant CMV
Fluoroidoaracytosine (FIAC)	HSV, VZV, CMV, EBV
Bromovinyldeoxyuridine (BVDU)	HSV-1, VZV
(S)-9-(3-hydroxy-2-phosphonylmethoxy-propyladenine) (HPMPA)	Broad spectrum DNA and retroviruses

References

1. Whitley HJ (1988) Herpes simplex virus infections of the central nervous system. Am J Med 85: 61–67
2. van der Meer JW, Guit HF, van den Broek PJ (1984) Infections in bone marrow transplant recipients. Sem Hematol 21: 123–140
3. Champlin RE, Gale RP (1984) The early complications of bone marrow transplantation. Sem Hematol 21: 101–108
4. Winston DW, Pollard RB, Howell CL et al. (1980) Cytomegalovirus infections associated with leukocyte transfusions. Am Intern Med 97: 671–675
5. Holland GN, Pepose JS, Pettit TH et al. (1983) Acquired immune deficiency syndrome – ocular manifestations. Ophthalmology 90: 859–873
6. Shepp DH, Dandliker PS, Meyers JD (1986) Treatment of varicellazoster virus infection in severely immunocompromised patients. A randomized comparison of acyclovir and vidarabine. N Engl J Med 314: 208–212
7. Schaefer HJ, Beauchamp L, de Miranda P et al. (1978) 9-(2-hydroxy-ethoxymethyl)guanine activity against viruses of the herpes group. Nature 272: 583–585
8. Meyers JD, Reed EC, Shepp DH et al. (1988) Acyclovir for prevention of cytomegalovirus infection and disease after allogenic marrow transplantation. N Engl J Med 318: 70–75
9. Wade MS, Newton B, Mclaren C et al. (1982) Intravenous acyclovir to treat mucocutaneous herpes simplex virus infection after marrow transplantation. Ann Intern Med 96: 265–269
10. Corey L, Spear PG (1986) Infections with herpes simplex viruses. N Engl J Med 3!4: 686–691
11. Hirsch MS, Schooley RT (1989) Resistance to antiviral drugs: the end of innocence. N Engl J Med 320: 313–314
12. Erlich KS, Mills J, Chatis P et al. (1989) Acyclovir-resistant herpes simplex virus infections in patients with acquired immunodeficiency syndrome. N Engl J Med 320: 293–296
13. Chatis PA, Miller CH, Schrager LE et al. (1989) Successful treatment with foscarnet of an acyclovir-resistant mucocutaneous infection with herpes simplex virus in a patient with acquired immunodeficiency syndrome. N Engl J Med 320: 297–300
14. Öberg B (1983) Antiviral effects of phosphonoformate (PFA). Pharmacol Ther 19: 387–415
15. Walmsley SL, Chew E, Read StE et al. (1988) Treatment of cytomegalovirus retinitis with trisodium phosphonoformate hexahyrate (foscarnet). J Inf Dis 157: 569–572
16. Cheng YC, Huang ES, Lin JC et al. (1983) Unique spectrum of activity of DHPG against herpes virus in vitro and its mode of action against herpes simplex virus type 1. Proc Natl Acad Sci USA 80: 2767–2770
17. Tyms AS, Davis JM, Jeffries DJ et al. (1984) BWB 759 U, an analogue of acyclovir, inhibits human cytomegalovirus in vitro. Lancet II: 924–925
18. Collaborative DHPG treatment study group (1986) Treatment of serious cytomegalovirus infections with 9-(1,3 dihidroxy-2-propoxymethyl)guanine in patients with AIDS and other immunodeficiencies. N Engl J Med 314: 801–805
19. Erice A, Chou S, Birron KK et al. (1989) Progressive disease due to ganciclovir-resistant cytomegalovirus in immunocompromized patients. N Engl J Med 320: 289–293

20. De Clercq E (1985) Problems and new aspects of antiviral treatment Herpesvirus infections in immunosuppressed patients. In: Jehn U (ed) Infections in cancer patients. Zuckschwert Munich, pp 91–114
21. Tricot G, De Clercq E, Boogaerts MA et al. (1986) Oral bromovinyldeoxyuridine therapy for herpes simplex and varicella-zoster virus infections in severely immuno-suppressed patients. J Med Virol 18: 11–18
22. De Clercq E, Holy A, Rosenberg J et al. (1986) A novel selective broad spectrum anti-DNA virus agent. Nature 323: 464–467

Prevention, Early Detection, and Management of Oncologic Emergencies

D.K. Mayer

Institute of Health Professions, MGH, 15 River Street, Boston, MA 02118, USA

Introduction

Oncologic emergencies are complications related to a cancer or its treatment which require immediate action to prevent the suffering and increased mortality associated with them. An oncologic emergency may present as an acute or chronic process and may be mild or severe. Although documentation is difficult, an increase in oncologic emergencies is anticipated since many more individuals are being treated and are living longer with their cancers. Many of the signs and symptoms of oncologic emergencies are common problems experienced by individuals with cancer, such as nausea, pain, irritability and headache. Treatment of these symptoms may mask an impending oncologic emergency, preventing early detection at a time when treatment may be most effective. It is the purpose of this paper to provide an assessment framework to evaluate the person with cancer and to present information about the most common oncologic emergencies.

Assessment

The key to the prevention and early detection of oncologic emergencies is in maintaining a high degree of suspicion and in conducting an organized and systematic assessment of the individual with cancer (Wood 1985). The frequency and completeness of this assessment depends upon how often the individual is seen and at risk or how symptomatic he or she is. Questions to guide what assessment to conduct should include:

1. "Is this individual *at risk* for developing an oncologic emergency from his/her cancer or treatment? If so, what can be done to prevent it from developing?" The associations between certain tumors and specific oncologic emergencies are outlined in Tables 1, 2 and 3. Patients with these tumors should be

Recent Results in Cancer Research, Vol. 121
© Springer-Verlag Berlin · Heidelberg 1991

screened for symptoms related to the potential oncologic emergency: for example, patients with bone metastases from breast cancer or myeloma should be questioned about back pain. If this has been experienced, the patient should be evaluated for spinal cord compression and prophylactically treated (e.g., by radiation). Patients should also be educated to report such problems. Certain emergencies are preventable, if anticipated, such as tumor lysis syndrome. The high risk patient should be well hydrated and treated with allopurinol and have his or her electrolytes monitored closely. By identifying high risk patients much can be done to prevent the suffering experienced with presentation at an advanced stage.

2. "Is this individual exhibiting any *signs or symptoms* that may be related to an oncologic emergency? What should be done to diagnose and treat it?" Since many of the presenting signs and symptoms may be common problems, such as vomiting or pain, these problems should be viewed with a degree of suspicion as "tips of the iceberg," and be followed by a careful evaluation. A family member may complain that the patient seems a little confused; the patient may be on narcotics for pain control but may also have hypercalcemia. A patient with ovarian cancer who is vomiting may be reacting to chemotherapy or may have a bowel obstruction from previous surgery and radiation therapy.

Education of patients and families about preventative measures (e.g., mobility and hydration in hypercalcemia), what signs or symptoms should be reported, and when (e.g., back pain in spinal cord compression), is a major nursing responsibility. Family members are more apt than professional staff to detect subtle changes in the patient such as irritability or lethargy. Questions should elicit this type of information from both the patient and family. Working collaboratively with the physician and other health team members to explore these compliants will speed diagnosis and improve the patient's prognosis.

Oncologic Emergencies

Oncologic emergencies are categorized by their mechanism of action as obstructive, metabolic, and infiltrative. The more common emergencies will be presented here; however, one must keep in mind that any acute, life threatening condition of the patient with cancer should be evaluated as an oncologic emergency.

Obstructive emergencies include spinal cord compression, superior vena cava syndrome, increased intracranial pressure, cardiac tamponade and bowel obstruction. Table 1 outlines the populations at risk and the signs and symptoms and management of these problems. Many of these emergencies can be anticipated by relating tumor site to possible site of obstruction (e.g., superior vena cava syndrome in a patient with an intrathoracic lymphoma). Prophylactic treatment of the tumor bulk through chemotherapy, radiation, or surgery

Table 1. Obstructive emergencies

Spinal cord compression

High risk populations:	Breast, lung, and prostate cancers, lymphoma, bone metastases
Signs/sympotoms:	Back pain, sensory and/or motor loss, autonomic dysfunction, hyperactive reflexes, positive Babinski sign
Management:	Radiation therapy or surgery, analgesics, steroids, physical therapy
Comments:	Prognosis correlated with degree of impairment and rapidity of onset at presentation.

Superior vena cava syndrome

High risk populations:	Lung cancer, intrathoracic lymphomas or other cancers
Signs/symptoms:	Venous distention, edema of face and upper extremities, dyspnea, cyanosis, headache, chest pain, drowsiness, lethargy, visual disturbances, Horner's syndrome
Management:	Radiation therapy, treatment of underlying malignancy, oxygen therapy, diuresis
Comments:	Recurrence may be experienced in 20% of patients

Increased intracranial pressure

High risk populations:	Lung and breast cancer, melanoma, leukemia
Signs/symptoms:	Headache, weakness, mood changes, mental status changes, aphasia, seizures, ataxia, hemiparesis, papilledema, vomiting, vital sign changes
Management:	Radiation therapy, surgery or intrathecal chemotherapy, steroids, anticonvulsants
Comments:	Primary treatment determined by cause of increased cranial pressure

Cardiac tamponade

High risk populations:	Breast and lung cancer, melanoma, lymphoma, mesothelioma
Signs/symptoms:	Dyspnea, cough, mental status change, pulsus paradoxus, hypotension, faint heart sounds, tachycardia
Management:	Immediate pericardiocentesis to prevent cardiac collapse
Comments:	Long-term control with pericardial window or instillation of sclerosing agent or pericardectomy

Bowel obstruction

High risk populations:	Colon, gynecologic and any pelvic cancers
Signs/symtoms:	Nausea, vomiting, abdominal distention and/or pain, decreased bowel sounds, obstipation
Management:	Fluid and electrolyte replacement, antibiotics, bowel rest, surgical decompression
Comments:	If complete obstruction, mortality increases if aggressive management not instituted with 24 h

---

Table 2. Metabolic emergencies

Hypercalcemia

High risk populations:	Breast and lung cancer, myeloma, hypernephroma
Signs/symptoms:	Nausea, vomiting, constipation, confusion, polyuria, lethargy, stupor→coma, arrhythmias
Management:	Hydration, calcium-lowering drugs, diuretics, mobility
Comments:	10%–20% of all cancer patients experience this; 50% mortality if hypercalcemic crisis occurs

Tumor lysis syndrome

High risk populations:	Lymphoma, leukemia
Signs/symptoms:	Weakness, confusion, irritability, muscle cramping, arrythmias, seizures, hyperuricemia, hyperkalemia, hyperphosphatemia, hypocalcemia, increased serum creatinine
Management:	Prevent with hydration, allopurinol
Comments:	Carefully monitor patients with bulky lymph node or abdominal disease for 48–72 h after initiating anticancer treatment

Syndrome of inappropriate antidiuretic hormone (SIADH)

High risk populations:	Lung and pancreatic cancer, lymphoma
Signs/symptoms:	Weight gain, irritability, weakness, lethargy, muscle cramps, nausea, confusion, seizures
Management:	Fluid restriction $\pm$ other medications, monitor intake and output, weigh patients
Comments:	Often subclinical presentation (e.g., abnormal electrolyte levels but asymptomatic)

Disseminated intravascular coagulation (DIC)

High risk populations:	Leukemia, adenocarcinoma, septicemia
Signs/symptoms:	Bleeding, bruising, tachycardia, hypotension, headache, decreased prothrombin time, increased partial thromboplastin time, decreased platelets
Management:	Treat underlying triggering mechanisms, give blood products $\pm$ heparin
Comments:	May be subclinical; mortality $\geq$ 50%

Septic shock

High risk populations:	Neutropenia, leukemia, lymphoma, myeloma
Signs/symptoms:	Fever, chills, tachycardia, hypotension, tachypnea, altered mental status, decreased urine output
Management:	Antibiotics, aggressive fluid replacement, inotropic agents
Comments:	20% Gram-negative infections lead to septic shock; overall mortality 70%; could precipitate DIC

Table 3. Infiltrative emergencies

Carotid artery erosion	
High risk populations:	Head and neck cancer
Signs/symptoms:	Change in wound appearance and/or drainage, bleeding from wound
Management:	Adequate nutrition, wound care to promote healing, "carotid precautions"
Comments:	18%–50% Mortality, associated with inadequate nutrition, previous radiation therapy, wound infections
Leukostasis	
High risk populations:	Leukemia (WBC > 100 000)
Signs/symptoms:	Mental status changes, headache, seizures
Management:	Leukopheresis, hydroxyurea, cranial irradiation
Comments:	Should be anticipated and is preventable
Hemorrhage	
High risk populations:	Thrombocytopenia, gastrointestinal cancers
Signs/symptoms:	Hematemesis, melena, tachycardia, hypotension, change in mental status
Management:	Intervention based on site and cause of bleeding
Comments:	If related to decreased platelet count, risk related to level and rapidity of decrease

should decrease the risk of these emergencies developing. Unfortunately, this kind of emergency may be the initial presentation of the tumor.

Metabolic emergencies include hypercalcemia, tumor lysis syndrome, syndrome of inappropriate antidiuretic hormone (SIADH), disseminated intravascular coagulation (DIC), and septic shock. Table 2 outlines the populations at risk and the signs and symptoms and management of these problems. With the exception of septic shock, these may be subclinical in nature: laboratory tests give abnormal results but the patient is asymptomatic.

Infiltrative emergencies include carotid artery erosion, leukostasis, and hemmorrhage. Table 3 outlines the populations at risk and the signs and symptoms and management of these problems. These emergencies are less frequent and occur in more clearly defined high risk patients (e.g., carotid artery erosion only in head and neck cancer patients).

Summary

The prevention and early detection of oncologic emergencies is critical in caring for the person with cancer. Although many will not develop an oncologic emergency during the course of their illness, the approach outlined in this paper will contribute significantly to the prevention and relief of suffering in those individuals who may develop them.

References

DeVita V, Hellman S, Rosenberg S (ed) (1985) Cancer principles and practice of oncology. Lippincott, Philadelphia, pp 1855–1906

Findley J (1987) Nursing management of common oncologic emergencies In: Ziegfeld C (ed) Core curriculum for oncology nursing. WB Saunders, Philadelphia, pp 321–332

Johnson B, Gross J (1985) Handbook of oncology nursing. Wiley, New York

Mayer D (1986) Oncologic emergencies. In: Baird S (ed) Decision making in oncology nursing. Decker, Philadelphia, pp 194–20

McNally J, Stair J, Somerville E (eds) (1985) Guidelines for cancer nursing practice. Grune and Stratton, New York

Wood H (ed) (1985) Acute complications of cancer. Semin Oncol Nursing, 1 (4): 229–301

Relief from Respiratory Distress in Advanced Cancer Patients

P. Drings and I. Günther

Abteilung für Innere Meidzin und Onkologie, Thorax-Klinik, W-6900 Heidelberg, FRG

Introduction

Not only patients with primary bronchogenic tumors but also patients with extrathoracic tumors and metastases of the lung and pleural cavity are at an ever increasing risk of developing respiratory failure and potential respiratory emergencies (Spain and Whittlesey 1989).

With the onset of local tumor growth and invasion, lung cancer can give rise to typical signs and symptoms. These relate to the location of the primary tumor – central, endobronchial, or peripheral – in addition to whether or not regional spread has occurred. With centrally located tumors, symptoms such as cough, wheezing, stridor, deep chest pain, hemoptysis, dyspnea caused by obstruction, with or without post-obstructive pneumonitis are so severe that they can threaten life. Peripheral lesions lead to pain, cough, and dyspnea caused by restriction, due to chest or pleural wall involvement. The intrathoracic spread of lung cancer, either by direct extension or by lymph metastases, produces regional symptoms: tracheal obstruction, lymphatic obstruction with pleural effusion, and lymphatic spread through lungs with hypoxemia and dyspnea.

Patients with lung cancer often have other medical problems: for example, chronic obstructive pulmonary disease related to smoking, chronic bronchitis and emphysema, cardiac problems related to coronary artery disease, and pulmonary diseases.

The tumors may cause an acute obstructive and restrictive ventilation disorder. This respiratory distress can be life-threatening or lead to permanent functional impairement (Drings 1988; Schuster and Marion 1983).

The occurrence of respiratory distress in the advanced stages of cancer could be caused by

- Tumor with obstruction or compression of the tracheobronchial tree or bleeding from tumor tissue
- Pleural effusion compromising lung volume

−Pneumothorax, tension pneumothorax, pulmonary edema of non-cardiac origin
−Diffuse pulmonary infiltrates
−Previous antineoplastic therapy
−Chronic underlying pulmonary or cardiac disease
−A combination of the above

Diagnosis

The definite diagnosis in patients with respiratory distress is made on the basis of the patient's history, physical examination, laboratory findings, chest X-ray, tomography, sputum examination, serologic tests, pulmonary function tests (e.g., spirometry), and arterial blood gas analyses. Invasive procedures are bronchoscopy, thoracoscopy, pleural biopsy, pulmonary and bronchial angiography, and mediastinoscopy. Bronchoscopy is the most common invasive procedure used for diagnosis and follow up in patients with respiratory distress. This is performed to investigate the cause of medically resistant chronic chest symptoms and signs. By means of bronchoscopy we can determine the site, extent, and cause of acute changes such as hemoptysis, acute inhalation injury, and regional abnormality on the chest X-ray (Becker 1990). Bronchoscopy is an essential tool in the evaluation of patients for thoracic surgery. It helps to evaluate the tracheobronchial tree for tumors, rule out metastases, obtain tissue and specimens, and determine the presence and exact level of tracheobronchial esophageal fistula (Becker 1990).

Treatment of Central Airway Obstruction

The treatment of respiratory failure consists of two simultaneous processes: (a) maintaining an acceptable level of oxygenation and ventilation and (b) reversing any airway obstruction removing secretions, and instigating antibiotic treatment of infection.

The management must be based upon as complete knoweldge as possible of the degree of obstruction, the extent of disability, and the degree to which the patient's disease is reversible. Restoration of ventilation and oxygenation is the main task in order to relieve the patient from respiratory distress (Brodsky et al. 1985; Ewer et al. 1986); therefore therapeutic bronchoscopy is indicated (Becker 1990) (Tables 1, 2).

Complications of a tumor process in the central tracheobronchial system cause life-threatening symptoms which must be relieved before the patient can undergo further therapy. The most common complication is airway stenosis which may threaten asphyxia or lead to dyspnea due to disturbed ventilation or to pneumonia due to infected retained secretions. With slow-growing and inoperable tumors, clinical symptoms arise if the residual bronchial lumen is

Table 1. Indication for endoscopic tumor therapy

Tumor complication

 - central airway stenosis
 - atelectasis, poststenotic pneumonia
 - hemoptysis
 - retained secretions
 - bleeding
 - ventil mechanism

Long-term palliation of slow growth (inoperable)
Tumors of central bronchial system
Afterloading (endobronchial radiotherapy)

Table 2. Technical possibilities of the therapeutic bronchoscopy

Suction

 - fiberscope
 - stiff bronchoscope

Mechanical instruments
High frequency diathermy
Cryosurgery
Laser application
Endoluminal radiotherapy
Application of adhesives
Implantation of tubes and catheters

5 mm or less. Extreme obstruction of the central airway is a dramatic event. Here laser therapy is indicated, provided that the ventilation is sufficient (Arabian and Spagnolo 1984; Becker 1990; Gelb and Epstein 1984).

Slow-growing tumors such as adenoid cystic carcinomas, carcinoids, and hypernephroma metastases can be treated endoscopically. (Becker 1990). A new form of treatment is endoscopic placing of the tubes for endoluminal radiation with the after-loading technique. This therapy (endobronchial radiotherapy) is curative in nature. Airway obstructions which cannot be relieved by removing tissue or scar strictures after therapy, or compression due to extrabronchial tumors, can be opened with the bronchoscope tube and stretched with bouginage or, rarely, internally splinted with endoscopic placement of an endoprosthesis (Becker 1990; Spain and Whittlesey 1989).

Hemoptysis

Massive hemoptysis is most frequently encountered in patients with pulmonary tuberculosis, bronchiectasis, lung abscess, or bronchogenic carcinoma (Panos et al. 1988). Infection developing behind an obstructing tumor promotes vascular rupture. In patients with a primary bronchogenic tumor, fatal hemoptysis was frequently associated with a necrotic squamous cell carcinoma (Miller and McGregor 1980). The management of massive hemoptysis draws on general medical principles as well as more specific diagnostic and therapeutic considerations.

Surgical resection remains the optimal management of massive hemoptysis (Panos et al. 1988). Contraindications depend upon the nature and extent of the disease producing hemorrhage as well as on prior treatment. Radiation therapy with the maximal dosage had been administered to many of these patients.

Hemoptysis can be stopped with hemostatics, thermocoagulation of the tissue, or removal of the exophytic part of the tumor. Bleeding from a peripheral tumor lesion or a poststenotic pneumonia can be blocked by an endoscopic balloon-tipped catheter (Fogarty) which can remain in position until embolization of the bronchial artery or thoracic surgical intervention has been carried out (Becker 1990; Remy et al. 1977; Uflacker et al. 1983).

Diffuse Pulmonary Infiltrates

Pulmonary hemorrhage, pulmonary emboli, pulmonary edema of cardiac or noncardiac origin, chemotherapy- and/or radiation-induced lung injury or lymphangitis carcinomatosa can each produce febrile pneumonitis with or without infectious varieties of pneumonia (Rubin 1988). The symptoms and signs associated with each category of disease are nonspecific. Diagnosis of the specific disease requires a histologic or bacterial culture documentation. For estimating the likely etiologies of pulmonary infiltrates, guidelines exist which rely on characterization of the underlying neoplastic disease and its treatment (Spain and Whittlesey 1989). Therefore a diagnostic procedure of high technical standard is indicated. The radiographic appearance may indicate a specific disease process, showing highly suggestive or at least more features. Diffuse interstitial infiltrates represent a larger diagnostic problem, with greater probability of opportunistic or noninfectious etiology. Bronchoalveolar lavage appears most helpful in diagnosing opportunistic infection. The organisms most often diagnosed via lavage are *Pneumocystis carinii*, cytomegaloviruses and mycobacteria (Stover et al. 1984; Stover 1987).

Supportive Management

Advanced cancer patients in respiratory distress need oxygen when they are severely hypoxic (Brodsky et al. 1985). Oxygen must be used, even at the lowest concentration possible, in order to obtain a PaO_2 in the 55 mmHg range, while the patients PaO_2, pH balance, and clinical status are carefully monitored. It is best to begin using nasal prongs with an oxygen flow of 1–2 l/min. If the initial level was low, even a small increase in PaO_2 results in significant increase in arterial oxygen content. Some increase in $PaCO_2$ can be expected and should not cause alarm if the patient is alert (Schuster and Marion 1983). If CO_2 narcosis is present and the respiration is so depressed by the CO_2 itself that the patient no longer reacts to the rapidly worsening hypoxemia, the only alternative is to intubate the trachea and provide mechanical ventilation support (Ewer et al. 1986; Schuster and Marion 1983).

Maintaining oxygenation and ventilation serves to save time while secretion removal, bronchial dilatation, and treatment of infection are instituted. Removal of secretions is accomplished by urging the patient to cough or by passing suction catheters into the trachea (Becker 1990).

Bronchodilators are often quite helpful for alarming symptoms. There are three categories of bronchodilator: the methylxanthines, the β_2-sympathomimetics, and anticholinergics. The methylxanthine theophyllin can be given orally, rectally, or parenterally. It additionally stimulates respiration and has cardiotonic and diuretic properties. Selective β_2-stimulating drugs (fenoterol, terbutaline, salbutamol) can be given orally and by aerosol with rare cardiac side effects. The anticholinergic agent ipratropiumbromide is also an effective bronchodilator.

The use of glucocorticosteroids is based upon very little scientific data. These agents have dose-related side effects. We give these agents only when administration of bronchodilators at maximum dosage and bronchopulmonary drainage have failed (Spain and Whittlesey 1989).

The use of antibiotics is more controversial in the setting of acute respiratory failure than in mucopurulent relapse without failure. Broad-spectrum antibiotics should be added to the therapy regimen if no microorganism is isolated. Erythromycin can be applied if the presence of *Legionella* or mycoplasmas is suspected (Spain and Whittlesey 1989).

Complications arising in the course of treatment for acute respiratory failure are cardiac arrhythmias, left ventricular failure, pulmonary emboli, and gastrointestinal hemorrhage due to stress ulceration. Cardiac arrhythmias resulting from a rapid drop in oxygenation or a rise in pH due to overventilation can be readily avoided. Improvement in lung function and oxygenation often reverses the pulmonary hypertension and right ventricular failure and induces diuresis.

Pulmonary emboli are suspected to be common in the setting of acute respiratory failure but are difficult to detect, because signs of cor pulmonale fluctuate with the degree of lung dysfunction. Low-dose heparin prophylaxis should be employed to prevent this complication (Spain and Whittlesey 1989).

Respiratory Failure Due to Cancer Involving the Pleural Wall

Many cancer patients develop pleural effusions during the course of their disease. Malignant effusions occur in 26%–49% of patients with breast cancer,

10%–24% of those with lung cancer, 6%–17% of those with ovarian neo-plasmas, and 13%–24% of those with malignant lymphomas. Patients with pleural effusions commonly present with dyspnea, cough, or chest pain, but 23% of patients are asymptomatic at presentation (Drings 1988). Pleural effusions cause respiratory embarrassment by mechanical impairment of lung expansion, and the resultant reduction in lung volume may predispose patients to atelectasis and recurrent infection.

The movement of pleural fluid is dependent on capillary and interstitial hydrostatic pressure, the plasma protein, and interstitial protein osmotic pressure. A disturbed equilibrium may be the result of changes in hydrostatic or osmotic pressure or of an increase in capillary permeability. Intrathoracic malignancies can affect these factors in several ways. Direct involvement of the pleural surface by tumor and the associated inflammation may lead to increased capillary permeability. Obstruction of lung or pleural lymphatic channels impairs reabsorption of fluid and protein. Obstruction of the pulmonary veins by tumor increases the capillary hydrostatic pressure, thus reducing the gradient between the parietal and visceral pleura. This may occur in patients with endobronchial obstruction, with atelectasis, or with postobstructive pneumonitis (Drings 1988). Severe hypoproteinemia may also impair the reabsorptive process.

Cell counts of the pleural effusion should be performed and cytologic examination carried out. Via thoracocentesis and thoracostomy-guided biopsy, a diagnosis of malignancy can be made in 94% of patients (Drings 1988).

The primary goal of treatment of malignant pleural effusions is relief of symptoms. A symptomatic, massive pleural effusion can be evacuated by effective systemic antineoplastic therapy is available, e.g., for patients with small cell lung cancer, breast cancer, or malignant lymphomas, in which case the systemic cytostatic treatment will prevent a reaccumulation of fluid in the pleural space. Most patients, however, suffer a recurrence of pleural effusion within a short period of time. These patients are treated with closed drainage thoracotomy and instillation therapy (Branscheid et al. 1988; Drings 1988). The aim of local therapeutic measures is obliteration of the pleural space. This prevents reaccumulation of fluid. The effectiveness of an intracavitary agent depends primarily on its ability to produce mesothelial fibrosis and pleural sclerosis, rather than on its specific antineoplastic activity. Pleurodesis is indicated provided that the pleural effusion is persistent, progressive, and has recurred within a short space of time, severe symptoms are present. lung expansion is possible, the performance index of the patient is sufficient, and the life expectation is longer than 2 months (Head 1983).

Complete evacuation of the pleural space is the first step. Various agents – cytostatics, such as 5-fluorouracil, thiotepa, doxorubicin, bleomycin, and other drugs, tetracyclines, quinacrine, talc powder, or radioactive isotopes – have been instilled intrapleurally to diminish the recurrence of pleural effusions (Drings 1988).

Intrapleural administration of tetracycline has been employed with very good results and few side effects. This agent acts solely by means of its sclerosing properties. Intrapleural administration of tetracycline has resulted in reduction of effusions in 72% of 141 patients (Drings 1988; Gravelyn et al. 1987); no additional therapy was required following administration. The survival of patients treated intrapleurally with tetracycline varied from 6 weeks to 34 months, compared to 2–3 months in the control group (Drings 1988).

Pleuritic pain is the only significant side effect reported with the use of tetracycline. The procedure for instilling tetracycline includes performing a closed-tube thoracotomy in the eighth or ninth intercostal space at the posterior axillary line and attaching a water-seal drainage with gentle suction for at least 24 h or until drainage has stopped.

After administration of tetracycline, the different response rates in various studies relate to the carefulness of technique, the extent of pleural tumor invasion, whether there is atelectasis, and the possibility or otherwise of opposing the pleura visceralis and parietalis (Gravelyn et al. 1987; Head 1983).

Administration of quinacrine or instillation of talc or radioactive isotopes are only of historical importance. The response rates after all intracavitary cytostatics were lower than the response rate after tetracycline. Instillation of fibrin adhesives has results similar to tetracylines (Drings 1988).

In cases where local and systemic measures are ineffective and severe symptoms are present, pleurectomy with decortication of the tumor is indicated. This is the last chance to save a lung overwhelmed by pleuritis carcinomatosa (Branscheid et al. 1988). The success rate of this surgical intervention is approximately 90% and it has a good long-term effectiveness. Complications occur frequently; persistent pneumonia and empyema appear in nearly 20% of patients postoperatively (Branscheid et al. 1988).

A special situation is the pleural effusion in patients with diffuse malignant mesothelioma. The treatment of this rare tumor is very difficult since there is no specific therapy available. Radical surgical resection is possible only in a few cases.

Reexpansion pulmonary edema (RPE) occurs as a rare complication when a chronically collapsed lung is rapidly reexpanded by evacuation of large amounts of air or fluid, usually with application of high negative intrapleural pressure. This often occurs when the lung is reexpanded without suction following pneumothorax, pleural effusion or atelectasis (Mahfood et al. 1988). The onset of RPE is immediate or within 24 h of intervention. The clinical manifestation varies from roentgenographic findings to mild or severe cardiorespiratory insufficiency, shock, coma, and death.

The degree of resulting hypoxia depends on the extent of ventilation/ perfusion mismatch and the resultant intrapulmonary shunting. Hydrothorax or pneumothorax, especially when chronic, should be evacuated slowly and pleural suction only applied after the lung is mostly reexpanded (Mahfood et al. 1988).

Spontaneous pneumothorax can be produced by metastasis from osteogenic sarcoma, Ewing's tumor, Wilms' tumor, melanoma, endometrial adenocarcinoma, and metastatic carcinoma of the rectum (Sharma and Rajani 1988). Surgical intervention is indicated here.

Respiratory Failure Related to Previous Antineoplastic Therapy

The lung is a common site of toxicity of cancer drugs. For a diagnosis of drug-induced pulmonary damage, the patient must have a history of drug exposure without other diseases known to cause pulmonary damage, and the absence of *Pneumocystis carinii* organisms, viral inclusions or, other signs of infection not be documented by lung biopsy. The problem of diagnosis occurs because the pathologic changes are often not specific (Drings 1988; Ginsberg and Comis 1984; Johnson et al. 1985).

The list of drugs that have been reported to cause pulmonary toxicity includes some of the major drugs used in cancer treatment. The drugs may be placed into two groups: those in which the pulmonary toxicity manifests itself as diffuse interstitial pneumonitis (bleomycin, busulfan, cyclophosphamide, chlorambucil, BCNU, mitomicyn, methotrexate, procarbazine) and those in which it does not (cytosine-arabinoside, azothioprine, mercaptopurine) (Ginsberg and Comis 1984; Muggia et al. 1983).

Drug-induced interstitial pneumonitis usually presents with dyspnea clinically, and sometimes with an unproductive cough. The chest X-ray may show a pattern of diffuse interstitial markings but can also be within normal limits, even in patients with significant pulmonary damage. The arterial blood gas analysis shows hypoxia with hypocapnia and respiratory alkalosis. The most sensitive pulmonary function test is the carbon monoxide diffusion capacity measurement, which typically becomes abnormal before the onset of clinical symptoms (Drings 1988; Ginsberg and Comis 1984; Muggia et al. 1983).

The clinical presentation of bleomycin toxicity is classic for interstitial pneumonitis. The histologic findings of bleomycin toxicity include an acute inflammatory infiltrate in the alveoli with both interstitial and alveolar edema and pulmonary hyaline membrane formation. The incidence of pulmonary toxicity from bleomycin is related to total dose; it is about 5% in patients who have received less than 450 mg/m². However, severe pulmonary fibrosis has been seen in patients who have received less than 100 mg/m² (Drings 1988; Ginsberg and Comis 1984).

Clinical symptoms are dry cough, dyspnea, tachypnea, fever, and cyanosis, which can still occur 1–3 months after administration of bleomycin.

At present there is no specific therapy to treat this pulmonary toxicity or to prevent it developing. Discontinuation of bleomycin therapy should therefore be considered in patients who have a rapid decline in pulmonary function. A synergistic toxic effect of previous bleomycin treatment and subsequent oxygen ventilation is assumed. When supplemental oxygen is used in a bleomycin-treated patient, therefore, the oxygen should be limited to the amount necessary to keep the arterial PO_2 above 60 mmHg (Drings 1988; Muggia et al. 1983).

The incidence of these complications after using alkylating agents appears to vary widely. In the case of busulfan 2%–11% of the patients exhibit abnormalities of pulmonary function and 12%–45% give histologic evidence of pulmonary injury. With BCNU the incidence has been related to total dose administered, reaching 50% for those who have received more than $1500 \, \text{mg/m}^2$ (Ginsberg and Comis 1984).

The incidence after treatment with cyclophosphamide or chlorambucil is difficult to determine, since these alkylating agents are so widely used.

The onset of mitomycin-C-induced pulmonary damage is not clearly related to total dose. This toxicity appears to respond well to corticosteroids. The incidence has been reported to be between 5% and 12% (Ginsberg and Comis 1984).

The clinical presentation of methotrexate-induced pulmonary toxicity is one of a prodrome of headache, malaise, dyspnea, and dry cough followed by bilateral development of diffuse infiltrate visible on the chest X-ray.

Procarbazine can provoke an allergic reaction with the development of pulmonary infiltrates, the patient presenting with a syndrome of fever, chills, arthralgia, urticaria, and peripheral eosinophilia. If the diagnosis "procarbazine lung" is made, procarbazine treatment should be discontinued and corticosteroids administered (Muggia et al. 1983).

Cytosine-arabinoside, azothioprine, and mercaptopurine are not associated with drug-induced interstitial pneumonitis. However, in the literature cytosine-arabinoside is described as a causal agent in patients who develop unexplained pulmonary edema within 30 days of the last drug dose (Muggia et al. 1983).

The clinical expression of radiation damage to lung can be divided into two temporally distinct syndromes (Gross 1977). Acute radiation pneumonitis occurs within 2–3 months after completion of thoracic irradiation; symptoms are insidious onset of exertional dyspnea, a dry cough, and radiologic changes of increased interstitial markings confined to the previous radiation portals (Gross 1977; Slanina et al. 1977). Late radiation fibrosis becomes clinically evident 9–12 months after irradiation. It is characterized as a restrictive pulmonary disease (Gross 1977).

The total radiation dose, daily fraction size, and volume of lung within the high-dose region are the major variables of radiation injury to lung. Radiation injury occurs in patients with primary lung tumors, mediastinal tumors, or malignant lymphomas who received high-dose irradiation ($> 40 \, \text{Gy}$) including a significant amount of surrounding lung tissue (Brodsky et al. 1985; Drings 1988; Johnson et al. 1985).

Modern treatment planning should result in symptomatic acute or late injury in only a low percentage of patients. In Hodgkin's disease patients with massive mediastinal involvement have an incidence of acute pneumonitis of approximately 20%, even with careful treatment planning. Symptoms such as non-productive cough, low- or high-grade fever, and mild or severe dyspnea should raise the suspicion of acute radiation pneumonitis. A follow-up chest X-ray is necessary during the 2–3 months after radiation therapy to reveal progressive interstitial changes confined to the previous radiation fields (Reynolds 1987; Johnson et al. 1985; Scheulen 1987).

In patients with mild symptoms, no treatment is required once an infectious process has been ruled out. Such patients need to be observed closely; if symptoms worsen, a course of oral steroids is recommended. The interval for resolution of acute radiation pneumonitis is quite variable: it may be only a few days or may last for many weeks or even months (Evans et al. 1987; Scheulen 1987).

Severe cases of pneumonitis occurs in less than 5% of patients receiving high-dose lung irradiation. These patients require hospitalization with aggressive supportive care. Intravenous steroids are recommended; once symptomatic improvement has occurred, the dosage steroids should be tapered down slowly to avoid a recrudescence of the pneumonitis (Evans et al. 1987).

Drugs such as bleomycin and busulfan can result in an acute pneumonitis similar to that induced by radiation. The concomitant or sequential use of these drugs and radiation may result in increased pulmonary toxicity. Complications of late fibrosis are related to the extent of the restrictive lung process and secondary infections. There is no effective treatment of late radiation fibrosis other than symptomatic treatment of the associated complications (Adamson and Bowden 1983; Drings 1988; Johnson et al. 1985).

The occurrence of respiratory distress symptoms and signs in advanced cancer patients can be anticipated and prevented by appropriate prophylactic measures or can be reversed if recognized and promptly treated. Early recognition and treatment of the symptoms of distress may make it possible to prolong survival and improve the quality of life.

In recent years the array of antineoplastic interventions has widened, with new approaches introduced by therapeutic bronchoscopy and its technical possibilities, e.g., endobronchial laser therapy, endobronchial radiotherapy, cryosurgery, high-frequency diathermy, applications of adhesives, and implantation of tubes and catheters. The basis on which these therapeutic advances rest is the improvement in anesthetic management for the treatment of acute respiratory failure, with continuous monitoring, oxygenation, and the versatility of modern ventilation support (Brodsky et al. 1985; Ewer et al. 1986; Schuster and Marion 1983).

References

Adamson IYR, Bowden DH (1983) Endothelial injury and repair in radiation induced pulmonary fibrosis. Am J Pathol 112: 224–230

Arabian A, Spagnolo S (1984) Laser therapy in patients with primary lung cancer. Chest 86: 519–523

Becker HD (1990) Möglichkeiten und Grenzen der endoskopischen Therapie beim Bronchialkarzinom. In: Drings P, Vogt-Moykopf I (eds) Thoraxtumoren. Springer, Berlin Heidelberg New York

Branscheid D, Bischoff H, Vogt-Moykopf I (1988) Chirurgie der malignen Pleuraergüsse einschließlich des malignen Pleura-mesothelioms. In: Hossfeld DK, Gatzemeier U (eds) Maligne Ergüsse. Beitr Onkol Karger, Basel, pp 81–87

Brodsky JB, Shulman MS, Swan M, Mark JB (1985) Pulse oximetry during one-lung ventilation. Anesthesiology 63: 212–214

Brooks BJ, Seifter EJ, Walsh TE et al. (1986) Pulmonary toxicity with combined modality therapy for limited stage small cell lung cancer. J Clin Oncol 4: 200–209

Drings P (1988) Die Therapie von Pleuraergüssen. In: Hossfeld DK, Gatzemeier U (eds) Maligne Ergüsse. Beitr Onkol Karger, Basel, pp 43–51

Drings P (1988) Kardiorespiratorische Spätfolgen nach Chemo- und Radiotherapie. Med Klin 83: 408–416

Evans ML, Grahan MM, Mahler PA et al. (1987) Use of steroids to suppress vascular response to radiation. Int J Radiat Oncol Biol Phys 13: 563–567

Ewer MS, Ali MK, Atta MS et al. (1986) Outcome of lung cancer patients requiring mechanical ventilation for pulmonary failure. JAMA 256: 3364–3366

Gelb AF, Epstein JD (1984) Laser in treatment of lung cancer. Chest 86: 662–666

Ginsberg SJ, Comis RL (1984) The pulmonary toxicity of antineoplastic agents. In: Perry MC, Yabro JW (eds) Toxicity of chemotherapy. Grune and Stratton, New York, pp 227–268

Gravelyn TR, Michelson MK, Gross BH (1987) Tetracycline pleurodesis for malignant pleural effusion. Cancer 59: 1973

Gross NJ (1977) Pulmonary effects of radiation therapy. Ann Intern Med 86: 81–92

Head JM (1983) Treatment of malignant pleura effusion. In: Choi (ed) Thoracic oncology. Raven, New York, p 353

Johnson BE, Ihde DC, Bunn PA et al. (1985) Patients with small-cell lung cancer treated with combination chemotherapy with or without irradiation. Ann Intern Med 103: 430–438

Mahfood S, Hix WR, Aaron BL, Blaese P, Watson DC (1988) Reexpansion pulmonary edema. Ann Thorac Surg 45: 340–345

Miller RR, McGregor DH (1980) Hemorrhage from carcinoma of the lung. Cancer 46: 200–205

Muggia FM, Louie AC, Sikic BI (1983) Pulmonary toxicity of antitumor agents. Cancer Treat Rev 10: 221–243

Panos RJ, Barr LF, Walsh TJ, Silverman HJ (1988) Factors associated with fatal hemoptysis in cancer patients. Chest 94: 1008–1013

Remy J, Alain A, Fardon H, Giraud R, Voisin C (1977) Treatment of hemoptysis by embolization of bronchial arteries. Radiology 122: 33–37

Reynolds HY (1987) Lung inflammation Normal host defense or a complication of some diseases? Ann Rev Med 8: 295–323

Rubin R (1988) Pneumonia in the immunocompromised host. In: Fishman A (ed) Pulmonary diseases and disorders, vol 3. McGraw-Hill, New York, pp 1745–1760

Scheulen M (1987) Reduction of lung toxicity. Cancer Treat Rev 14: 231–243

Schuster DP, Marion JM (1983) Precedents for meaningful recovery during treatment in a medical intensive care unit: outcome in patients with hematologic malignancy. Am J Med 75: 402–408

Sharma S, Rajani M, Aggarwal S, Puri S, Bajal VN (1988) Spontaneous pneumothorax and pneumomediastinum in metastatic lung disease. Indian J Chest Dis Allied Sci 30: 125–132

Slanina J, Musshoff K, Raghner T, Stlasny R (1977) Long-term side effects in irradiated patients with Hodgkin's disease. Int J Radiol Oncol Biol Phys 2: 1–19

Spain RC, Whittlesey D (1989) Respiratory emergencies in patients with cancer. Semin Oncol 16: 471–489

Stover DE, Zaman MB, Hajdu SI et al. (1984) Bronchoalveolar lavage in the diagnosis of diffuse pulmonary infiltrates in the immunosuppressed host. Ann Inter Med 101: 1–7

Stover DS (1987) Diagnostic approach to life-threatening pulmonary infiltrates. In: Turnbull A (ed) Surgical emergencies in the cancer patient. Yearbook Medical, Chicago, pp 140–151

Uflacker R, Kaemmerer A, Meyes C et al. (1983) Management of massive hemoptysis by bronchial artery embolization. Radiology 146: 627–634

Treatment and Support in Confusional States

L.M. Lesko and S. Fleishman

Memorial Sloan-Kettering Cancer Center (MSKCC), New York, NY, USA

Introduction

In patients with cancer, delirium occurs both as a transient central nervous system complication of disease and as a side effect of treatment. Dementia, while much less common, is a far more devastating complication because of its irreversible course. Both are mistaken for depression or an emotional response to stress. Prompt and early recognition of the symptoms and a thorough workup to establish the cause and treatment can prevent progression of delirium to coma and death, and the progression of dementia may be slowed. Recognizing diagnostic symptoms and signs and managing the psychologic and behavioral consequences are crucial to good patient care.

This manuscript will review important issues in regard to delirium and dementia in general, then as they apply in cancer, with the greater emphasis placed on delirium. The following topics will be covered: diagnostic criteria, prevalence, etiology, and clinical evaluation and management.

Definition and Diagnosis

Bonhoeffer (1910) was among the first to describe transient delirious states as "toxic" psychoses, suggesting their exogenous or organic (nonfunctional) origin. Engel and Romano (1959) emphasized that delirium is the clinical picture resulting from global impairment of mental function accompanied by diffuse slowing of EEG patterns, and it can result from a range of pathophysiologic causes which disrupt normal mental function. Later, Plum and Posner (1972) described delirium as a state characterized by clouded consciousness, disorientation, suspiciousness, fears, irritability, misperception of sensory stimuli, and, often, delusions and visual hallucinations.

Lipowski (1980, 1983) has provided the most scholarly review of organic mental syndromes. He proposed an organization (Table 1) of delirium and

Table 1. Organic mental disorders. (Modified from Lipowski 1980)

Global cognitive impairment:
   Delirium
   Dementia

Selective or circumscribed cognitive abnormalities:
   Amnestic syndrome
   Organic hallucinosis

Disorders resembling functional disorders:
   Organic delusional syndrome
   Organic affective syndrome

---

dementia based on presenting mental symptoms, signs, and behavior; these categories served as the basis for the current DSM-III classification (Table 2). He suggested that there are two types of *global* cognitive impairment: delirium and dementia. Other forms of impairment appear in which there is selective memory loss, as seen in the *amnestic syndrome* and in *organic hallucinations*. In the latter disorder mental functions are largely intact but exist in the presence of visual, tactile, or auditory hallucinations. Such disorders are seen most often in drug-induced toxic or withdrawal states (e.g., alcohol, steroids). Another type of dysfunction is characterized by relatively intact cognition and symptoms that closely resemble those· of a functional or psychological disorder: *organic delusional syndrome* (seen in drug or metabolic or psychologically induced states) or *organic affective syndrome*, in which mood is the predominantly changed aspect of mental function, with symptoms of depression or mania.

Table 2 a – f gives the DSM-III diagnostic criteria used for differentiating the symptoms of the above-mentioned organic brain syndromes. They all represent

Table 2a. Diagnostic criteria for delirium (DSM-III; APA 1980)

A. Clouding of consciousness (reduced clarity of awareness of the environment), with reduced capacity to shift, focus, and sustain attention to environmental stimuli.
B. At least two of the following:
   1. Perceptual disturbance: misinterpretations, illusions, or hallucinations
   2. Speech that is at times incoherent
   3. Disturbance of sleep-wake cycle, with insomnia or daytime drowsiness
   4. Increased or decreased psychomotor activity
C. Disorientation and memory impairment (if testable).
D. Clinical features that develop over a short period of time (usually hours to days) and tend to fluctuate over the course of a day.
E. Evidence, from the history, physical examination, or laboratory test, of a specific organic factor judged to be etiologically related to the disturbance.

Table 2b. Diagnostic criteria for dementia (DSM III; APA 1980)

A. A loss of intellectual abilities of sufficient severity to interfere with the social or occupational functioning.
B. Memory impairment.
C. At least one of the following:
   1. Impairment of abstract thinking as manifested by concrete interpretation of proverbs, inability to find similarities and differences between related words, difficulty in defining words and concepts, and other similar tasks
   2. Impaired judgement
   3. Other disturbances of higher cortical function, such as aphasia (disorder of language due to brain dysfunction), apraxia (inability to carry out motor function), agnosia (failure to recognize or identify objects despite intact sensory function), "constructional difficulty" (e.g., inability to copy three-dimensional figures, assemble blocks, or arrange sticks in specific designs)
   4. Personality change, i.e., alteration or accentuation of premorbid traits
D. State of consciousness not clouded (i.e., does not meet the criteria for Delirium or Intoxication, although these may be superimposed).
E. Either 1 or 2:
   1. Evidence from the history, physical examination, or laboratory tests, of a specific organic factor that is judged to be etiologically related to the disturbance
   2. In the absence of such evidence, an organic factor necessary for the development of the syndrome can be presumed if conditions other than Organic Mental Disorders have been reasonably excluded and if the behavioral change represents cognitive impairment in a variety of areas

Table 2c. Diagnostic criteria for amnestic syndrome (DSM-III; APA 1980)

A. Both short-term memory impairment (inability to learn new information) and long-term memory impairment (inability to remember information that was known in the past) are the predominant clinical features.
B. No clouding of consciousness, as in Delirium and Intoxication, or general loss of major intellectual abilities, as in Dementia.
C. Evidence, from the history, physical laboratory, or laboratory tests, of a specific organic factor that is judged to be etiologically related to the disturbance.

Table 2d. Diagnostic criteria for organic hallucinosis (DSM-III; APA 1980)

A. Persistent or recurrent hallucinations are the predominant clinical feature.
B. No clouding of consciousness, as in Delirium; no significant loss of intellectual abilities, as in Dementia; no predominant disturbance of mood, as in Organic Affective Syndrome; no predominant delusions, as in Organic Delusional Syndrome.
C. Evidence, from the history, physical examination, or laboratory tests, of a specific organic factor that is judged to be etiologically related to the disturbance.

Table 2e. Diagnostic criteria for organic delusional syndrome (DSM-III; APA 1980)

A. Delusions are the predominant clinical feature.
B. There is no clouding of consciousness, as in Delirium; there are no significant loss of intellectual abilities, as in Dementia; there are no prominent hallucinations, as in Organic Hallucinosis.
C. There is evidence, from the history, physical examination, or laboratory tests, of a specific organic factor that is judged to be etiologically related to the disturbance.

Table 2f. Diagnostic criteria for organic affective syndrome (DSM-III; APA 1980)

A. The predominant disturbance is a disturbance in mood, with at least two of the associated symptoms for manic or major depressive episode.
B. No clouding of consciousness, as in Delirium; no significant loss of intellectual abilities, as in Dementia; no predominant delusions or hallucinations, as in Organic Delusional Syndrome or Organic Hallucinosis.
C. Evidence, from the history, physical examination, or laboratory tests, of a specific organic factor that is judged to be etiologically related to the disturbance.

mental changes which are the results of different patterns of impaired perception of the environment, faulty processing, storage, and retrieval of information, and impairment of insight and judgment.

At times it is difficult to differentiate between delirium and early dementia, which has a profound impairment of memory. Delirium is characterized by fluctuating levels of consciousness (attention) and disordered orientation, with symptoms worsening at night. Dementia appears in a relatively alert individual and is associated with a less profoundly disordered sleep-wake cycle with impaired memory, judgment, and abstract thinking. In older individuals who are physically ill, both delirium and dementia may be present. Liston (1984) has outlined the major diagnostic differences in the clinical picture of delirium and dementia. (Table 3). The differential diagnosis of disorders of cognition, in older patients, is the presence of depression, which represents a pseudodementia (Wells, 1979).

Prevalence in Cancer

Transient delirium often occurs in hospitalized cancer patients undergoing active and palliative treatment; dementia is relatively uncommon. Eleven studies of organic mental disorders in cancer patients note a prevalence of delirium ranging from 8% to 85% (Derogatis et al. 1983; Fleishman and Lesko 1989). It is readily apparent from the populations evaluated in these studies that there are three subgroups in particular at risk for increased incidence of delirium: patients

Table 3. Clinical features of delirium and dementia. (Adapted from Liston 1984)

Feature	Delirium	Dementia
Impaired memory	+ + +	+ + +
Impaired thinking	+ + +	+ + +
Impaired judgment	+ + +	+ + +
Clouding of consciousness	+ + +	−
Major attention deficits	+ + +	+
Fluctuation over course of a day	+ + +	+
Disorientation	+ + +	+ +
Vivid perceptual disturbances	+ +	+
Incoherent speech	+ +	+
Disrupted sleep-wake cycle	+ +	+
Nocturnal exacerbation	+ +	+
Insight	+ +	+
Acute or subacute onset	+ +	−

+ + + Always present; + + usually present; + present sometime; − usually absent.

under treatment in the hospital, those in older age groups (Seymour et al., 1980), and those with more advanced or terminal disease. Hospitalized patients in general are at especially high risk of developing a narcotic or steroid-induced confusional state, or a metabolic encephalopathy related to consequences of disease or treatment. At MSKCC Posner (1979) estimates that 15%–20% of patients in medical oncology units may be experiencing some degree of cognitive impairment, usually not recognized unless it becomes severe or is accompanied by behavioral changes. The prevalence of dementia, usually from unusual remote effects on the central nervous system (CNS), or from radiation, is so low that no similar studies have been carried out.

Etiology of Delirium and Dementia

The causes of delirium and dementia are outlined briefly in Table 4. Posner (1978) outlines two main etiologies of CNS complications: (1) *direct effects* related to primary brain tumor or metastatic spread by local extension or by hematogenous or lymphatic routes, which may result in both delirium and permanent intellectual loss or dementia; and (2) *indirect effects*, far more frequent, and more commonly causing delirium, as a consequence of metabolic encephalopathy, vital organ failure, electrolyte imbalance, drug or radiation side effects, infection, vascular complications, nutritional changes, and paraneoplastic syndromes.

Table 4. Etiologies of delirium in cancer patients. (Adapted from Posner 1978)

Direct:
Primary brain tumor
Metastatic spread

Indirect:
Metabolic encephalopathy due to vital organ failure
Electrolyte imbalance
Treatment side effects from
   narcotics
   anticholinergics
   chemotherapeutic agents; steroids
   radiation

Infection
Hematologic abnormalities
Nutrition
Paraneoplastic syndromes

Failure of an organ, particularly liver, kidney, lung, thyroid and adrenal, is a common source of mental status change in patients with advanced disease. Among treatment side effects, narcotic analgesics are a common cause of clouded consciousness and psychotic states. Anticholinergic drugs can produce psychotic states as can commonly used drugs in cancer: amphotericin, cimetidine and acyclovir (Table 5). Among the chemotherapeutic agents, steroids are the worst offenders (Table 6), producing organic affective syndromes and psychosis. Transiently altered mental function with altered attention, level of consciousness, cognition, and mood change are seen at times with particular cytotoxic agents: including methotrexate (given intrathacally or at high dose), 5-fluoro-uracil, the vinca alkaloids, bleomycin, cisplatin, L-asparaginase, and procarbazine (Young and Posner 1980).

Cranial radiation produces mild to severe immediate side effects and may also be associated with delayed effects. Radiation effects can range from time-limited "somnolence syndromes" to a mild to moderate cognitive loss (seen in children given CNS prophylaxis for acute lymphocytic leukemia), to dementia (seen in some patients who receive radiation for brain tumors or CNS prophylaxis for lung cancer). Infections of the CNS produce an encephalopathy secondary to bacterial, viral, or fungal invasion of the brain. Some of the nutritional deficiencies seen in cancer and associated with mental status changes are thiamine deficiency, which produces Wernicke/Korsakoff syndrome, and folic acid and vitamin B_{12} deficiency, which can also produce progressive cognitive impairment and dementia. Paraneoplastic syndromes are the rare clinical abnormalities caused by cancer but not resulting from direct invasion of the organ involved. While this definition implies any nonmetastatic effect of cancer

Table 5. Drugs with anticholinergic effects used in cancer treatment

Antiemetics:	Prochlorperazine metaclopramide	Narcotic analgesics:	Codeine Hydromorphone Levodromoran
Antihistamines:	Diphenhydramine Hydroxyzine		Meperidine Methadone
Antiparkinsonians:	Benztropine Trihexyphenidyl		Morphine
Antipsychotics:	Chlorpromazine Thioridazine Haloperidol	Tricyclic antidepressants:	Amitriptyline Nortriptyline Imipramine Desipramine Doxepin Maprotoline
Atropine			Trazodone
Antispasmodics:	Clinidium Diphenoxylate Hyoscyamine	Scopolamine	

Table 6. Common psychological changes with steroids administration

During treatment:
Sense of well being or mild depression
Optimism
Increased appetite; weight gain
Insomnia

During withdrawal:
Mild depression
Irritability
Anorexia
Headache and myalgias

on the nervous system, it is usually used to refer to the remote effects of cancer (e.g., multifocal leukoencephalopathy, cerebellar degeneration) and the effects on mental and neurologic function of the hormone-producing tumors (e.g., lung, adrenal).

Clinical Evaluation

Subtle changes in mental status are apt to go unnoticed or be attributed to the stress of illness. These changes may continue unnoticed if the patient's behavior remains quiet and unobtrusive. Overt behavioral and personality changes often must occur before the possibility of a delirium is recognized. Table 7 outlines the early signs and symptoms of delirium and those which appear late, when severely disordered mental function has developed. The earliest signs are often readily identified from the nurses' progress notes about behavioral changes at night: unaccustomed restlessness and episodes of disorientation. Anger, irritability, and temper outbursts may be noted during the day; withdrawal and refusal to speak to staff or relatives is seen and forgetfulness, previously absent, becomes apparent.

When the delirium develops further and obvious mental changes occur, symptoms may resemble those of a functional psychotic state, with compromise of compliance to treatment and, at times, risk of harm to self or others. The person may become uncooperative, angry, abusive, and demanding, and may attempt to leave the hospital if not detained. Perceptual misconceptions (illusions) of persons and objects usually have a suspicious, paranoid association; delusions resulting from misinterpretation of events, again, usually reflect fears of being harmed, especially when associated with auditory and visual hallucinations. Patients can at times incur serious injury, requiring close monitoring of their behavior. While such a psychological state in a physically healthy person would be treated in a psychiatric unit, the level of physical illness in cancer patients often precludes transfer to a psychiatric unit.

In summary, the clinical picture of delirium must be evaluated by comparing it to the patient's prior level of mental function, obtained by outside history from family members and from the patient's medical chart, which will indicate mental state on prior visits or admissions. Review of notes from social work or nurses

Table 7. Behavioral symptomatology of delirium in cancer patients

---

Early, mild symptoms:
Change in sleep pattern with restlessness and transient periods of disorientation
Increased irritability, anger, temper outburst
Withdrawal, refusal to talk to staff or relatives
Forgetfulness not previously present

Late, severe symptoms:
Refusal to cooperate with reasonable requests
Angry, swearing, shouting, abusive
Demanding to go home; pacing corridor
Illusions (misidentifies staff, visual & sensory clues)
Delusions (misinterprets events, usually paranoid, fears of being harmed)
Hallucinations (visual and auditory)

---

may pick up changes noted by relatives. This review must include obtaining a history of prior drug or alcohol abuse and mental illness.

When delirium is suspected, the patient's mental state should be tested by conducting a full mental status examination. The clinical examination covers four major areas: the patient's appearance and behavior, mood and affect, thought content, and intellectual function. Several assessment scales of mental status have been developed to screen for the presence of deficits and to provide a more standardized clinical measure. The Cognitive Capacity Screening developed by Jacobs (1977) and the Mini-Mental State Exam by Folstein et al. (1984) have been widely used. However, they must be interpreted in light of the patient's educational level and language. They often pick up gross changes but miss subtle ones which are important for recognition of mild delirium and dementia.

The advantages to routine use of these tests, nevertheless, are several. They assure testing in all areas and provide a quantitative evaluation that helps in monitoring changes in mental state. They require only a few minutes to administer, can be given by any staff member, and encourage obtaining a record of baseline mental status of patients at time of admission.

Pauker et al. (1978) developed a rapid method of assessment using a handheld tachistoscope which measures reaction time to a visual stimulus. While this is simple and fast, it too will fail to identify early defects. When discret deficits need to be assessed, by far the most preferable approach is to refer a patient for neuropsychological testing, in which the areas of dysfunction can be delineated and the level of global dysfunction specified.

Management

The management of delirium is directed to determining the underlying cause. Since the cancer patients who develop delirium are likely to be the most seriously ill, transfer to a psychiatric unit is usually not possible and the ability of the oncology staff to handle both emergency and the more common nonemergency situations is important. Table 8 gives the principles of management (Fleishman and Lesko 1989).

Table 8. Management of delirium

1. Prompt recognition and diagnosis
2. Prompt treatment of underlying cause
3. Psychiatric consultation – *early*, not late
4. One-to-one nurse or companion
5. Oral neuroleptics, when needed
6. Alert all nursing shifts about changes in behavior e.g., often worse at night

Treatment of a Mild Confusional State

When a patient shows signs and symptoms of a *delirium with mild behavioral changes*, prompt diagnosis, with treatment of the underlying medical cause, is crucial. Environmental manipulation, the judicious use of oral antipsychotic medication, and staff and family instruction in management all help to calm the patient and reassure family members.

Environmental manipulation is important, since patients with delirium are especially sensitive to their environment. Rooms should be quiet and well lit during the daytime. A night light will reduce the disorientation that worsens during the evening and night hours when visual cues are reduced. Frequent, short contact with a supportive family member or a familiar staff member who speaks in a calm, reassuring voice sets a quiet and orderly tone. One or two family members who consistently visit the patient provide an added sense of continuity and stability for the patient.The addition of a calendar, clock, and even a few small, familiar objects from home help reorient a forgetful, mildly confused patient. Sensory input should not be excessive. Many different individuals entering the room with requests or procedures enhance the patient's sense of confusion. The one-to-one companion or nurse becomes the monitor of both the patient and the environment, providing a stable day/night schedule and explaining noises or unfamilar equipment. Encouragement of walking, reading, and participation in personal care promotes awareness of reality and reduces the response to delusional ideas.

Oral antipsychotic medications are the drugs of choice, since other sedatives (benzodiazepines, barbiturates, antihistamines) can worsen confusion. Hospitalized cancer patients usually respond to low doses, such as 0.5 mg haloperidol or 10 mg thioridazine or chlorpromazine given two or three times daily. Haloperidol and chlorpromazine can be given in several forms: tablet, liquid concentrate, or parenteral for intramuscular or intravenous injection. Antipsychotics are not commercially prepared in suppository form, but they can be prepared by a hospital pharmacist on request. Absorption, however, is not reliable. Haloperidol, having a higher drug potency than the other medications mentioned, gives less orthostatic hypotension and anticholinergic effects per milligram equivalent of antipsychotic activity, although patients with only *mild symptoms of a delirium* will rarely need the faster acting parenteral route. Nausea and vomiting from chemotherapy, gastric tumors, *non per os* orders, malabsorption states, or immediate postoperative treatment may require that medication be given.

Monitoring the patient's behavior several times a day is essential. Visits at different times of the day are helpful, particularly if medication dosage is being titrated against the patient's behavior. Any psychotropic drug should be given at the lowest effective dose. A progress note indicating the time the mental status was assessed helps to convey this information to staff on all shifts. Integration of nurses' and physicians' progress notes is particularly valuable when managing patients with neurologic complications of cancer, to assure easy and frequent review of changes in mental state. Use of standardized mental status scales, such as the Mini-Mental State or Cognitive Capacity Screening examination, provide a charted record of standardized observations.

Outpatient follow-up of patients who have had an acute delirium while being treated in the hospital is essential. Patients often fear that they "lost their mind" in the hospital and feel distress at having "lost track" of a period of time. They need to discuss their recall of events and be assured that their medical illness or treatment was the cause. The family too is reassured by such information and by being included in visits with the patient. Emergency situations can serve the purpose of making the transition to the home environment easier. If a psychotropic drug was given, it must be monitored and slowly tapered at home.

Emergency Management of Severe Delirium

While emergency situations happen infrequently, they are highly distressful to the fearful patient and to other patients and their visiting family members. The ability of staff on a unit to optimally manage a delirious patient is related to their tolerance towards patients whose behavior is unpredictable, frustrating, and at times frightening. It is helpful to identify one or two staff members on a unit who are interested in psychiatric problems and disturbed patients. However, all staff members should know the legal and ethical issues, as well as how to handle a patient in a psychiatric emergency situation when behavior is unpredictable. For this reason, it is important to have a plan, known to staff, by which a situation can be effectively and rapidly contained with maximal patient safety and minimal disrupting of the floor activities. Such a situation most often arises when a confused patient becomes belligerent, assaultive, and cannot respond to reasonable requests. The first step is to call the psychiatrist, who evaluates the situation and organizes, if needed, a team composed of the floor staff. Assistance of a security officer or guard is requested if there is a danger of extremely belligerent behavior. Security staff receive instruction in their training about sensitive management of patients in these situations. They may be asked only to be present unobstrusively in case the situation escalates, or if a dangerous staircase or exit poses a hazard.

Every effort must be made to assure the patient that he is safe and secure. Explanation to the family members present is important to ensure their understanding and cooperation with a request to remain in the room as persons trusted by the patient. The hospital room is familiar and if a trusted staff member can be brought to the room this is helpful; otherwise, moving the patient to a quiet area away from others is desirable and often sufficient to induce a calmer state in which one-to-one observation by a nurse can be instituted. The room should be cleared of potentially dangerous objects if the risk warrants it.

If necessary, the patient should be encouraged to take an oral sedative in the form of a liquid concentrate, which allows rapid absorption. If the patient refuses oral medication, or if the oral route is inadvisable for medical reasons, e.g., low platelet count, parenteral medication should be considered (Adams 1984). Haloperidol is used because it rarely induces hypotension, gives minimal sedation, and has a relatively short half-life, allowing close titration of dose with behavior (Donlon et al. 1979). The use of intravenous or intramuscular haloperidol 0.5–2.0 mg is recommended as an initial dose; by the intravenous route, it is given at 1 mg/min. The physician should monitor behavior carefully after the initial dose and determine if additional doses are needed. A repeat dose may be given in 60 min if agitation has not subsided. Usually, one to three doses are sufficient. When the acute agitation resolves, the aptient should be switched to an oral form of haloperidol at a dose of about half to one-and-a-half times the intravenous or intramuscular dose. Extrapyramidal side effects are not common at these dose levels. They are usually controlled by intravenous or oral diphenhydramine 25–50 mg twice daily, or benztropine 0.5 to 1 mg p.o. or i.v. twice daily.

Most patients can be calmed by environmental changes, others can be encouraged to take medication. However, it is occasionally necessary to temporarily restrain the patient to prevent harm (e.g., the assaultive patient who has thrombocytopenia). If needed, minimal restraint is applied to each extremity while the medication is given.

When any physical restraint is used, the "least restrictive" type is indicated. Occasionally a "posey" nylon vest or limb restraints composed of loosely applied cotton padding and soft gauze are used to prevent a confused patient from removing catheters or tubes. Nylon mesh "sheets" that attach to the fixed parts of a hospital bed are a safer and less restrictive method of restraint. Use of any restraint should be for the shortest possible period and accompanied by careful and close monitoring of vital signs, behavior, intake, and output by a companion in constant attendance. Restraint of cancer patients requires special consideration in the presence of thrombocytopenia, fever, or dehydration. We find that one-to-one nursing observation is adequate in almost all situations, rather than physical restraint.

Special Diagnostic and Management Issues

Steroids

Corticosteroids are used frequently in cancer therapy: as primary chemothera-peutic agents as a means to reduce edema associated with brain and spinal cord lesions, and, increasingly, as an antiemetic in combination with metaclopramide, haloperidol, diphenhydramine, or lorazepam.

The behavioral response to steroids is independent of the dose used: more severe effects are seen with higher doses, but they can also occur at small doses. While a sense of well being and increased appetite are useful initial side effects, obesity and proximal motor senses are adverse effects which occur over time, along with insomnia, restlessness, hyperactivity, and depression. When steroids are withdrawn, mild depression or irritability may be noticeable (See Table 6).

Severe mood disturbances are far less common than those outlined above. They are characterized by mania, severe depression, or delirium with affective changes. These drug-induced changes, termed organic affective syndromes, may be accompanied by frank hallucinations and delusions and may be clinically indistinguishable from a primary affective illness. The actual frequency of covert mental changes is not known, since few systematic studies have been undertaken in patients with cancer. It appears that some patients experience illusions and hallucinations but do not report them, recognizing that they are drug-related. Severe mood disturbances usually occur when the steroid dose is abruptly changed, either increased, tapered, or discontinued. During withdrawal, myalgias or arthralgias appear which help to confirm the physiologic effects of the dosage reduction.

A history of drug abuse, alcohol dependence, or prior psychiatric illness is not a reason to withhold steroids from a patient. Mood and mental status should be carefully monitored; an antidepressant and/or antipsychotic should be given if early affective signs appear. We have not found that lithium given prophylactically prevents affective complications. Treatment of steroid-induced psychosis involves the same management as deliriums of other causes, utilizing the same psychotropic drugs. The exceptions to this are reactions relating to a rapid tapering off of the steroid; in this instance the treatment, as for other withdrawal states in relation to barbiturates or narcotics, may be to raise the steroid dose and lower it again gradually, while also instituting antipsychotic medication if symptoms are severe.

Anticholinergics

A wide range of drugs with anticholinergic properties, blocking cholinergic neurotransmission, are used in cancer patients (see Table 5). Antihistamines, antiemetics, antiparkinsonian drugs, antipsychotics, narcotic analgesics, atropine to dry respiratory secretions during surgery, scopolamine, and tricyclics are used often in cancer. An anticholinergic delirium can arise from any of these drugs. However, the more common problem in cancer patients occurs when several drugs with these properties have been given for different reasons. The potential for additive anticholinergic side effects must be kept in mind. It is particularly important to watch for this complications in the postoperative period when several of the agents may have been ordered concurrently. The picture is characterized by a delirium accompanied by hyperpyrexia, mydriasis, dehydration, vasodilatation, hypertension, tachycardia, constipation, and urinary retention.

Treatment is to discontinue or tapper *all* anticholinergic agents when possible. The use of physostigmine, a reversible *peripheral* anticholinesterase, is required when tachycardia or resulting arrythmias make the situation life-threatening.

Physostigmine is administered intramuscularly or intravenously at 0.5–1.0 mg, at a rate of no more than 1.0 mg/min, repeated at 10- to 30-min intervals. It is administered only when resuscitation equipment is available in case of cardiac arrest or respiratory failure due to obstruction by a sudden overabundance of secretions.

If sedation is necessary, antipsychotic medication at the lowest doses and with the lowest anticholinergic properties (haloperidol) or short-acting barbiturates (sodium amytal) or benzodiazepine (intravenous lorazepan) should be used. Caution must be used since these agents themselves may worsen behavioral signs and symptoms in a paradoxical fashion, or make clinical assessment of the anticholinergic state more difficult. Environmental alteration, physical restraint, and constant observation are best used until the anticholinergic drugs are metabolized.

References

Adams F (1984) Neuropsychiatric evaluation and treatment of delirium in the critically ill cancer patient. The Cancer Bulletin of the University of Texas MD. Anderson Hospital and Tumor Institute 36: 156–160

APA (1980) Diagnostic and statistical manual III. APA, Washington DC

Bonhoeffer K (1910) Die symtomatischen Psychosen in Gefolge von akuten Infectionen und inneren Erkrankungen. Deuticke, Leipzig, p 94

Derogatis LR, Morrow GR, Fetting J, Penman D, Piasetsky S, Schmale A, Henricks M, Cornicke CL Jr (1983) The prevalence of psychiatric disorders among cancer patients. JAMA 249: 751–757

Donlon PT, Hopkin J, Tupin J (1979) Overview: efficacy and safety of the rapid neuroleptization method with injectable haloperidol. Am J Psychiatry 136: 273–278

Engel GL, Romano J (1959) Delirium: a syndrome of cerebral insufficiency. J Chron Dis 9: 260–277

Fleishman SB, Lesko LM (1989) Delirium and dementia. In: Holland JC, Rowland JH (eds) Psychooncology: psychological care of the patient with cancer. Oxford University Press, New York, pp 342–355

Folstein MF, Fetting JH, Lobo-A, Niaz U, Capozzoli K (1984) Cognitive assessment of cancer patients. Cancer 53: (suppl 15): 2250–2255

Jacobs JW (1977) Screening for organic mental syndromes in the medically ill. Ann Intern Med 86: 40–46

Lipowski ZJ (1980) A new look at organic brain syndromes. Am J Psychiatry 137: 674–678

Lipowksi ZJ (1983) Transient cognitive disorder (delirium, acute confusional states) in the elderly. Am J Psychiatry 140: 1426–1436

Liston EH (1984) Diagnosis and management of delirium in the elderly patient. Psychiatry Ann 14: 109–118

Pauker NE, Folstein MF, Moran TH (1978) The clinical utility of the hand-held tachistoscope. J Nerv Ment Dis 166: 126–129

Plum F, Posner JB (1972) The diagnosis of stupor and coma, 2nd ed. Davis, Philadelphia, p 4

Posner JB (1978) Neurologic complications of systemic cancer. DM 25: 1–60

Posner JB (1979) Delirium and exogenous metabolic brain disease. In: Beeson PB, McDermott W, Wynaarden JB (eds) Cecil textbook of medicine. Saunders, Philadelphia, pp 644–651

Seymour DG, Henschke PJ, Cape RD, Campbell AJ (1980) Acute confusional states and dementia in the elderly: the role of dehydration/volume depletion, physical illness and age. Age Aging, 9: 137–146

Wells CE (1979) Pseudodementia. Am J Psychiatry 136: 859–900

Young DF, Posner JB (1980) Nervous system toxicity of the chemotherapeutic agents. In: Viken PM, Bruyn GW (eds) Handbook of clinical neurology, vol 39. Neurological manifestations of systemic diseases Part II. Elsevier, New York

Palliative Care: A New Reality in Medicine

V. Ventafridda

Division of Pain Therapy and Palliative Care, National Cancer Institute, Milan, Italy

Introduction

Cancer is, today, one of the greatest problems for the world's population. Globally, 8% of all deaths are caused by cancer [1], and in the developed countries this percentage is even higher: in Europe, for example, it is over 22% [2]. Each year there are approximately 7 million new cancer patients worldwide and about 5 million people die [3, 4]. About half of the people suffering cancer are in developing countries. In the literature it is estimated that there are currently about 14 million people living with cancer [4–6]. In the developed countries 67% of the male and 60% of the female cancer patients die as a result of their disease. In developing countries cancer mortality is even higher and, because of the increasing longevity of the population, cancer mortality will increase by about 40% between now and the year 2000.

For three of the eight main forms of cancer – lung, mouth, and liver cancer – primary prevention is adequate to lower the incidence of the disease. In another three kinds of cancer – breast, cervix, and mouth cancer – patients can be cured by specific treatment if the disease is diagnosed early enough. Palliative care, the main priority of which is pain control, is effective in every type of advanced cancer [7].

WHO Guidelines on Cancer Pain Relief

With a brief to prepare guidelines for relief of cancer pain, a WHO Consultation in 1982 brought together in Milan, Italy, a group of experts in the management of cancer pain from the fields of anesthesiology, neurology, neurosurgery, nursing, oncology, pharmacology, psychology, and surgery. The consensus reached in formulating these guidelines using a limited number was that pain relief using a limited number of drugs was a realistic target for the majority of cancer patients throughout the world.

The subsequent important work done by the WHO resulted in the publication of *Cancer Pain Relief* [8], which was produced by the participants of a WHO meeting on the comprehensive management of cancer pain held in Geneva in 1984. Among the participants were experts on cancer pain management, on national and international legislation concerning the regulation of opioid drugs, on health care delivery, on health education, and on pharmaceutical research and manufacturing, as well as representatives of several international non-governmental organizations. The method of pain relief is based on a three-step ladder from nonopioids, via weak opioids, to strong opioids and drugs administrated, usually orally, on an hourly basis. At each step adjuvant drugs (steroids, psychotropic drugs, etc.) may be added if necessary.

At the initiative of the WHO and the WHO Collaborating Center for Cancer Pain Relief at the National Cancer Institute, Milan, since 1985 many countries with different health care systems have undertaken studies on the applicability and the effectiveness of the guidelines [9–13]. The number of patients treated ranged from 20 in one field-test to 1229 in another study. A total of 1642 cases have been reported. In each of the studies it has been shown that, for the majority of terminal cancer patients, pain can be either reduced considerably or completely controlled by the use of analgesics alone or combined with adjuvant drugs.

The Meaning of Palliative Care

In the terminal phase of the disease, the patients are generally no longer responsive to anticancer therapies. It is at this time that palliative care becomes necessary to support the patient through a period of physical and psychosocial suffering that is absolutely neglected by the traditional oncological establishment.

With palliative care a new medicine has been born, with aims and methods completely different from the intensive or invasive attitudes, often unwanted by patients, which are usual in these clinical situations. Palliative care aims to give the patient and his or her the highest quality of life possible. It consists in a global approach to controlling the patient's suffering and is carried out by a multidisciplinary team composed of physicians, nurses, social workers, and volunteers.

The following are the main characteristics of this new field of medicine:

– It affirms life and regards dying as a normal process.
– It neither hastens nor postpones death.
– It provides relief from pain and other distressing symptoms.
– It integrates the psychological and spiritual aspects of patient care.
– It offers a support system to help the family cope during the patient's illness and in bereavement.
– Investigations are kept to a minimum and treatment is directed to symptom control and psychosocial support and not to the underlying disease process.

– Radiotherapy, chemotherapy, and surgery have a place in palliative care. They are used, however, in such a way to ensure that the symptomatic benefits of treatment clearly outweigh the disadvantages [14, 15].

The center of attention is the human being, his or her personality and subjective feelings, and not just the illness or the nociception but the total suffering which it causes and the impact it has on the family. The unit of care is the family rather that just the patient. The family's active participation in care is expected and their enquiries are encouraged. This kind of approach means that continued monitoring of the patients, either in hospital care or in the home setting, is needed. The latter is regarded as the better option, taking into consideration that the patient's home is the best place for him or her to live and that the family is a very important part of the team.

The Care Givers

The basis of care in the home setting is continued professional supervision. The involvement of a variety of health care workers is necessary and they must be trained to evaluate patient's needs and resources; educate and advise patients and families; provide psychological support for both; and know how to use drugs in pain and symptom control.

The major role in the team is played by the nurses, as they have particular responsibilities in providing the patient and the family with information, counselling, and education. They facilitate the continuity of care between home and hospital as well as ensuring that contact with the treating physician is maintained and that he or she is kept constantly informed. It is the nurse who has the closest contact with the patient and who can best monitor and evaluate the pain and other symptoms. This is why they must have the authority to adjust the dosage of drugs, within prescribed ranges, to give the necessary relief at any given time. Voluntary helpers are also important in the team to provide sufficient care for the patients. They may be found through associations or may be friends and neighbors.

Palliative Care Organizations

Fully developed palliative care programs include the following components:

1. *Home care.* Palliative care stresses that the primary setting of care is the home. In contrary to traditional medical care and funding, which are based on an institutional model, the institutions are not the focal point of the program but act as a backup resource, the center point for organizing the teams.
2. *Consultation service.* Specially trained health-care workers provide a consultation service for patients in hospital and in the community and for their families. This includes the referral of patients to the agencies that, in some countries, offer financial assistance to patients with advanced cancer.

3. *Day care*. The institutions also serve as palliative care day centers that can be attended by patients living alone two or three times a week. Day-care centers also supply support for the families, alleviating the demands home care places on them.
4. *Inpatient care*. Hospitalization concentrates on controlling pain and other manifestations of physical and psychosocial distress in cases where home care is not practicable.
5. *Beravement support*. Trained health-care workers or volunteers may also support people needing help to cope with their bereavement.

Recent Developments

The movement initiated by a small group of experts under the patronage of the WHO is now spreading in many developed countries. In recent years, palliative care has become established in an increasing number of countries, and academic posts have been created in various countries such as Australia, Canada, and the United Kingdom. This is the context in which the European Association of Palliative Care, several national associations, and journals for palliative care have been founded.

Hospices and palliative-care units or home-care units are the practical results. Studies have demonstrated that a palliative-care center results in raised standards of care in neighboring general hospitals [16, 17].

Besides the initiative of the WHO, since 1986 there have been other major developments:

- The introduction of a policy for Cancer Pain Relief in the Indian states of Gujarat, Karnataka, Kerala [18], Maharastra, and Tamil Nadu was the result of the National Cancer Control Plan for India [19]. This included provision for training professional health workers, and has made oral morphine available for the first time in these states.
- In the USA the State of Wisconsin established a Cancer Pain Initiative, to serve as a WHO demonstration project [20].
- The French government [21] and Japan [22] have adopted a policy for care of the terminally ill.
- The governments of Australia, Sweden [23], and Japan [22] have adopted a policy for pain control.
- In Italy the prescription of oral opioid drugs has been allowed by an official decree [24].

Conclusions

Nothing would be more effective in improving the quality of life of the world's advanced cancer patients and their families than implementing the knowledge that exists about pain and symptom control in cancer. Although for most terminal cancer patients palliative care is the only realistic solution, few of the cancer control resources go to palliative care and, in general, there is little or no training for health-care workers in this type of care. All too often palliative care is ignored or seen as something that comes at the very end of the list of treatment options. Curative care and palliative care are not mutually exclusive. However, for many cancer patients curative treatment is not effective, and for them it would be of great benefit to have access to palliative care. It is thus important to make the public more aware about the existence and the potential benefit of palliative care.

References

1. World Health Organization (1984) Cancer as a global problem. Weekly Epidemiol Rec 59: 125–126
2. Commission of the European Community (1988) Europe against cancer. Luxembourg, Office of Official Publications of the European Community
3. Parkin DM, Laara E, Muir CS (1988) Estimates of the worldwide frequency of twelve major cancers. Int J cancer 41: 184–197
4. World Population Trends (1983)
5. Aoki K, Sugenoya J, Ohno Y, Kobayashi H, Kawaguchi T (1981) Estimated point prevalence of cancer in Japan, 1977. In: Seg M, Tominaga S, Aoki K, Fujimoto I (eds) Cancer mortality and morbidity statistics. Japan and the world. Japan Scientific Societies, Tokyo, pp 117–120
6. Hanai A (1987) Estimation of the number of cancer survivors according to site in Japan. Jap J Cancer Res 78: 537–546
7. Stjernswärd J, Stanley K, Koroltchouk V (1986) Quality of life of cancer patients – goals and objectives. In: Ventafridda V, van Dam FS, Yancik R, Tamburini M (eds) Assessment of quality of life and cancer treatment. Excerpta Medica, Amsterdam, pp 1–8
8. World Health Organization (1986) Cancer pain relief. World Health Organization, Geneva
9. Rappaz O, Tripiana J, Rapin CH, Stjernswärd J, Junod JP (1985) Soins palliatifs et traitement de la douleru cancereuse en geriatrie. Ther Umschau/Rev Ther 42: 843–848
10. Takeda F (1986) Results of field-testing in Japan of the WHO draft interim guidelines on relief of cancer pain. Pain Clin 1: 83–89
11. Ventafridda V, Tamburini M, Caraceni A, De Conno F, Naldi F (1987) A validation study of the WHO method for cancer pain relief. Cancer 59: 851–856
12. Walker VA, Hoskin PJ, Hanks GW, White ID (1988) Evaluation of WHO analgesic guidelines for cancer pain in a hospital-based palliative care unit. J Pain Symptom Management 3: 145–149
13. Zech D, Grond S, Schug S, Meuser T, Stobbe B, Lehmann KA. Pain control according to WHO guidelines in 1140 cancer patients
14. Bates TD (1984) Radiotherapy in terminal care. In: Saunders CM (ed) The management of terminal disease. Edward Arnold, London, pp 133–138
15. Bates TD (1989) Radiotherapy, chemotherapy and harmone therapy in the relief of cancer pain. In: Swerdlow M (ed) Relief of intractable pain, 4th edn. Elsevier, Amsterdam

16. Parkes CM, Parkes J (1984) Hospice versus hospital care: reevaluation after ten years as seen by surviving spouses. Postgrad Med J 60: 120–124
17. Kane RL, Wales J, Bernstein L, Leibowitz A, Kaplan S (1984) A randomized controlled trial of hospice care. Lancer I: 890–894
18. Nair K (1988) Ten year action plan for cancer control in Kerala. Trivandrum, Kerala
19. Government of India (1984) National cancer control plan for India. Director General of Health Services, Ministry of Health and Welfare, New Delhi
20. Joranson DE, Dahl JL, Engbert D (1987) Wisconsin initiative for improving cancer pain management: progress report. J Pain Symptom Management 2: 111–113
21. Ministére des Affaires Sociales et de l'Emploi, Ministére Chargé de la Santé et de la Famille (1988) Soigner et accompagner Jusqu'au bout soulager la souffrance. Paris
22. Ministry of Health and Welfare and Japan Medical Association (1989) Manual of care for terminally ill cancer patients. Tokyo (1989)
23. Swedish National Board of Health and Welfare (1989) General recommendation: the management of pain in the terminal stage of life. Stockholm
24. Ministero della Sanità (1989) Decreta Art 1. Gazetta ufficiale della Republica Italiana. Rome

Cure and Care: Interaction Between Cancer Centers and Palliative Care Units

N. MacDonald

University of Alberta, Palliative Medicine, Edmonton, Alberta, Canada

At the turn of the century a diagnosis of invasive cancer was tantamount to a death sentence. Since then, improved understanding of the basic mechanisms of the disease accompanied by the introduction of rational surgical, radiotherapeutic, and medical therapies has radically changed the outlook for newly diagnosed patients with malignant disease. Today, in North America, slightly less than 50% of patients may expect to be alive and free of disease five years after diagnosis. In the developing countries, the statistics are far less favorable – only 20%–30% of patients will be cured because of delays in diagnosis and problems with access to therapy.

Oncologists, both in the laboratories and at the bedside, are optimists and, because of demonstrated success in certain areas of cancer, may have overestimated our rate of progress. Now, it appears that there are boundaries which limit the success of current approaches. Pending the introduction of fundamentally new management techniques, we may anticipate that, for some years to come, the majority of cancer patients in the world will die of their disease following a period of illness characterized by the presence of pain, physical disability, and varying degrees of emotional and spiritual distress. The incidence of cancer continues to increase throughout the world, particularly in those areas where tobacco use continues to expand. Today, approximately 5 million people die of cancer each year. In 20 years, unless a change in ethical standards and improvements in health education occur, the expected increase in tobacco-related cancers will mean that the estimated death toll will rise to over 8 million people per year.

Even though most of their patients will die of their disease, cancer centres have not assigned a high priority to the needs of dying cancer patients and their families, nor to studies on the mechanisms and treatment of the symptoms which bedevil their final days. As cancer research flowered, large interinstitutional groups developed, but the thrust of clinical research was directed towards assessing aspects of disease progression, such as survival and objective tumor response, while evaluation of the impact of cancer therapies on pain, other physical symptoms, and on psychosocial parameters was assigned a low priority [1].

Thus, an imbalance in the "care–cure equation" existed. Efforts to balance this equation did not arise from the traditional oncology leadership but, rather, through the initiatives of a group of concerned physicians, nurses, and motivated volunteers, the majority of whom were not connected with cancer centres. Thus, parallel but separate from progress in other aspects of cancer care, the palliative care movement developed, initially in Britain, and latterly in North America, the Antipodes, and the Western European continent.

Although both groups were ultimately concerned with the lot of cancer patients, in many places their activities were not coordinated and a state of "two solitudes" existed. The line of division was not absolute – for example, the Royal Marsden Hospital in London had set aside beds for advanced cancer patients for many years and, indeed, oral morphine (the use of which is a tenet of the palliative care movement) was used there for some years before the birth of the palliative care movement in the mid-1960s. Similarly, the Sloan Kettering Cancer Institute in New York had a small but excellent pain research group, while the Mayo Clinic Cancer Center carried out a series of excellent analgesic studies in the late 1960s and early 1970s. Nevertheless, the thrust of most cancer centres was towards therapy designed to impact on the trajectory of illness. Patients who were not suitable for interventional trials would often be returned to the care of community physicians.

Clearly, there is a need for coordination between cancer centres and community based palliative care programmes. The principles upon which each is based can with profit be introduced to the other organization. Indeed, in view of the numbers of advanced cancer patients and the lack of available therapies for many of their problems, cancer centres must increasingly recognize their responsibility to introduce palliative care programs within their own institutions and to study the impact of anticancer therapies on the symptoms and quality of life of patients enrolled in clinical trials.

Cancer Centres: Lessons to Be Learned from the Palliative Care Movement

The suffering of advanced cancer patients is a compound of physical distress, fear, loneliness, concerns about the meaning of illness, the anguish of the unknown, and the concern of the dying for the loved ones who will be bereaved and their well being. Cancer centres deal with large volumes of patients. In the course of assessment and therapy, patients and their families may be exposed to flotillas of attending staff, residents and nurse specialists, each concerned with a special facet of care. It is often difficult to engineer a comprehensive pattern of care, with attention to physical, social, and emotional problems, in the course of extremely busy outpatient visits.

The training criteria for medical oncologists demand that they develop skills in the comprehensive care of their patients [1]. However, while training, they are stimulated to direct their energies to studies on the pathophysiology of cancer and associated cancer therapies; relatively less emphasis is placed on developing skills and managing problems associated with advanced cancer. Lack of interest is sometimes tangibly expressed when patients are discharged from follow-up in cancer centres when deemed to be no longer responsive to anti-tumour treatments. They may be returned to family physicians from whom they may have lost contact while in the course of treatment at the cancer centre, or who, by experience, training, and lack of community support systems, may be unable properly to help the patient and family.

When introduced into cancer centres, the principles of palliative care can clearly improve the care of patients and families. Comprehensive palliative care programmes are normally characterized by the following features [3]:

Interdisciplinary Care

The traditional hierarchical medical model whereby the physician directs therapy and carrys out treatments, sometimes with assistance from others, is discarded and replaced by a collegial team approach. While the team may usually, though not always, continue to be led by a physician, it is recognized that other health professionals and, increasingy, volunteers have specific roles to play. This feature improves staff morale and reduces stress. Authority matches responsibility, resulting in increased job satisfaction.

Relaxation of Bureaucratic Regulations

Instead of moulding the patients and families to fit the system, the system is adjusted to the needs of the patients. For example, on a palliative care ward visiting hours are flexible, pets may be taken on the wards, and any activity is accepted as long as it does not embarrass or disturb the other patients. The maintenance of patient dignity is stressed – dignity is enhanced when personal freedom is maintained.

Hierarchy of Problems

The importance of problems as perceived by patients, families and medical attendants may differ considerably at any given point in time. For example, the oncologist may be primarily concerned with the response of the cancer to therapy, the patient at that moment may be primarily concerned with psycho-logical-spiritual issues and the control of distressing symptoms, while the family members may be primarily concerned about financial problems. The interest of palliative care physicians and nurses is more geared to what patients and families may regard as their most important difficulties.

Maintenance of Hope

Many patients and families enter palliative care programmes having been told either formally or by implication that nothing more can be done for them. They may feel that they have been expelled from the human family prematurely. In the palliative care programme, hope is reinstituted; even though patients may recognize that they are going to die, they can experience short-term relief of distressing symptoms. Patients and families develop an attitude of preparing for the worst but expecting the best.

Conservative Investigations

Investigations are kept to a minimum, while the therapies are directed primarily towards symptom control and psychosocial counselling rather than reversal of the basic disease process. Most palliative treatments leave the patient with an immediate sense of relief and not with an intensification of symptoms. An admirable paradox exists: acute care medicine is offered in an environment of relative tranquillity.

Physical Environment

Care is offered in a ward environment where ambience is judged to be important, aesthetic standards are high and patient and family autonomy are maintained.

Integration of Complex Therapies in a Home–Hospital Setting

Patients may obtain pain relief following the application of a complicated (for the patient and family) pharmacologic or non-pharmacologic plan. In order for this success to be maintained, it is essential that hospital-based therapies can be applied in the home and that problems, as they arise, can be rapidly assessed and corrected. Cancer patients often take a array of compounds with a mixed profile of benefits and potential side effects which must constantly be adjusted. They may benefit from the application of technical procedures (such as subcutaneous infusion or intraspinal procedures) which are readily maintained in a hospital setting but less certainly so in the home. Palliative care programmes provide the vehicle through which the complexities of hospital care can be maintained in a home setting without loss of efficacy.

All of the above aspects of palliative care are not unique to a special field. They simply are elements of humane medical care in any setting. Cancer centres can introduce these principles, and are doing so, but a reassessment of priorities is required.

Palliative Care: Lessons to Be Learned from Cancer Centres

Self-criticism

The palliative care movement has certain messianic features. Movements run the risk of accepting unsubstantiated dogma and becoming self-congratulatory. It is important to reevaluate tenets and move beyond the established base to improve the approaches to care currently in vogue. Oncology programmes are normally characterized by a questioning of, sometimes even cynical approach to claims of therapeutic success. The application of a rigid intellectual analysis of palliative care tenets will benefit the movement.

Increased Emphasis on Quality Research

Following the emergence of medical oncology as a discipline, leaders in the field recognized that progress could only be made through the design of impeccable clinical studies and the adoption of common standards for classifying and assessing disease which would provide a common language for interpretation of results. Large multi-institutional study groups came into existence. Consequently, proven therapeutic advances could be introduced for the benefit of the community while other unproven therapies were tested and discarded.

Considering the extraordinary expansion of the palliative care movement, it is surprising that a proportional research base for the field did not develop. Research in cancer pain is carried out by relatively few isolated groups and, aside from psycho-oncology, multi-institutional studies are rarely noted. For example, a review of 25 recent consecutive studies in cancer pain that were published in either *Pain* or the *Journal of Pain and Symptom Management* showed that only 12 of them were conducted in a blinded fashion. Patient numbers were modest, the mechanism of the pain syndrome was identified in only seven trials, and only three of them described in any detail the previous analgesic treatment which the patients had received [4]. Levine and Sackett [5] have outlined six requirements for analgesic studies:

1. Was the assignment of patients to the different opiates randomized?
2. Were all clinically relevant outcomes reported?
3. Were the patients recognizable?
4. Were both clinical and statistical significance considered?
5. Was the opiate regimen feasible in routine clinical practice?
6. Were all patients who entered the study accounted for at its conclusion?

These requirements are rarely fulfilled in cancer pain studies.

It is very difficult to interpret the cancer pain literature because of the lack of an accepted classification for cancer pain or of a system for reporting study endpoints and the utilization of therapy over the long-term.

Our group has recently introduced a staging system which combines clinical epidemiological features of cancer pain with anatomical definition [6]. The system considers seven features of the patient pain:

1. Mechanism of pain
2. Presence of incident pain
3. Level of prior narcotic requirement
4. Cognitive function
5. Psychological distress
6. Rate of development of tolerance
7. Past history of alcohol or drug abuse

We studied 56 consecutive patients with cancer pain using this classification system. The patients came from either an advanced breast cancer clinic or from our Pain and Symptom Control Group. All patients are treated following the usual standard procedures for the treatment of cancer pain. All patients were receiving a narcotic analgesics and had access to rescue doses for breakthrough pain.

The variable with the highest correlation for poor pain control was development of rapid tolerance. This group presumably includes people, who for unknown reasons, had an as yet unexplained aberrant physiological response to narcotics or had an undiagnosed pain syndrome less responsive to narcotics. Other correlates for poor pain control included patients who were rated to have psychological distress, neuropathic pain, and those with impaired cognitive function. Previous opioid exposure, incident pain, or a history of drug dependence had a lower correlation with poor pain control but the subset numbers were small.

The purpose of this study was to identify a population of patients who do poorly with the best available therapy and to develop a system for accurately communicating pain research results to other colleagues. We are currently attempting to refine the system with input from several other groups. Ultimately we hope that a common "lingua franca" will emerge which will enable us to interpret our literature and facilitate the conduct of large interdisciplinary trials.

Anti-Cancer Intervention for Symptom Relief

A risk arising from the existence of "two solitudes" relates to the possibility that on either side of the hospice–cancer centre interface, patients may not have full access to the full range of therapies which may alleviate their suffering. The misunderstanding of the use of opiates in acute care hospitals has been well documented [7]. Less clearly delineated is the count of patients enrolled in hospice programmes who could have responded to, but did not receive, palliative radiation therapy, palliative chemotherapy, or preventive surgical procedures.

The role of radiation therapy in the management of localized distressing symptoms is well established. Less clearly established is the concept of palliative chemotherapy for pain and symptom relief in the absence of measurable objective remission. Certainly, symptom control is enhanced in patients with advanced cancer if they have an objective remission to chemotherapy [8]. It is less apparent whether these agents improve pain control in the absence of measurable tumour regression. Regardless of its effects on the tumour, as chemotherapy has a profound inhibitory effect on host lymphocytes and granulocytes, and on the products of these cells, it is theoretically possible that they could produce analgesia through modification of the milieu surrounding tumour tissue. For example, non-steroidal anti-inflammatory drugs are believed to act primarily at the periphery through the inhibition of prostaglandins. Prostaglandin synthesis is, in turn, stimulated by a lymphokine, interleukin 1. Methotrexate, a drug commonly used by rheumatologists to control inflammatory pain, has a profound inhibitory effect on interleukin 1. At the present time, methotrexate has not been studied as an analgesic agent in cancer patients.

Alkylating agents have been reported to have analgesic properties when used in regional infusion protocols. Some of the earliest trials of chemotherapy involved the administration of high-dose cytotoxic agents to specific regions of the body. Some of these studies reported the occurrence of pain relief without tumour remission. As alkylating agents and other chemotherapeutic agents cause demyelination and axis cylinder fragmentation, it is possible that modification of peripheral nerve function by cytotoxic drugs can influence transmission of sensory stimuli [9].

Recently, medical oncologists have been studying diphosphonates which may have a role in actually preventing the development of pain in patients with bone metastasis. Metastatic tumours invading bone advance through a process involving reabsorption of normal bone adjacent to the tumour. Activation of osteoclasts by multiple tumour- or host-produced factors is a likely mechanism of bone resorption with metastatic bone tumours. Diphosphonates have a direct inhibitory effect on osteoclast function and also may act through interfering with osteoclast contact with bone.

A number of diphosphonates have demonstrated benefit in the treatment of Paget's disease and the hypercalcaemia of malignancy. A recent open-label trial concluded that the oral use of one of these agents produced a significant decrease in bone pain and pathologic fractures in the treatment group which consisted of a group of women with metastatic breast cancer [10]. It remains to be determined whether these agents are effective in other cancers metastasizing to bone or whether their efficacy can be proven in large multi-institution double-blind trials.

The cachexia–anorexia syndrome is the most common untreatable symptom complex in advanced cancer. Medical oncologists have recently delineated the role of corticosteroids in the treatment of this syndrome [10] and have documented that progestational agents can serve as powerful appetite stimulants [11, 12].

These studies are examples of potentially important therapeutic advances dependent upon involvement of large volumes of patients within cancer centres, using clinical research techniques commonly used by oncologists. Clinical research is difficult to conduct at the end of life. For both humane and scientific reasons, access to patients at an early time in their trajectory of illness is important. This can only be achieved if cancer centres and palliative care programmes are integrated, or if cancer centres develop strong internal palliative medicine groups.

Palliative Medicine: The Fourth Phase of Preventive Oncology

As we approach the end of the twentieth century, numerous countries are engaged in a review of their cancer control programmes for the year 2000. Cancer centres have stressed the importance of primary prevention, early diagnosis (secondary prevention) and the treatment of invasive cancer once established (the tertiary phase of cancer prevention). It is reasonable to think of prevention of suffering as a fourth phase of cancer prevention and to provide it with a priority within cancer centre planning. Its priority ranking should be reflected in improved funding for care of advanced cancer patients, the development of palliative care teams within cancer centres, and increased emphasis on research relevant to palliative medicine. Cancer centres accept the need for subspecialty development in endocrinology, neurology, and other fields of oncology; it is therefore eminently reasonable that special groups concerned with the management of patients with advanced disease should be formed in cancer centres.

As in other areas of cancer control, prevention of a problem is preferable to reaction to an established problem. Evidence exists that the principles of palliative care (including giving psychosocial support), if applied early in the course of illness, in conjunction with anti-cancer treatment, will result in improvement in patient symptoms and possibly even survival [12]. The prevention of suffering is a principal tenet of the palliative care movement and should be viewed as the fourth phase of cancer prevention. Ideally, palliative care is an exercise in forward planning and not a model of crisis intervention. This view is admirably reflected in the World Health Organization Cancer Program, which assigns a high priority to the alleviation of cancer pain throughout the world. The plan emphasizes pain prevention in contrast to continuous reaction to the presence of distress.

While progress has been made in the management of cancer pain, many questions remain to be addressed, particularly in reference to the study of the asthenia–anorexia–cachexia syndromes. The increasing integration of palliative care programmes in cancer centres with their fundamental emphasis on research and large patient volume will provide an intellectual stimulus for palliative care. For example, the components of tumour biology which result in some patients developing pain and not others, and give rise to the profound loss of weight and asthenia which are now the most devastating symptoms of patients with advanced cancer, have not been studied in an integrated fashion by any group. The benefits of integrating the activities of basic science studies with clinical colleagues have been demonstrated in other fields of cancer research. A similar approach is advocated for research on pain, anorexia–cachexia, and other physical and psychological problems poorly addressed with current therapies.

Advances are dependent on the willingness of cancer centres to consider a redistribution of financial resources and to base their decisions on ethical considerations in addition to the financial concerns which can dominate health planning. While great strides have been made towards balancing the care–cure equation, the next step is dependent upon the dissolution of the "two solitudes" which split the palliative care movement and cancer centres apart from each other, and the consequent full integration of responsibility for the study and care of patients with advanced cancer into the cancer centre organizational pattern.

References

1. MacDonald N (1989) The role of medical oncology in cancer pain control. In: Hill Jr CS, Fields WS (eds) Advances in pain research and therapy. Raven, New York, pp 123–130
2. Kennedy BJ (1990) Medical oncology: the past, present and future. Ann R Coll Phys Surg Can 23: 39–44
3. MacDonald N (1984) The hospice movement: an oncologist's viewpoint. Ca-A cancer J clin 34: 179–82
4. MacDonald N, Bruera E (1990) Clinical trials in cancer pain research. In: Foley KM et al. (eds) Advances in pain research and therapy, vol 16. Raven, New York, pp 443–449
5. Levine M, Sackett D (1986) Heroin vs morphine for cancer pain. Arch Intern Med 146: 353–356
6. Bruera E, MacMillan K, Hanson J, Macdonald N (1989) The Edmonton staging system for cancer pain: preliminary report. Pain 37: 203–209
7. Marks R, Sachar F (1973) Undertreatment of medical inpatients with narcotic analgesics. Ann Intern Med 78: 173–181
8. Osoba D, Rusthoven J, Turnbull K et al. (1985) Combination chemotherapy with bleomycin, etoposide, and cis-platin in metastatic non-small cell lung cancer. J Clin Oncol 5: 1470–1485
9. MacDonald N (1990) The role of medical and surgical oncology in the management of cancer pain. In: Foley KM (ed) Advances in pain research and therapy, vol 16. Raven, New York
10. Vanholten Verzantvootat TA, Bijvoton OLM, et al. (1987) Reduced morbidity from skeletal metastases in breast cancer patients in long-term biphosphonate (ADP) treatment. Lancet II: 983–985
11. Bruera E, MacMillan K, Hanson J, MacDonald N (1989) A double-blind trial of megestrol acetate (MA) on appetite (A), caloric intake (CI), nutritional status (NS) and other symptoms in patients (PTS) with advanced cancer. ASCO Annual Meeting, May 21–23
12. Spiegel D, Blume JR et al. (1989) Effects of psychosocial treatment on survival of patients with metastatic breast cancer. Lancet ii: 888–891

Optimizing Palliative Nursing Skills by Education

J. Webber

Cancer Relief Macmillan Fund, 114 Kingsley Road,
Maidstone, Kent ME15 7UP, United Kingdom

Over the last 20 years there has been an increasing emphasis on the role of education in preparing health care professionals to work in the field of palliative care. As a result, a huge variety of educational initiatives have come into being. For example, it is estimated that in the United States alone, more than 10 000 courses and seminars are held every year in relation to dying and death (Eddy and Alles 1983). Similarly a recent study in the United Kingdom revealed that all schools and colleges of nursing now include teaching on palliative care in basic and continuing education programmes (RCN, in press).

Despite this growing emphasis however, the value of educational programmes about palliative care is still largely unknown, as very few initiatives have been described and even fewer systematically evaluated.

Of studies which have been carried out, most have focused on the effects of education on attitudes towards death, and death-related anxiety (Murphy 1986). Results however, are unclear. Although some studies have demonstrated a reduction in death anxiety, or an improvement in attitudes towards death (Caty and Tamlyn 1984), others have shown no such effect (Yarber et al. 1981), or have had equivocal results (Lev 1986). In addition, little work has been done to determine what effect death-related anxiety in the carer has on the care delivered to the patient. It is therefore by no means clear that a reduction in death anxiety is a useful educational goal.

A few studies have looked at other educational outcomes, including the development of communication skills (McGuire 1988) and the capacity of the nurse to manage stress and personal feelings (Conboy-Hill 1986). One area where the effects of education have been clearly demonstrated is that of expansion of the knowledge base (Llewelyn and Fielding 1988). Although it can be argued that knowledge alone is insufficient to engender positive attitudes towards the care of dying patients, it has been demonstrated in at least one study that nursing students perceived themselves to be more at ease with dying patients after their knowledge base had been expanded (Wagner 1964). It is also undoubtedly true that *lack* of knowledge will not contribute to positive attitudes.

A review of the literature indicates that few, if any, researchers have focused specifically on the impact of education on problems which nurses themselves identify when entering courses about palliative care. As a nurse educator, I firmly believe that, if they are to be successful, educational activities must begin by addressing the perceived problems and needs of the student in relation to the tasks for which he or she is being prepared. In this paper therefore, I would like briefly to describe the results of a study which I undertook to evaluate the outcomes and effectiveness of a short course for nurses caring for patients with advanced cancer. By doing this I hope to demonstrate that palliative nursing skills can be enhanced through education.

Aims of the Research

The study addressed the following two questions:

1. What are the problems which nurses encounter when caring for patients with advanced cancer?
2. Are these problems capable of modification by means of an educational intervention specifically designed to address the needs of nurses working in this field?

The course was of 10 days' duration and was attended by 25 nurses of various ages and experience, working in community or institutional settings. Two thirds operated in, or from, a specialist cancer or palliative care centre and the remainder in non-specialist settings. The evaluation was designed to assess the effects of the course over a period of 1 year.

Using questionnaires, interviews and critical incident analysis, the nurses' problems, satisfactions and coping strategies when caring for patients with advanced cancer were elicited immediately prior to, 6 months after, and then 1 year after the course. The results were analysed under a number of headings and overt and covert themes were identified. This enabled a comparison to be made between pre- and post-course themes. During the remainder of this paper I would like to describe and discuss some of these.

Pre-course Themes

In the pre-course phase of the study, two major themes emerged: the need to identify "solutions", and the need to maintain control.

The Need to Identify "Solutions"

This theme related to the need of the nurse to feel that a patient's situation was in some way improving and moving towards a good outcome. It had two main components:

1. *Solving problems*. The nurse needed to believe that he or she was solving problems for patients and families and in some way resolving difficulties. If this was not possible then frustration and anger arose. Two areas were viewed as particularly important in this connection: the ability to control pain and symptoms, and the skills to solve relationship problems within families.

2. *Seeing patients get better*. Even though most of the nurses were working in settings dedicated to the care of terminally ill patients, visible deterioration in physical status created problems. Once physical improvement as a goal of care was recognised as non-viable, many nurses were unable to identify their professional role.

For example, one nurse commented: "I worry about not having any answers for them (i.e. patients and families). I mean what really can you do when someone isn't going to get better? At times I find myself literally at a loss for words or actions. I can't see what is appropriate to plan for in their care and I just don't seem to have a goal."

It seems that, despite the development of models for nursing with goals oriented towards care and adaptation rather than cure, our move away from the traditional cure-oriented medical model is still not complete. I believe this needs to be taken very seriously. Baider and Porath (1981) found that if a nurse cannot realise her professional goals whilst caring for terminally ill cancer patients, then frustration, anger and malaise manifest themselves, and ultimately the nurse will develop an attitude of submission to routine and resigned indifference.

The Need to Maintain Control

The second theme which emerged from the pre-course data concerned the need to maintain control over specific situations: conversations, the expression of emotions, and the manner of a patient's dying.

1. *Conversations*. Many nurses described how they deliberately kept conversations with patients at a superficial level, to preclude the possibility of being asked difficult questions. For example, one commented: "If patients try to talk to me about the future or their feelings I just pass it off, otherwise I don't know where it might lead. I'm constantly worried in case I get out of my depth."

2. *Expression of patients' and families' emotions*. If patients are facing death, it seems reasonable that they may express sadness, anxiety or anger. To the nurse, however, this poses a threat to the sense of control which is so crucial. Almost two thirds of the sample in the study described the possibility of patients or relatives "getting upset" as a major problem.

3. *The manner of a patient's dying*. Thirdly, there was a need to maintain control over the manner of a patient's dying. For many of the nurses in the study, the way in which a patient handled the dying process was crucial and was used as a criterion against which to measure the quality of the care which he or she

provided. At least three elements appeared to be essential if a death was to be labelled "good".

Firstly, good quality of life immediately prior to death had to be apparent. If it was perceived as absent, many nurses became anxious, depressed and angry.

Secondly, communication within the family had to be harmonious, open and effective. As one nurse explained: "If there are problems of relationships between patients and families, I feel very stressed. I feel there is no way of making the death peaceful or dignified if they can't all share together."

Thirdly, death had to be accepted by the patient and family. This was the element which, if absent, generated the most anxiety, and well over two thirds of the nurses identified this as their major problem. One summed up the views of most in the following comment: "I feel worried and upset when the patient won't accept his death. It means you can't make it peaceful for him and it upsets the family and the staff. I just don't know how to get them to accept the inevitable. It's a real problem to me."

These then were the two major themes which emerged strongly from the pre-course data.

Post-course Themes

In order to demonstrate the benefits derived from the educational intervention I would now like to contrast the pre-course themes with those which emerged 6 months after and 1 year after the course.

It was noteworthy that very few of the problems identified before the course were mentioned at this later stage and, consequently, when it was analysed the data revealed no major negative themes. Instead two positive themes and one potentially positive theme emerged.

Confidence and Empowerment

The first theme was one of an increased sense of confidence and empowerment in the work situation and, in particular, a recognition of the ability of the nurse to influence events and improve the quality of care offered to patients. There was also evidence of a greater capacity to tolerate unsatisfactory outcomes and handle the expression of strong emotions. Indeed, several nurses described situations where, for the first time ever, they had allowed patients to control conversations and ask difficult questions. Describing such an incident, one nurse concluded: "Before the course I would not have thought of letting the conversation get so deep. But I had confidence to believe I could handle that awful situation and bring something to it. It gave me a tremendous sense of satisfaction." Most marked of all within this area was the emergence of confidence and enhanced ability to identify professional goals for patients, even when it was recognised that their physical condition was deteriorating.

Self-Awareness and Self-Acceptance

Analysis also revealed that the nurses had developed more insight into their own personal needs and motivations, and that this was of particular importance to them when dealing with patients' questions concerning diagnosis and prognosis. Several nurses described incidents where they had recognised that their own anxiety, rather than the needs of the patient, was the factor influencing the use of avoidance and blocking strategies in conversations. This self-knowledge enabled them to contain their own anxieties in order to meet the needs of the patients. There was also a greater acceptance of personal limitations and less internal pressure to solve every problem for every patient and family. Similarly, patients' expressions of anger or depression were less likely to be viewed as an indication of personal failure. This was well expressed by one who concluded the description of a difficult interview with a very angry patient and distressed family by commenting: "I came out of the room and I just sat down and thought back to the things we'd talked about on the course. That we're only human, not perfect, and can only do our best. I realised I couldn't make everything okay for him and I couldn't blame myself because I'd come up against a problem that couldn't be put right for the family."

Another nurse looking back over the year following the course, commented: "Mostly, I think it has made me much more aware of my feelings and beliefs and helped to see that although I'm a nurse, I am also a person; and sometimes being a person seems more important than being a nurse."

It seems that greater self-awareness enabled the nurses to be more comfortable with their humanity.

Patient Advocacy

A cluster of problems which had scarcely emerged in the pre-course phase of the study, became an important theme at this stage. They concerned the rights of patients, and focused particularly on the need for early and appropriate referrals to specialist services, the importance of true "informed consent", and anger over the misuse of anti-cancer treatment in the terminal phase of the disease. It seems that by raising awareness, the course, although reducing many problems, actually created a small number of new ones. However, these were definitely "positive" problems.

Conclusion

By comparing the major themes which emerged from the pre- and post-course data collection in this study, I hope I have been able to demonstrate that the skills and knowledge which enhance the care of patients with advanced cancer can be developed and improved through education. However, there is much that could be of assistance in planning effective educational programmes in this field, which we still do not know. For example, which teaching methods are most effective and what content areas are most appropriate? What is the optimal length for courses and how should they be structured? Should they be theory-based, practice-based, or a mixture of both? Most important of all, do the beneficial effects of education in palliative care remain stable over time? These are all questions to which we have no clear answers.

Most nurses acknowledge the importance of education in improving palliative care, and this is clearly good. However, true commitment to education must go further than simply planning or participating in courses. If this highly effective tool is to be maximised to the full, then our commitment must be extended to research into the effects of education.

We have made a start on this, but much remains to be done. Only when we have done it, will we be able to echo the title of this paper and truly speak with confidence of the *optimisation of palliative nursing skills through education*.

References

Baider L, Porath S (1981) Uncovering far: group experience of nurses in a cancer ward. Int J Nurs Stud 18: 47–52

Caty S, Tamlyn D (1984) Positive efforts of education on nursing students' attitudes towards death and dying. Nurs Papers 16: 41–52

Conboy-Hill S (1986) Terminal care: their death in your hands. Professional Nurse 2 (2): 51–53

Eddy J, Alles W (1983) Death Education. Mosby, Toronto

Lev EL (1986) Effects of course in hospice nursing: attitudes and behaviours of baccalaureate school of nursing undergraduates and graduates. Psychol Rep 59: 847–858

Llewelyn S, Fielding G (1988) Am I dying, nurse? Nurs Mirror 20: 30–31

McGuire P (1988) The stress of communicating with seriously ill patients. Nursing: 32

Murphy P (1986) Reduction in nurses' death anxiety following a death awareness workshop. J Cont Ed: 12 (4)

Royal College of Nursing (1990) A report of the Working Party of the R.C.N. Palliative Nursing Forum. (in press)

Wagner B (1964) Teaching students to work with the dying. Am Nurs J 64: 1281–1310

Yarber W, Gobel P, Rublee D (1981) Effects of death education on nursing students anxiety and locus of control. J Sch Health 51: 367–372

Education and Palliative Care: A Different Approach

J.F. Forbes[1] and D. Allbrook[2]

[1]Department of Surgical Oncology, University of Newcastle, Newcastle Mater
  Misericordiae Hospital, Wararah, NSW 2298, Australia
[2]Department of Palliative Care, University of Newcastle,
  Newcastle Mater Misericordiae Hospital, Wararah, NSW 2298, Australia

Education in palliative care for both undergraduates and graduates requires emphasis on special areas. Not only is it important to impart new knowledge and factual data, as for most other disciplines, it is in addition essential to focus on efficient communication, management of poor prognosis patients, and the involvement of a community-based team for optimal care. Education must also involve input from key paramedical staff who have crucial roles in patient care.

The Medical Faculty at the University of Newcastle embraces important innovations in its undergraduate teaching programme which are pursued throughout the course for all disciplines, including oncology in general and palliative care in particular. These innovations are considered first with a description of the Medical School and then in application to teaching palliative care. The use of community practitioners for teaching is a particular feature of the Medical Faculty, which we believe allows a unique contribution to palliative care education for both undergraduates and practising doctors.

Medical Education in Australia

Australia has ten medical schools, the oldest, at the Universities of Melbourne, Sydney and Adelaide, having been established in the nineteenth century. Newcastle, the youngest, had its first student intake in March 1978. The older schools have used a traditional course structure, with emphasis on pre-clinical basic science teaching and subsequent clinical teaching based in university teaching hospitals. Although these older schools have had reviews of course structure, the basic format remains.

Entry to medical schools is restricted and is largely based on academic performance – students must gain marks in the top 1%–2% of their State to be considered. A small number gain entry under special criteria. Most courses are of 6 years' duration after secondary school, and most students are about 18 years old at entry and 24 years old at graduation. About 50% of graduates are women.

Recent Results in Cancer Research, Vol. 121
© Springer-Verlag Berlin · Heidelberg 1991

In 1986 1350 students graduated from the ten schools (the Australian population is about 16 million). Graduates must complete a compulsory pre-registration intern year.

Newcastle Medical School

The Newcastle Medical School was established to provide a different approach. The Foundation Dean of the Faculty, Professor David Maddison, ensured that this occurred at every level of education, and his successor Professor John Hamilton has continued this.

Student Entry

The School is one of three in the State of New South Wales and offers 64 places each year. Because of concern that academic ability alone may not guarantee the skills needed by a doctor, an alternative admission system was developed. This has two entry streams – one a demanding academic stream and the other less demanding academically. Entry to both is based on academic achievements, aptitude testing and structured interviews.

Academic Stream

Students are admitted according to their academic performance and usually must be in the top 1%–2% at their final secondary school examinations (Higher School Certificate, HSC). They must still complete their aptitude test and interview. There are no special subject pre-requisites.

Alternative Stream

Students must be in the top 10% in their HSC or have a credit average at alternative tertiary studies. They may be aged up to their mid to late 30s. They complete the same aptitude test as the academic stream and go through the same interview process. In addition, a fixed number of places are allocated for Aboriginal students.

Interview Process

An objective structured interview has been refined over several years to aid selection. By the end of 1986, 1600 applicants had been interviewed from 13 000 applicants and 584 were admitted to the course. The interview has been shown to be an independent predictor of student's ability to complete the course and their ability to gain honours (Powis et al. 1988).

Table 1. Characteristics assessed at interview

---

1. Compatibility with the innovative style of studies at the University.[a]
2. Perseverance: the ability to persist in the face of setbacks and frustration.
3. Tolerance of ambiguity: acceptance of the reality that decisions and actions may be necessary in the face of uncertainty.
4. Supportiveness: the ability to lend strength to others under pressure or in time of need, or both.
5. Motivation: personal realistic desire to become a doctor.
6. Self-confidence: ability to communicate with others without excessive shyness or diffidence and to formulate views and communicate them clearly.

Note: Characteristics 1–5 are rated on a "best" to "worst" scale, five points, and characteristic 6 is assessed overall.
[a] Engel CE, Clarke RM. (1979) Medical education with a difference. Programmed Learning and Educational Technology 16: 70–87.

The interview is conducted by two people – one Faculty member and one non-Faculty member of the community. Students are initially scored independently by each interviewer, and a final score is then jointly agreed and assigned. It is unusual for interviewers to disagree markedly.

The interview assesses six characteristics in the student (Table 1). The list of qualities sought was developed after wide discussion at the outset and is comparable to that of Ben Gurion University of the Negev at Beer Sheva, Israel (Powis et al. 1988). The interview lasts about 45 minutes.

The interview at entry level aims to identify motivated and capable students who might otherwise be denied entry into Medical School. We believe it also addresses characteristics likely to be of particular importance in a caring doctor who will be able to contribute within palliative care. Interviewers receive training and instructions designed to aid them in interviewing efficiently. Candidates are made to feel that the Faculty is genuinely concerned about their personal views and feelings. In addition, an atmosphere is aimed for which is friendly, which allows focus on candidates' views and feelings, and which ensures that discussion topics are adequately covered.

The process is discussed in detail by Powis et al. (1988), who have reported a high level of agreement between assessors.

Undergraduate Teaching

Students complete a 5-year course which integrates basic science and clinical teaching from the outset. The full-time academic staff (about 50) are supported by more than 500 local practitioners, allowing integration of teaching with the community's medical services throughout the entire course. Close links are also maintained with the regional Department of Health. There is no separation into

Table 2. Undergraduate curriculum: education objectives (Domains) for all facets including palliative care

Domain I:	Professional Skills
	Skills necessary to practice medicine, including history taking and clinical examination.
Domain II:	Critical Reasoning
	The ability to gather information and analyse, interpret and evaluate it. The application of scientific method to clinical practice.
Domain III:	Identification, Prevention and Management of Illness
	An understanding of health, normal mechanisms of the pathophysiology of disease and its manifestations, the principles of investigation and management of disease and the principles of health promotion and maintenance.
Domain IV:	Population Medicine
	The application of the principles and practice of individual medicine to the community and to the population; and an understanding of the incidence and prevalence of disease and the organisation and efficiency of health care delivery.
Domain V:	Self-Directed Learning
	The ability to take responsibility for evaluating one's own performance, implementing one's own education and contributing to the education of others.

Note: All aspects of communication skills are considered throughout the course.

pre-clinical and clinical components as in other Australian Medical Schools. Students take part in small group problem-solving sessions from their 1st year and consider both real and simulated clinical problems. The aim is to focus not just on the biological and conventional medical aspects of disease, but to also explore social and psychological aspects of health and disease. This is particularly important for palliative care.

Particular attention is given to work in small tutorial groups with a tutor as a guide rather than an expert. to encourage students to learn problem solving for themselves.

The 5 years of the course have discrete blocks each year. Throughout all years, however, attention is given to five particular areas of learning, or Domains (Table 2), that we believe are important for the graduate, and of particular relevance to palliative care education.

Palliative Care Education in Newcastle

Undergraduate Education

Cancer services in the Hunter Valley in New South Wales are based at the Newcastle Mater Misericordiae Hospital, where The Mater Oncology Centre, one of three Comprehensive Cancer Centres for the State, is located. This Centre has separate departments for Surgical, Medical and Radiation Oncology, as well as Cancer Education, Pharmacy, Cancer Research, Biological Therapy and Palliative Care.

Students from the Medical Faculty receive oncology teaching throughout their 5-year course and are all attached full time to the Oncology Centre for $3\frac{1}{2}$ weeks during their 5th (final) year, with students attending in groups of four to six at a time. During this time they are exposed to all components of oncology care.

Undergraduate Palliative Care teaching is focused on this full time attachment and is structured so as to be integrated with the teaching of other components of oncology and to highlight the principles on which the Medical School is based. Students are instructed in the philosophy of the Department and follow a planned programme.

During their 1st week, students meet staff of the Department and learn more of the scope of palliative care services. They receive a copy of the Department's Symptom Control Guide and the importance of developing special skills (Domain I) in symptom control is emphasized. A selected bibliography is also provided, and the session is completed with a video on basic principles of pain control in advanced cancer. Emphasis is given to the importance of a team approach, integrating palliative care into overall care, and the role of the community medical resources in delivering palliative care.

For the 2nd week, students visit a patient's home with a nurse or become involved with ward visits, after which an in-depth discussion is held on the patient concerned, with the emphasis on the uniqueness of the person and on the social unit and the observed roles of all the people encountered. The students discuss the role that they would play if they were the family general practioner and are encouraged to organise their thoughts in a detailed plan prior to discussion. This allows application of the teaching Domain principles, in particular the Critical Reasoning Skills (Domain II) and Population Medicine (organisation and efficacy of health care delivery, Domain IV).

The 3rd week in Palliative Care allows for a follow-up visit to the student's patient, with emphasis on assessment of quality of life and changes in this for the patient. Particular attention is paid to ways of measuring quality of life and the many aspects of medical illness, social unit and, particularly, therapy that can affect it. This focus extends the traditional teaching on Management of Illness (Domain III) and encourages students to broaden their perspective and understanding of all disease management to embrace the principles important to palliative care.

Students take part in the regular review of patients under care in the Department, and can attend the weekly Department meetings and observe the workings of an interprofessional team. Professional Skills (Domain I) are enhanced by having students integrated into the Department's activities. The demands of history taking and the physical examination needed to provide palliative care can be demonstrated.

Throughout the students' attachment, Self-Directed Learning (Domain V) is fostered. Students can work through parts of the bibliography provided, and they have access to Department papers, journals, tapes (audio and visual) and selected reprints. Staff are available for discussion of material that students choose to pursue.

Students may elect in-depth studies at selected intervals during the curriculum. For example, in the final year students may elect a 5-week research and in-depth clinical experience in palliative care and prepare this for publication or presentation to Faculty.

As students are concurrently involved with other Departments within the Oncology Centre, there are many opportunities to consider the unique and overlapping roles of different disciplines within the area of oncology. They can observe the limitations of each, as discussed by staff, and also the unique features of, e.g., Surgery and Medical Oncology, and the Dietitian's and Social Worker's roles. An appreciation of the importance of each person's understanding the role of others is stressed: the surgical oncologist must appreciate and provide palliative care for most patients, often from the time of first contact, but is not always well trained in care of the dying and grief management; the palliative care specialist has an awareness of the important palliative role of surgery for many patients, but does not operate (Forbes 1988).

Of course, the students are also exposed to a considerable degree to the personal philosophy of the teacher (Allbrook 1983, 1989, 1990a, 1990b; Forbes 1988). This is "superimposed" on 4 years of education with emphasis on Critical Reasoning Skills (Domain II), so we have some confidence that unreasonable, inappropriate or irrelevant personal philosophies will be rejected.

Communication

All areas of medical practice rely on efficient communication for their success, and palliative care is no exception. During the Palliative Care and Surgical Oncology part of the course we pursue the Faculty's emphasis on communication skills both verbal (writtern and oral) and non-verbal.

Students are provided withguidelines, and examples from these are highlighted as they occur during the Oncology course block. The problems and disadvantages of poor communication, the need for conveying reassurance at times of uncertainty, and practicing this as well as stating it by non-verbal means, are stressed. The methods for constructively using non-verbal communication are considered, including frequency of visits, use of a patient's name, eye contact, physical contact (hand shaking), introduction of oneself, physical positioning with a patient, types and sequences of questions that reflect attitude as well as factual enquiry, examination style and sequence, and listening ability.

The verbal communication skills that are discussed do not differ from those taught throughout the course, but, as in many other disciplines (e.g., Geriatrics and Paediatrics), their importance is highlighted in Palliative Care. The stress of illness, the diagnosis of cancer, stressful and often complex therapies and exposure to a large number of medical and paramedical staff all demand that verbal communication be understanding, kindly and efficient. When the prospect of terminal illness and new fears are added, the special demands placed on verbal communication are acute. Tragic despair and anxiety may be only a "simple misunderstanding" away. Opportunities to mislead are widespread. We believe that attention to training in communication skills is essential to produce a capable doctor. It is also essential for the provision of palliative care – for the patient and the members of the social unit. Efficient communication also forms the foundation of a capable, confident and efficient team of people.

Student Guidelines for Verbal Communication

Guidelines are provided for all students and are illustrated by practical examples throughout the course block. They include the following:

- The doctor's responsibility is to "nudge" the patient in the direction of reality, but never to force him.
- Always endeavour to explain the reasons for the patient's symptoms.
- "Listen before you leap" is a useful guiding principle, especially in the later stages of the patient's illness.
- It is often necessary to give the patient permission to talk. "Are you worried about yourself?" "How is your family affected by your illness?"
- Generally, patients who want to know more about their condition will ask, if given the opportunity.
- Generally, patients who do not want to know will not ask.
- Truth has a broad spectrum with gentleness at one end and harshness at the other. Patients always prefer gentle truth.
- Euphemism is legitimate if used to express truth gently; it is wrong if used to deceive.
- The doctor–patient relationship is founded on trust. It is fostered by honesty but poisoned by deceit.
- It is always wrong to lie. Lord Justice Denning's (1959) judgement that "there is something wrong with a morality which proclaims that it is right to tell a lie even in a good cause" is apposite.
- The aim is to make dying a little easier, not to apply the dogma of always divulging the truth". (Hinton 1967)
- Do not compromise the doctor–patient relationship by making unwise (and unethical) promises to the relatives.

Postgraduate Education

The Medical School benefits from extensive teaching involvement by community doctors, including general practitioners and specialists in many disciplines. Throughout the course students have opportunities to continue their education within the medical practice of these doctors. This is not just encouraged, it is an essential part of the teaching programme and ensures that the Newcastle medical graduate understands from personal experience how the Teaching Hospital is integrated into the community.

We also have integration of regional (Government) Department of Health resources with the Department of Palliative Care in the Hunter Oncology Centre. The palliative care service for the region has an Outreach Team with six contributing physicians and five palliative care nurses to provide a 24 h a day, 7 days a week service. The service also works with the Departments of Psychiatry and Anaesthesia.

The service has a community profile that is familiar to all doctors in the region, as individual patients' doctors are involved in the delivery of palliative care in discussion with and under the guidance of individual team members. This process allows the community practitioners to be aware of current treatment plans by regular and personal experience. The education process works because the practitioners are involved in management of their own patients.

Palliative care is regularly a subject of postgraduate education programmes, including hospital-based medical meetings and particular initiatives of the region's Postgraduate Medical Society. Consequently, there is an expectation by doctors that palliative care will form part of postgraduate education activities on an equal footing with other disciplines.

Conclusion

The Newcastle University Medical School has a commitment to training doctors not only in traditional skills and medical knowledge, but also in those additional areas that contribute to making a complete doctor – critical reasoning skills, population medicine, communication, and self-directed learning. The under-graduate course emphasises these throughout and integrates teaching with the delivery of medical services in the community. Education in palliative care highlights the course objectives. The aims are to produce a caring doctor, well informed in the requirements for palliative care, a high quality service for patients and the community, and integration of postgraduate education into regular medical activities.

References

Allbrook D (1983) Torture and the teaching of medical ethics. Med J Aust 2: 206–207
Allbrook D (1989) Cure versus care? Or is it all care? J Palliative Care 5 (3): 44–46
Allbrook D (1990a) Who owns palliative care? Med J Aust 4: 170–171
Allbrook D (1990b) Education in palliative care: ten years of innovative medical education. Newcastle NSW Faculty of Medicine, University of Newcastle. (in press)

Forbes JF (1988) Principles and potential of palliative surgery in patients with advanced cancer. In: Senn H, Schmid L (eds) Supportive care in cancer patients. Springer, Berlin Heidelberg New York, pp 134–142 (Recent results cancer res, vol 108)

Hinton J (1967) Dying. Penguin, Harmsworth

Powis DA, Neame RLB, Bristow T, Murphy LB (1988) The objective structured interview for medical student selection. Br Med J 296: 765–768

Palliative Care in German Hospice: The Medical and Psychological Concept of the Christophorus-Haus

T. Flöter

Christophorus-Haus, Roßmarkt 23, W-6000 Frankfurt 1, FRG

The Christophorus-Haus in Frankfurt was opened as a model project in 1988. This new facility offers additional medical and psychological assistance, care and support to chronically ill persons, in particular cancer patients. Every year more than 200 000 persons are affected by cancer, and roughly the same number die of this disease in the Federal Republic of Germany. About two thirds of the patients suffer from chronic pain once the illness has reached an advanced stage. The Christophorus-Haus focuses most of its attention on these persons.

The aim of the Christophorus-Haus is to comfort, strengthen and lend support to chronically ill people. As the Munich psychotherapist Almuth Sellschop put it, "The aim is not only to help people survive but above all to help them remain active in life".

The philosophy of the Christophorus-Haus focuses on outpatient treatment and support of the patients by our team and on nursing and care at home as well as on pain control, psychotherapy and social guidance. Other major tasks of the Christophorus-Haus are to accompany the patient on his way to death and assist the family during the period of mourning.

The idea of this institution was developed by Ingeborg and Jörg Harmsen with reference to the experience gained by English and American hospices, and put into practice with the collaboration of the Schmerztherapeutischen Kolloquium e.V., a registered association in Frankfurt with a membership of about 1500 doctors and psychologists. The work is carried out only on an outpatient basis with a small day-clinic. For medical and organisational reasons it will be necessary to add a small inpatient ward.

The medical and psychological programme is based on a holistic, psychosomatic view of disease which pays particular attention to the patient's social context. The programme concentrates on the patient himself and his quality of life. In addition to medical treatment by family doctors and oncologists, the Christophorus-Haus offers complementary medical and psychological assistance and care: medical guidance, pain control, psychological advice and therapy, home nursing, and social and pastoral support.

Recent Results in Cancer Research, Vol. 121
© Springer-Verlag Berlin · Heidelberg 1991

The objective of the Christophorus-Haus is to give all cancer patients and their families every possible kind of support, to build up hope, to help those suffering from cancer, and to strengthen their self-respect and confidence in their ability to help themselves. With doctors, nurses, psychologists, social and pastoral workers functioning as a team, the aim is to open up to patients the possibility of

- Being rehabilitated
- Speaking about their disease and related anxieties
- Living free of symptoms, especially free of pain
- Pursuing personal activities more
- Being nursed at home
- Being looked after at home when dying

The first phase (day clinic) of the Christophorus-Haus programme comprises four main activities:

1. Medical pain therapy, complementary medical guidance and support
2. Psychological pain therapy, psychological guidance, help in coping with stress and fear
3. Guidance on general daily living, nutrition, health training, family involvement
4. Day clinic and home nursing

A telephone information service is also available, and training seminars, advanced training and Balint groups are held for patients, family members, any interested persons and the staff of the Christophorus-Haus. Our medicopsychological, socio-ecological cancer help programme is regarded as complementary to, not as competition to, traditional medical treatment being given at the same time.

Pain therapy does not simply mean giving analgesics but has many other aspects. Drugs that are administered have to be taken regularly and in sufficient quantity, under constant medical supervision. As a rule, oral administration is better for cancer patients than injections. There are other methods of pain therapy, such as local anaesthesia, acupuncture, transcutaneous electrical nerve stimulation, hypnosis, psychotherapeutic methods to ease pain ("fakir" techniques), etc.

Nutrition plays a major role for patients with pain. Our nutritional programme is based on vegetarian wholemeal food on the model of the Bristol diet, i.e. apart from a sufficiency of vitamins, minerals and trace elements, the essential aspect of this diet is that the organism is supplied with as many vital substances from untreated, natural foodstuffs as possible, in order to activate and strengthen the defence mechanisms of the body.

Psychological methods, such as the Bochum health training described by Simonton (1978), are directed to exercising a positive outlook on life and developing a positive imagination, which will promote health and alleviate disease. For cancer as for other diseases, the great chance for rehabilitation lies in psychological stimulation of the immune system.

The difficulties of an hospice working in Germany can best be explained by giving a few figures. At present we employ 6 full-time nurses, 20 part-time nurses on call, 2 psychologists and 2 social workers. The Christophorus-Haus further works on a regular basis with 6 doctors and with 15 voluntary helpers, 1 pastoral adviser and two honorary managing directors. In our first year in action we cared for 59 patients at home; on a monthly basis this means 20–30 patients continuously. We had 40 cancer patients and 19 others. Of the 430 day clinic patients the majority (305) came for pain therapy. Forty patients came for psychotherapy, 25 for guidance on nutrition and 20 for visualization.

Other activities of the Christophorus-Haus have included producing information leaflets, poster campaigns, training seminars, congresses, charity bazaars, discussions for family members and Balint groups. The main components of our PR work have been individual and group visits, media activities and providing personal information to politicians and public figures. Despite the managing directors' personal financial commitment, despite the money reimbursed by the health insurance and despite the financing of doctors and psychologists, which is independent of the Christophorus-Haus, there is an annual shortfall of DM 250 000 for material and staff expenses for home care.

There are thus not only organisational reasons standing in the way of a broad hospice movement in Germany, but also simple financial reasons. The main trouble is that hospices have no defined place in German health care and it is nearly impossible to link out- and inpatient care. We hope that through the particular work we do in the Christophorus-Haus we have been able to point out the lack in our health care system so that this crucial gap can soon be closed.

Reference

Simonton C (1978) Wieder gesund werden. Rowohtt, Reinbek

Parental Death: A Preventive Intervention

G.H. Christ and K. Siegel

Department of Social Work, Memorial Sloan Kettering Center, 1275 York Avenue, New York, NY 10021, USA

Introduction

The loss of a parent during childhood is a profound psychological trauma which threatens a child's normal social and emotional development [1]. At Memorial Sloan-Kettering Cancer Center (MSKCC), a comprehensive cancer treatment and research center, parents turned to our staff for help in dealing with their own and their children's reactions to the presence of cancer in one of the parents. Our clinical experiences with these parents led us to hypothesize that the terminal stage and death of a parent contain the most stressful and traumatic experiences during the course of the disease [2]. In this presentation we will limit ourselves to a description of an ongoing study that specifically addresses the question: Can psychoeducational parent guidance intervention prevent or lessen the deleterious effects on children of the terminal stage and death of a parent from cancer?

Background

MSKCC is a 565-bed cancer treatment and research hospital located in the center of New York City. Approximately 7000 new patients are referred each year, 80% from New York and the greater metropolitan area, an additional 15% from the rest of the United States, and 5% from other countries.

The department of social work has 35 members who provide the majority of the psychosocial services for MSKCC patients and their families, and 12 members who are involved in psychosocial research. We provide two general classes of psychosocial services:

1. *Support services*, which range from finding affordable housing for patients and their families from outside New York City, arranging transportation to and from the hospital, arranging home care services for patients leaving the hospital or for those treated on an outpatient basis, and so on, to assisting with financial needs.

Recent Results in Cancer Research, Vol. 121
© Springer-Verlag Berlin Heidelberg 1991

2. *Counselling services*, which range from developing patient, family, and staff support groups, and providing counselling and therapeutic interventions to patients and their families, to developing post-treatment services for cancer survivors.

It was in the context of our counselling services that patients and/or their spouses asked our help with the reactions of their children. In collaboration with our research staff, we monitored the services we provided in response to these requests, developed training films for use with staff and parent groups, and tried a number of different interventions as part of a service delivery–exploratory hypothesis generating effort. We were interested in determining the efficacy of providing a service that might prevent future difficulties for both children and the surviving spouse.

Rationale for This Study

It has been documented that the loss of a parent [3, 4] and of a spouse have profound psychosocial effects. Especially with children, the long-term consequences of this experience may be quite severe. Over the years we have been impressed with the great differences in coping abilities of different families. We postulated that some coping strategies lead to better, others to worse outcomes as the children mature. The next logical step was to develop interventions that might improve the quality of the parental interaction with the children. In summary, the underlying goals of the study were:

1. To understand the process of normal and pathological mourning of children and adolescents
2. To understand the short- and long-term sequelae of parental loss
3. To determine whether a psychosocial intervention during the terminal stages of an illness and for a few months after the death might improve the short- and long-term adjustment of the surviving spouse and children

Our Rationale for Intervention

From our clinical experiences and a review of existing clinical and research literature, we elected to develop a psychoeducational intervention that utilizes a parent guidance model. We further chose to develop an intervention beginning about 6 months before the death and continuing for about 6 months after the death of the parent. The intervention is only being offered to intact families fluent in English, with children between the ages of 7 and 16. Of 200 families who agree to participate in the study, we are randomly selecting 100 to receive the intervention, and provide only the standard social work services to the other 100 control families. We plan to follow these families for a number of years to determine whether there are differences between these two groups at different stages of the children's development that could be attributed to differences in the work of mourning. We will now describe the rationale for each of the study decisions that were made.

We chose a psychoeducational intervention based on a parent guidance model because in our experience we had found that a great many of the parents needed information and were able to make excellent use of it. We are a society of highly mobile small nuclear families, where most young adults have no experience with death and dying, so that parents generally have no background experience in helping youngsters deal with early death of a parent. In addition, over the years we have become impressed with the resilience and emotional strength of many of the patients and their spouses. Characteristically, parents are able to generalize: i.e., given some information and possible solutions, the parents can apply these findings to many other appropriate situations. In short, our experience was that most of the parents dealt well with a guidance model where they were given information and instruction, and then used it well.

However, we were also aware that the information needed to be given within a therapeutic context that recognized and provided support for the parents' own distress. Their own grief and emotional reactions to the serious illness and loss of a young spouse at times presented barriers to optimal parenting. Therefore, the intervention has a therapeutic, supportive component. The integration of the educational and supportive components present a significant therapeutic challenge to the clinicians.

We chose to target the child primarily through work with the parents because of our experience with the mourning process of children. Unlike adults, children do not have a sustained mourning experience. They move in and out of memories and affects related to the mourning process. The relationship between mourning and difficulties in some aspects of daily living, like school work, concentration, etc., may not be as clear for a child as for an adult, and is often best dealt with at those moments when the child is willing and able to talk about some aspect of the illness experience. In addition, since the overwhelming feelings may come up weeks or months after the death of the parent, it is logical that a parent may be the only one available to help the child deal with the emerging feelings. Especially with younger children, we find it is often very difficult to try to recapture the mood, the affect, and the situation hours or days later, as would be necessary to deal with it in a weekly child guidance session.

The intervention begins about 6 months before the death of the parent and continues for about 6 months after it for several reasons. Our experience had been that the terminal stage of the parent's illness is one of the most stressful and difficult ones for the well parent. Decisions that may seriously affect the children in later years are made: for example, it is not uncommon for younger children to be sent away to stay with relatives. This is a potentially highly traumatic experience. Similarly, hospital visits during the last days or weeks of the illness can be important both for the patient and for the children. Lack of advance planning for the children's care following the death of the patient can result in threatening disorganization, insecurity, and emotional deprivation in the family for weeks after the death. The physical and/or emotional withdrawal of the family members from each other during the terminal stage lends itself to mistaken interpretations by children. They may blame themselves or the well parent for some of the difficult events.

Finally, we felt we needed to establish a relationship with the family while it was still intact in order to optimize our chances of successfully engaging the family members in the intervention. In several previous follow-up studies we conducted we found it was more difficult to engage families in an intervention after the death if they did not already have a strong tie with us and an experience of us as being helpful. When we made contact with a surviving parent after the death of the spouse, we sometimes heard "Why weren't you there sooner, when I really needed your help?"

It was not easy to get family referrals 6 months before the death of a parent! Oncologists rightly denied their ability to foresee events that closely. Some initially feared that we would divulge information to patients and their spouses prematurely. We were more successful when we changed the definition of our request for referral of families to: referral when the ill parent's recurrence is no longer responding to available treatments. We introduced ourselves to the families as interested in doing a study to determine if we could help parents care for their children during a serious recurrence of the cancer.

In both the pre- and the post-death period, the interventionist meets with the well parent alone for about six sessions, with each child alone once or twice (as needed for a comprehensive psychosocial assessment of the child's adjustment to events), and with the well parent and children together once to facilitate mutual support and open communication.

In the pre-death period, during the first two sessions with the well parent, the interventionist conducts an illness-specific assessment of the family, identifies major concerns, prioritizes objectives for her work with the family, and initiates the educational and supportive process. During the third and (if necessary) fourth sessions with the child, she conducts an assessment of the children's adaptation to the stresses of the illness and reports the findings to the well parent in the next session. Sessions five and six focus on reinforcing the generic principles of increasing parenting competence, facilitating open family communication about the illness, and fostering stability in the children's environment. The interventionist also clarifies family members' concern and suggests possible solutions. In the last two sessions the interventionist addresses the preparation of the family for the death of the ill parent. During each session there is time for discussion of the handling of the children and dealing with specific problems or questions. Age- and developmental stage-specific information is also shared with the parent.

The post-death sessions start 2–4 weeks after the death of the parent and continues for about 5 months following the loss. The sequence of sessions is similar to the pre-death sequence, except that most of the sessions are held in the home. The focus now includes more discussion about the mourning processes and the new integration of the family. The interventionist assesses the families' management of the actual death and their immediate reactions to the loss during the first two post-death sessions. The children are reassessed individually in the third session. In the fourth session the interventionist reports her findings on the children to the parent and arranges for a joint meeting with the parent and children together in session five. She assists the parent in coping with the areas of greatest concern in session six; this usually focuses on clarifying the nature of the grief process in both the parent and the children and helping them sustain themselves through it. The process of termination is begun in session seven and completed in session eight, along with plans for follow-up contact.

Preliminary Findings

We are in the first 2 years of a 5-year study and have not yet begun the systematic analysis of the data comparing those who did with those who did not receive an intervention. We have, however, been impressed with a number of findings we would like to share with you.

First, about two thirds of the families approached agree to participate in a study without knowing they may receive an intervention. Families have spontaneously described the sessions as helpful, including those families who were initially reluctant to participate. Mothers tend to be more emotionally involved and more knowledgeable about the children than fathers. Fathers tend to feel more secure about their ability to handle the emotional reactions of the children. Men seem much less able to handle the emotional impact of the loss of their spouse. Further, the impact of being a small isolated nuclear family brings practical problems to fathers who are left with young children – problems that often seem insurmountable. In summary, our clinical impression is that surviving fathers have a harder course to follow, and generally do not handle their own and their children's reactions as well as surviving mothers.

By far the largest majority of the children and adolescents welcome the opportunity to talk openly about their experiences, and find the intervention helpful. A small minority, primarily those youngsters who have strong feelings of anger and rage at both the surviving and the dead parent, initially resist our approaches. Most of the youngsters struggle with some variant of unrealistic feelings of blame for the illness and death of the parent. In general, the younger children are concerned with some of the practical issues of ongoing family function. With surviving fathers, this takes the form of concern about meal preparation, being taken to and from after-school activities, shopping, etc. With surviving mothers, this takes the form of struggling with the impact of financial changes, concerns about disruptions consequent upon moving to cheaper quarters, etc. The older youngsters are often more preoccupied about possibly being overwhelmed by taking on some of the responsibilities of the dead parent and providing emotional support to the surviving parent or younger siblings, and about being able to pursue longer range plans such as going on to college, etc. In general, the older youngsters appreciate the opportunity to discuss these types of concerns with the interventionist, because they often feel guilty discussing these "selfish" preoccupations with the surviving parent.

Summary

The untimely death of a spouse and parent is extraordinarily painful and difficult. Whether a brief intervention such as the one we are exploring is enough to make a significant difference in the mourning process and future optimum survival has yet to be seen. To date we are gratified that the immediate response of most of the surviving spouses and children is that the intervention is a helpful experience.

References

1. Osterweis M, Solomon F, Green M (eds) (1984) Bereavement: reactions, consequences and care. National Academy, Washington DC
2. Siegel K, Christ G, Mresago F (1990) A preventive program for bereaved children. Am J Orthopsychiatry.
3. Berlinsky E, Biller HA (1982) Parental death and psychological development. Heath, Lexington MA
4. Furman RA (1964) Death and the young child: some preliminary considerations. Psychoanalytic study of the child, vol 19. International University Press, New York, pp 321–333.

Optimising Beravement Outcome: Reading the Road Ahead

A. Couldrick

Sir Michael Sobell House, Churchill Hospital, Headington, Oxford OX3 7LJ, United Kingdom

"Mourning is not forgetting, it is an undoing. Every minute tie has to be untied and something permanent and valuable recovered and assimilated from the knot." (Allingham 1952).

How we mourn and how our mourning will be resolved, will depend on

How we perceive the loss
Our age
The age of the person dying
How prepared we were
Our inner strengths and outer resources
Our relationship with the person who died

In this paper I want to consider the significance of the time with the dying person, the last weeks, days and hours.

Robbins (1983) stresses that "a gentle passage from life to death can only be achieved in a large measure by relieving any distressing symptom of mind, body and spirit". Terminal care does not end with the death of the patient – whose suffering is over. The suffering of the family may be beginning. Thomas Mann said, "A man's dying is more the survivor's affair than his own". So what is a good death experience for the survivors?

Nimocks suggests that "Goodness can be defined in terms of the extent to which the interactants accept the impending death, receive mutual emotional care and spiritual support, mitigate the dying person's discomfort and isolation and complete unfinished business" (Nimocks et al. 1987) Parkes and Cameron (1983) draw our attention to the fact that, where the patient suffered uncontrolled pain, the key carer suffered from the memory of that pain long after the death. They also suggest that, when the death was unanticipated, the bereaved become preoccupied by remorse and guilt.

Parkes and Cameron wrote this in 1983, and yet, as recently as this year, a widow wrote bitterly to a British newspaper, disclosing how she and her dying

Recent Results in Cancer Research, Vol. 121
© Springer-Verlag Berlin · Heidelberg 1991

husband had been denied the opportunity to share the knowledge that he was dying. (Herzberg 1990). The staff, despite appeals for information, had urged the couple to believe that the treatment was arresting the disease, until 5 hours before the husband's death, when they finally admitted that it could not.

Unanticipated bereavement, with shock, anger and persistent illusions that the dead person will return, is hard to bear, but may be alleviated where the patient has cancer. There is a need for accurate information abut the situation, together with emotional support that allows time for the impending loss to be taken in and the changes anticipated and prepared for. Ideally, the patient can be similarly informed and supported, so that the whole family is on the same wavelength and mutual sharing is possible. It takes time to break bad news, it takes time to believe what you have been told, but it is possible for a person's psychological state to improve whilst his physical condition is deteriorating. Stedeford (1988) maintained that this preparation has a significant effect upon the carer who has to come to terms with the illness, the death, and life without that person.

Reading the Road Ahead

For the last 3 years we have been evaluating the bereavement support service at Sobell House. Up to 150 key carers – that is, those who were perceived by the hospice team to be the most significantly affected by the patient's death – have been interviewed at 13 and 20 months after the death, to explore the physical and emotional effects precipitated by the death and the level of support they had received. The bereaved who felt the illness and the dying was managed well seem to be saying this:

Control

There is a need for someone to be *in control*, that is, to contain the situation for both the patient and the family. Sarton, in her book *A Reckoning*, speaks of the nurse being "streetwise in death", and reminds us that each death that a family experiences is unique for them. They simply do not know what to expect. They are lost and afraid and need to feel that someone has experienced it before and can guide them.

Mrs O., whose husband David died aged 40 years, said in her interview 13 months after his death, "The last year of his illness and the days before his death had an enormously significant effect upon the way I have felt in this last year; we managed to say everything we wanted to one another. I knew that although he was very weak, he had little pain and there was always someone to turn to."

What else does control mean? – That the symptoms were not unexpected to the professional and mostly could be alleviated, and that the person who was dying could remain in control of their environment.

Care

The relatives also identified the importance of the *care* given by professionals, that is, that the standards of medical and nursing care were "good enough". This was one typical comment from a relative recalling the time before the death:

"I knew that we were cared for. The nurses came when they said they would. The doctors never gave up on her. She wasn't always without pain but I knew the staff never stopped trying to get it right."

In simple ways the road ahead may be read. Care includes anticipating problems such as incontinence and loss of mobility. Measures such as having to hand a mackintosh to protect the bed and a commode may seem simplistic, but incontinence may precipitate a crisis which may be the last straw for the carer.
   Relatives said:

"The nurse showed me how to transfer him from the bed to the commode without hurting him."
"She taught me how to massage my mother so that I never felt helpless when she cried because her back hurt."
"The nurse taught us how to change wet sheets with my husband still lying in the bed."

Even more importantly, the professionals need to prepare the family for the changes that may occur in the last few days or hours and be accessible to reassure or advise about:

Confusional states which often herald death
Restlessness, perspiring, colour changes
Exacerbation of pain which may be controlled quickly when the family have been taught how to adjust oral analgesia
Altered states of consciousness which bring home the reality of impending death
Alteration in breathing patterns which may be interpreted as signs of distress

The *route* of medication can be planned. How many patients are admitted to hospital hours before death because the appropriate medication is not available or simply because the family had no one to turn to? The patient becomes restless, the colour changes, the breathing seems distressed. Tragically, the dying person may find himself living his last hours in an ambulance on his way to die amongst strangers. I would suggest that this can be avoided by good communication.

Communication

Communication with the family is essential if the patient is also to share the responsibility for the management of his illness and his death. He must be given honest information from which he may make choices. He may choose to die in hospital, but he cannot make that choice if all around him conspire to exclude him (Glaser and Strauss 1965).

Mrs D., deeply jaundiced and within days of her death, was told by her family that she would recover. Desperately sad and lonely in her hidden fear that she was mortally ill, she eventually plucked up courage to ask the nurse, "Am I dying?"

The nurse knew how strongly the family felt that she should *not* know and simply held her hands, without replying. Mrs D. understood and they wept together, and then the nurse said "If you knew that you were dying, what would you like to do?"

She sent for her family and told them that she wanted to come home to die. She then discussed and planned with her husband and sister the future care of her 6-year-old daughter.

In bereavement her family feel that she had *control* over her life and death, that she helped them to *care* for her, and that she enabled them to *communicate* at the deepest level with her and amongst themselves. They are proud of her and of themselves because they achieved what she wanted. Yes, they are sad, they mourn her, but their mourning is not complicated by regret and guilt.

Lastly, I want to consider children facing the loss of a parent. We can read a little of the road ahead for them. They need to be included and informed. There are clear indications that the loss itself of a parent is not as damaging as the bewilderment and the emotional climate of deprivation that may ensue (Elizer and Kaffman 1983, Hilgard et al. 1960). We can assist the parents to prepare and support the bereaved child.

Andrew's mother died one Christmas Eve when he was just 8 years old. His father wondered if he should send him away to loving grandparents; after all, Christmas is a time to be happy.

He talked it through with the nurse and the doctor and finally decided that the time left for his wife was precious for all three of them.

Andrew was with his mother when she died. He washed her hands and face and combed her hair, and together they kept vigil until daylight.

His father informed the school of the death and when his class resumed, Andrew returned to school. His teacher did not know what to say to him, but as was usual she asked the children to tell about their Christmas. To her horror, Andrew stepped forward.

He said simply to the class, "My mother died on Christmas Eve. I was there, I washed her and then we had a funeral".

The children were absorbed. "What did she look like?" they asked; "Where is she now?" Straightforwardly, he answered them and explained that she was in the ground now because she did not need her sick body any longer.

The teacher thanked him and he returned to his seat, but when they filed out for break, she noticed that the children gathered round him, and touched him. She felt that Andrew had opened the way for her by his honesty and openness. She could now acknowledge his loss, and check out with him how life is without a mother.

It is now 2 years since her death. Andrew talks about her comfortably. He has photographs by his bed and he cherishes what he calls "mum's box" which his mother prepared for him. In it is a favourite brooch, a book of poems, that she hoped he would learn to love, and many pictures of the family together. He rarely looks in it now but he never goes on holiday without it.

Reading the road ahead is not always easy. We cannot always foresee traumatic events but we have to try so that those who mourn do not have their mourning ties tangled by *our* indifference and ignorance.

"Mourning is not forgetting, it is an undoing. Every minute tie has to be untied and something permanent and valuable recovered and assimilated from the knot." (Allingham 1952).

References

Allingham M (1952) Tiger in the smoke, Chatto and Windus, London

Cameron J, Parkes CM (1983) Terminal Care: evaluation of effects on surviving family of care before and after bereavement. Postgrad Med J 59: 73–78

Elizer E, Kaffman M (1983) Factors influencing the severity of childhood bereavement reactions. Am J Orthopsychiatry 53: 668–676

Glaser BG, Strauss AL (1965) Awareness of dying, Aldine, Chicago

Herzberg E (1990) The bitterness of not knowing the worst. Independent 23 Jan 1990: 17 (London newspaper)

Hilgard J, Newman M, Fisk J (1960) Strength of adult ego following childhood bereavement. Am J Orthopsychiatry 30: 788–799

Nimocks MJA, Webb L, Connell JR (1987) Communication and the terminally ill: a theoretical model. Death Stud II: 323–344

Robbins J (1983) Caring for the dying patient and the family. Harper and Row, London, pp 141–142

Sarton M (1984) A reckoning. Women's Press, London

Stedeford A (1988) Essential psychiatry. Blackwell, Oxford, p 220

Rehabilitation of the Person with Cancer

D.K. Mayer

Institute of Health Professions, MGH, 15 River Street, Boston, MA 02118, USA

Introduction

This year approximately one million Americans will be diagnosed with cancer and five million will be alive with this disease (ACS 1990). It is also estimated that over 65% will be alive at least 5 years from diagnosis in the year 2000, an increase from the current 50%. Many of these individuals will be cured, but other long-term survivors will be alive with residual or recurrent cancer. As a result of the past, current, and projected progress in cancer care, a shift in current practice must occur to incorporate issues of rehabilitation and survivorship.

Rehabilitation is a process by which individuals are assisted to achieve optimal functioning in their environments within the limits imposed by cancer (Mayer and O'Connor 1989). Historically, rehabilitation has not been systematically or consistently integrated as a process in cancer care. This paper will briefly explore what is known and make recommendations to guide cancer care health professionals into the 21st century.

Scope of the Problem

Comprehensive reviews of the physiologic and psychosocial effects of surviving cancer have recently been published (Loescher et al. 1989; Welch-McCaffrey et al. 1989). These effects are influenced by the individual's age (current and at time of diagnosis), type of cancer, and the treatment received (see the list of references).

A variety of studies have been conducted evaluating the needs of longer term survivors of cancer. In a study conducted at Stanford University, over 400 patients with lymphomas were surveyed (Fobair 1986). Approximately one third of all patients continued to have some difficulties. Forty-two percent were experiencing problems at work, 37% had energy levels that had not returned to baseline, and 20% were complaining of decreased sexual activity. What is striking is that these patients had a 9-year mean follow-up after diagnosis.

Cella (1987) reviewed many of the psychosocial and public issues affecting cancer survivors. He identified "higher risk" patients in need of evaluation for additional interventions. These included those with a previous psychiatric history or diagnosis, a lack of social support system, or a poor prognosis. From 3% to 5% of cancer patients develop significant anxiety disorders (similar to post-traumatic stress syndrome) as a result of their treatment. These disorders are treatable and such patients (estimated at 500 000 over 10 years) should be referred for intervention. Many cancer patients are also at increased risk of a second malignancy as a result of their disease or treatment. There will be an increased need for follow-up of the previously treated cancer patient that can attend to the long-term sequelae (Meadows and Hobbie 1986). Certainly, age-related issues create added problems—for example, the needs of the developing child returning to school or the elderly adult coping with other chronic illnesses.

Interpersonal problems with family and friends and within the community have been found to be dependent on the pre-illness relationships (Cella 1987; Lewis 1986). About equal numbers (20%) find improvement while others note worsening relationships. Issues of role-shifting, financial burdens, fears of contagion and recurrence and infertility are just some of the stressors added to an existing social support system. About one third of patients find this a "sorting out" time, with some friends noting distancing while other friends become closer. In another study of over 600 patients, conducted through the Pennsylvania American Cancer Society, 59% had at least one major unmet need (e.g., money, social support, transportation) (Houts et al. 1988). These needs are not being identified on a regular or consistent basis in clinical practice.

Many children with cancer experience difficulties returning to and doing well in school (Ferguson et al. 1986; Koocher 1985). This has been studied and documented more carefully in pediatric oncology than for adults facing cancer. Young adults may also experience job rejection or other discriminatory practices based on their cancer histories. Occupationally, 80% of cancer patients return to work after their diagnosis. The majority of adults (60%–80%) experience at least one problem such as the need to work fewer hours, having less stamina, or having problems with coworkers. Many feel "locked in" to their present jobs by not being promoted or offered other jobs within their company or for fear of losing insurance coverage. Insurance may be terminated or premiums increased as a result of the diagnosis; transferring policies is often difficult due to "preexisting conditions" clauses.

If one projects these findings to the five million Americans alive today with cancer, their potential needs become enormous. Whether and how these needs are being identified and met on a consistent or systematic basis are not clear.

Existing Programs and Services

In a review of 36 cancer rehabilitation programs, the typical program consisted of a program director (usually a physician), nurse, social worker, physical therapist, occupational therapist, pharmacist, nutritionist, and speech-language therapist (Harvey et al. 1982). The success of these programs was dependent on referral patterns within the community and on team communication. A study at the University of California at Los Angeles identified the needs of patients and developed referral services and resources within the community on the basis of this assessment, instead of having a defined program (Polinsky 1987). They provided access to counselling, support groups, health care (physical therapy, nutrition etc.), life planning, and education/information This may be a more practical approach for many clinical sites. The American Cancer Society serves 500 000 individuals with cancer annually through their various rehabilitation programs. These are mostly focused on specific deficits (or "body parts") such as "Reach to Recovery" for women with mastectomies and "Lost Cords" for people with laryngectomies. These programs are admirable and provide a great service but may not address needs that other professional services might, since large groups of patients without such clearly defined needs are left with few resources. As yet, a rehabilitation model that is adaptable to a variety of needs in a variety of settings has not been successfully implemented on a wide scale in this country.

Barriers to Successful Rehabilitation

A conference sponsored by the Oncology Nursing Society (ONS) in 1988 had representatives from a variety of professional organizations to identify barriers to successful cancer rehabilitation. Barriers identified included: health care professionals' philosophy and education, the need for a broader and deeper scientific data base on the topic, the need for better coordination and collaboration amongst care providers, and adequate reimbursement for services. The coordination of long-term care in today's health care system is a major problem. Where will these patients be followed? By whom and for how long? Underlying all of these barriers was a persistent attitude amongst the public, patients, and health providers that cancer remains a terminal disease and to which an acute short-term treatment-focused orientation is appropriate.

Recommendations

As a result of this conference, the following ONS positions were developed and approved:

1. Rehabilitation services will be available to address the physical, psychological, spiritual, social, vocational, and educational potential of the individual.
2. Services will be provided according to the preventative, restorative, supportive, or palliative needs of the individual.
3. Individuals must achieve optimal functioning within the limits imposed by their cancer.

We must address the barriers to achieving these goals. More research should be conducted, health care professionals' curricula should include these topics, and reimbursement for services should be provided, to name just a few. One can begin to look at individual and institutional practices to incorporate the assessment and management of individuals with cancer. How often and in what way are these patients' needs evaluated? Most importantly, and, I believe, before many other issues are addressed, we must begin to broaden our focus of care from an acute, short-term, treatment-oriented approach to a long-term chronic illness model. Unless we can change our attitudes about the rehabilitation needs of the person experiencing cancer, little will be different in the 21st century. I challenge you to make these changes.

References

American Cancer Society (1990) Facts and figures ACS, Atlanta

Armstrong G et al. (1982) Multidimensional assessment of psychological problems in children with cancer. Res Nurs Health 5 (4): 205–211

Baranovsky A Myers M (1986) Cancer incidence and survival in patients 65 years of age and older. CA 36(1): 22–37

Barofsky I (1982) Job discrimination: a measure of the social death of the cancer patient. Cancer rehabilitation. Bull Publishing, Palo Alto pp 145-153

Bloom B, Knorr R, Evans A (1985) The epidemiology of disease expense – the costs of caring for children with cancer. JAMA 253 (16): 2393–3295

Broadwell D (1987) Rehabilitation needs of the patient with cancer. Cancer 60: 563–568

Cella D (1987) Cancer survival: psychosocial and public issues. Cancer Invest 5(1): 59–67

Dietz, J (1980) Adaptive rehabilitation in cancer: a program to improve quality of survival. Postgrad Med 68(1): 145–153

Devlin J, Maguire P, Phillips P, Crowther D, Chambers H (1987) Psychological problems associated with diagnosis and treatment of lymphomas part I: retrospective study, part II: prospective study. Br Med J 295: 953–957

Dudas S, Carlson C (1988) Cancer rehabilitation. Oncol Nurs Forum 15(2): 183–188

Ferguson J, Ruccione K, Hobbie W (1986) The effects of the treatment for cancer in children on growth and development. JAPON 3(4): 13–21

Fibair P, Hoppe R. Bloom J, Cox R, Varghese A, Spiegel D (1986) Psychological problems among survivors of Hodgkin's disease. J Clin Oncol 4(5): 805–814

Harvey R, Jellinek H, Habeck R (1982) Cancer rehabilitation: an analysis of 36 programs approaches. JAMA 247(15): 2127–214

Hoffman B (1989) Cancer survivors at work: job problems and discrimination. Oncol Nurs Forum 16(1): 39–43

Houts P, Yasko J, Kahn B, Schelzel G, Marconi K (1988) Unmet psychological, social and economic needs of persons with cancer in Pennsylvania. Cancer 58: 255–2361

Klopovich P (1983) Research on problems of chronicity in childhood cancer. Oncol Nurs Forum 10(3): 72–75

Koocher G (1985) Psychosocial care of the child cured of cancer. Pediatr Nurs 11(2): 91–93

Lewis F (1986) The impact of cancer on the family: a critical analysis of the research literature. Patient Educ Couns 8: 269–289

Loescher L, Welch-McCaffrey D, Leigh S, Hoffman B, Meyskensf (1989) Surviving adult cancers, part 1: physiologic effects. Ann Inter Med 111: 411–432

Mayer D, O'Connor L (1989) Rehabilitation of persons with cancer: an ONS position statement. Oncol Nurs Forum 16(3): 433

McMillan S (1989) The relationship between age and intensity of cancer-related symptoms. Oncol Nurs Forum 16(2): 237–241

Meadows A, Hobbie W (1986) The medical consequences of cure. Cancer 58: 524–528

Mor V (1987) Work loss, insurance coverage, and financial burden among cancer patients. Proceedings of the workshop on employment, insurance and the patient with cancer. American Cancer Society

Mulhern R, Wasserman A, Friedman A, Fairclough D (1989) Social competence and behavioral adjustment of children who are long-term survivors of cancer. Pediatrics 8(1): 18–25

Mullan F (1984) Reentry: the educational needs of the cancer survivor. Health Educ Q Spring Suppl 10: 88–94

Nerenz D, Love R, Leuenthal H, Easterling D (1986) Psychosocial consequences of cancer chemotherapy for elderly patients. Health Serv Res 20(6): 961–976

Polinsky M, Ganz P, Rofessaet-O'Berry J, Heinrich R, Schag G (1987) Developing a comprehensive network of rehabilitation resources for referral of cancer patients. Psychosoc Oncol 5(2): 1–10

Roth S (1989) Setting goals in rehabilitation. Oncol Nurs Forum 16(1): 106

Teta M (1986) Psychosocial consequences of childhood and adolescent cancer survival. J Chronic Dis 9: 751–759

Veronisi U, Martino G (1978) Can life be the same after cancer treatment? Tumori 64: 345–351

Watson P (1986) Rehabilitation philosophy: a means of fostering a positive attitude toward cancer. J Enterostom Ther 13: 153–156

Welch-McCaffrey D (1986) To teach or not to teach? Overcoming barriers to patient education in geriatric oncology. Oncol Nurs Forum 13(4): 25–31

Welch-McCaffrey D, Hoffman B, Leigh S, Loescher L, Meyskens F (1989) Surviving adult cancers, part 2. Psychosocial implications. Ann Intern Med 111: 517–524

Wetle T (1987) Age as a risk factor for inadequate treatment. JAMA 258(4): 516

Wheatley G, Cunnick W, Wright B, Van Keuren D (1974) The employment of persons with a history of treatment for cancer. Cancer 33(2): 441–445

Wofford L (1987) "Cured" . . . Now what? Pediatr Nurs 1(4): 252–254

Interdisciplinary Rehabilitation of the Laryngectomee

W. Lehmann[1] and H. Krebs[2]

[1]Clinic of Otolaryngology-Head and Neck Surgery, Cantonal University Hospital,
 1211 Geneva, Switzerland
[2]Kommunikations-und Publikumsforschung, 93 Geering-Straße, 8049 Zürich,
 Switzerland

Total laryngectomy – i.e., total removal of the larynx and the vocal cords – is today still the best treatment for certain types of cancer of the larynx. Nevertheless, it constitutes physically a severe mutilation and psychologically an extremely traumatic operation. The loss of speech and the existence of a hole in the throat are felt by those who have undergone a laryngectomy and their relatives to be a serious disability. This is aggravated by such other inconveniences as the loss of the ability to breathe through one's nose and the loss of the sense of smell, restrictions in bathing or showering, and the fact that teeth have often been extracted prior to radiation therapy.

The rehabilitation of a laryngectomee is a very complex process chiefly involving the head and neck surgeon, the hospital nurse, the logopedist, the social worker, the patient's physician, the patient's partner, and contact with other laryngectomees. With regard to the situation of the laryngectomees in Switzerland, we should like to present here some of the results of a patient opinion survey.

Method

With a view to the twentieth anniversary of the founding of the Union of the Swiss Associations of Laryngectomees (*Union Schweizerischer Kehlkopflosenvereinigungen*) the Swiss Cancer League contracted the Swiss Society for Practical Social Research in Zürich to perform a representative patient opinion survey. This survey, concerning the living situation of laryngectomees, was intended to provide information about the medical, social, psychological, work-related, and financial problems of laryngectomees.

The group about which this survey was to provide information was defined as all the men and women who had undergone total laryngectomy due to carcinoma of the larynx and who were living in Switzerland at the beginning of 1989. Only partial information exists concerning the total number of laryngectomees living in Switzerland, available from various sources. There are no overall statistics. On the basis of a variety of information, the total number is estimated at between about 600 and a maximum of 800. The majority of these are members of the Union of the Swiss Associations of Laryngectomees.

In order to conduct a representative survey, it was necessary to gather as many addresses as possible of the people concerned. The Union made membership lists available to the research institute, corrected to the end of 1988. Addresses of non-members were obtained with the help of the hospitals at which the operations had been performed.

A representative sample was extracted from the more than 520 addresses and the selected persons were contacted. The readiness to provide information was extraordinarily high. Only a few of those contacted refused an interview or felt in too poor physical or mental health for an interview.

Thirty experienced and specially trained interviewers conducted the interviews, which took an average of 50–60 min each. A good half of the interviews were conducted alone with the person concerned; in 4 out of 10 cases the spouse was present – rarely another person.

The Interviewes

Three hundred and thirty-two laryngectomees were interviewed personally using standardized, pretested questionnaires. The interviews took place during the first quarter of 1989. 55% of the interviewees live in the German-speaking part of Switzerland, 27% in the French-speaking part, and 18% in the Italian-speaking part, which has only 4% of the population of Switzerland. Nine out of 10 laryngectomees are men. Of the men, almost 80% are married, of the women only 40%. Women laryngectomees are frequently single and live alone.

As to ages, at the time of interview 6% of the interviewees were under 50 years old, and 44% between 50 and 64. About half were aged 65 or older. Only every fourth person interviewed was still in employment. On average, 7 years had passed since the operation.

At the time of operation, 22% of those interviewed were below 50 years of age, and 54% between the ages of 50 and 64. This means that three out of four freshly operated laryngectomees were still of employable age: only one in four was already above 65 years old at the time of the operation.

For those interviewed, the operation had taken place from 1 year to more than 20 years previously. The results of the interviews show how those affected today view their situation then, and the period immediately after the operation, and how they feel about their situation today.

Results

Preparation for the Operation

How do the persons interviewed today recollect the situation prior to their operation? 82% remember that they were prepared for the operation and informed about the consequences. 14% remember that they were informed insufficiently or not at all. 4% did not answer the question. The preparatory talks were almost always conducted by the physician. Only 7% stated spontaneously that they were also prepared by a logopedist.

It was also the physician who informed the spouse or other relatives of the patient concerned about the operation and its consequences prior to the operation. This was the case for seven out of ten patients. Here again, note the differences in the speech regions: in the Italian-speaking part of Switzerland, the relatives were informed in 82% of cases, in the German-speaking part in 72%, and in the French-speaking part in only 61% of cases.

How did the patients and their relatives react to the physician's notification of the operation? 45% of the patients said that they were calm and collected; 34% reported being frightened and shocked; 19% felt depressed and sad. The reactions of their relatives are described as follows: 20% characterized theirs as calm and collected; 48% said that the notification of the operation caused a shock. A good 30% stated that those around them reacted "positively" and provided support. It should be mentioned here that the large majority of those interviewed stated quite clearly during the interview that after an initial shock, their families showed a great deal of understanding for their new situation.

A good third of the patients (36%) were in touch with a laryngectomee prior to their own operation. 13% refused such a meeting; 42% were not even offered one. Where contact existed, the majority considered it to be useful: 69% of these patients stated that contact with a laryngectomee was helpful to them, while 23% said that this contact provided no advantages.

Treatment and State of Health

On average, patients were hospitalized for 3–4 weeks after a total laryngectomy; this period was longer for approximately a third of the patients. Almost all were satisfied with the care and treatment they received in the hospital. 27% were subjected to radiation treatment before the operation and another 54% after the operation; about half required dental treatment.

Today, seven out of ten patients still go to a hospital or see an otorhinolaryngologist for regular medical check-ups. The large majority considered their relationship with the physician to be good. Two thirds of the patients described their present state of health as good under the circumstances. Nevertheless, 43% reported considerable breathing disorders and 27% have swallowing disorders. Every second interviewee admitted occasionally having experienced fear of suffocation attacks, of breathing problems, of a relapse or a deterioration, of the loss of speech, or of psychological crises since the operation.

Speech Rehabilitation

The loss of speech after a total laryngectomy is the high price laryngectomees must pay to save their lives. An ideal solution to the problem of speech communication for all laryngectomees has not yet been found, as is confirmed by the data from out interviews. Nine of ten laryngectomees received speech therapy to learn the esophageal voice. This therapy was provided in 80%–90% of cases in the German- and French-speaking parts of Switzerland by logopedists; in the Italian-speaking part, only 24% were trained by a logopedist. It is interesting to discover that for the whole of Switzerland, approximately one fifth of laryngectomees received speech training from another laryngectomee; in the Italian-speaking part the figure was 80%.

The period between the operation and the start of speech therapy varied from 1 week to more than 12 weeks. Approximately half of the patients receiving speech therapy began during the first 6 weeks after the operation, most of the rest later. Usually, medical reasons were the cause of this relatively long waiting period, as air injection into the esophagus is only possible after the operation incisions have healed.

The duration of speech therapy also depended mainly on the postoperative anatomical situation as well as on age and mental condition. The average duration was 12 weeks, but the range was from 1 week to more than 1 year. An average of 20 lessons were received, but again the range was wide, from less than 10 to more than 50.

The most difficult period in all efforts at speech therapy is the period until a speech communication is possible with the outside world. Half of the laryngectomees took 1–3 months, 20% needed 4–6 months, and 15% took even longer. For 5% speech communication was still not possible at the time of interview. 65% were satisfied with the results of speech rehabilitation, 15% reasonably satisfied, 17% dissatisfied, 3% gave no answer. As for the relatives, two thirds of the interviewees said they had adapted well to the new method of communication; one third reported initial difficulties.

Up-to-date information about the methods of communication was provided by questions about the most frequently used means of communication. For 51% it is the esophageal voice, for 31% the electronic voice prosthesis, for 25% pseudomurmur (whisper), for 11% written communication, and for 2% gestures and mime. 20% frequently use two or more communication techniques.

There is, of course, no way of providing the laryngectomee with a normal voice. In those cases where the desired success had not materialized, at least the will and the effort from all sides were regarded as definitely worthy of praise.

Social and Work Environment

Laryngectomees are affected at a central area of social life: their speech, the most important means of establishing interpersonal contacts, is severely impaired.

Laryngectomees have to find the courage to learn to communicate in a new manner. In order to live with speech and nonverbal communication, they need relatives, coworkers, friends, neighbors, people on the street, on the telephone, in the shops, at their place of work, who are ready and able to accept this new method of communication.

Fortunately, two thirds of the interviewees stated that their relatives had been very understanding and had adjusted well to the new type of communication. In one third of cases, however, the process of adaptation had caused initial difficulties for the relatives – possibly because there was too little outside information and preparation.

Support from the environment is frequently necessary not only in the area of communication, but also during daily tasks at home and during personal hygiene (e.g., bathing). It is encouraging that a good three quarters of all interviewees were able to be independently in this area. Approximately 25% of the men and 40% of the women are dependent on the help of others. The men usually receive this from their wives, while women frequently complain of lack of support. It should be repeated that there are considerably more singles among the women than among the men, and single laryngectomees as a rule have more difficulties in all areas. This is substantiated by the answers from our interviewees. Clearly, they should receive more attention and support.

Help from neighbors and friends is very important. More than half of the interviewees was able to count on such help, but 12% knew no-one nearby to whom they could go for help. This is unsatisfactory, as laryngectomees should have recourse to social resources in the family, their circle of acquaintances, and in their neighborhood to help them to master their lot.

It can be regarded as a turning point in a person's life when, in consequence of an operation, he or she must completely or partially give up work or accept considerable reductions in working activity and material wellbeing. Prior to their operation, 70% of all the interviewees were employed, afterwards only 34%. Almost every fourth laryngectomee who was employable after the operation had to change jobs; every second laryngectomee had to reduce his or her working time. More than half felt restricted with regard to the performance of their work and their chances of promotion, and one quarter felt restricted with regard to their contacts at their place of work.

Free time activities are another aspect of social wellbeing. The great majority of the laryngectomees interviewed are still quite active in their free time: more than 90% had a hobby, more than half were active in sports. Other pastimes frequently mentioned were music, reading, gardening, needle-work, games, and TV and radio. Moving about in public and social life is not unproblematic for laryngectomees, as coughing and expectoration can be especially inconvenient when among people not familiar with these difficulties.

What are the limitations outside the home? Approximately half of those interviewed felt restricted in daily communication and around 40% during social gatherings, when going out or on vacation, or while travelling. Approximately a quarter reported limitations when out shopping.

Fears which keep returning after the laryngectomy also cause problems: fear of suffocation attacks, of loss of speech, and of the ability to communicate. Although the devotion on the part of the closest relatives on the whole is considerable, the need for friendship, love, and marriage of many of the interviewees was more difficult to meet after than before the operation.

The interviewees also stated definite wishes and their needs for improved and new services. In the social area, the list of wishes showed the following priorities:

- Most importantly, improved psychological preparation for the operation: partly from a practical point of view – e.g., to be able to try out a microphone and other aids – but also as a moral prop.
- Better and more frequent speech courses, refresher seminars and repeat courses. Also, speech courses should be conducted by laryngectomees.
- Improved possibilities for contact with laryngectomees: for example, visiting those freshly operated upon; more outings, congresses, group discussions after the operation; a contact person close to where one lives, something to alleviate the isolation of singles.
- Education of the general public, to make it easier to utilize social opportunities, leisure occupations, and public events. Improved public information about the illness and the communication capabilities of laryngectomees. Reduction of public prejudices.
- Special rehabilitation centers, aimed at care after the operation, medical treatment after the operation, and convalescence. Perhaps even a home for laryngectomees.

Reintegration into Working Life and Financial Status

The financial status of laryngectomees depends on whether they wish to or are able to continue employment after the operation. If they are not able to reintegrate into working life, their material existence depends essentially on insurance payments.

The principle of the Swiss federal insurance for disabled persons, namely, "reintegration before pension," also applies to laryngectomees. This maxim is especially valid in view of the age of the operated patients: approximately three quarters of those operated upon were below retirement age (65 or 62 years in Switzerland). Of these by far the majority, namely 70% of those interviewed, were employed at the time of the interview.

With regard to the return to work, it must be remembered that most laryngectomees already have several years or decades of active working life behind them. This ought to allow a favorable prognosis for a return to work. On the other hand, the results of the interviews show that only 34% of the laryngectomees were still completely or partially employed after the operation, and only 25% at the time of the interview. This result can only be partly explained by the fact that a number of patients have now reached the age of retirement.

One reason could be the absence of timely vocational guidance. This ought to be included in the rehabilitation plan at the time the decision to operate is made. Counseling should start as soon as the patient is able to care for him- or herself and speech and language training have begun. The success of the return to speech and of the return to work are heavily interdependent.

Only 30% of the interviewees expressed a wish for vocational counseling. Food for thought is provided by the fact that almost a third of this quite small number received no vocational counseling. Nevertheless, there are indications that the vocational guidance that took place made reintegration into working life easier, if the statements by the employed and by the unemployed are compared. Of those below 65 years of age today, approximately 40% wanted vocational counseling. The percentage of those that received counseling was clearly higher in the employed than in the unemployed group.

If efforts towards a return to work are unsuccessful, insurance payments take the place of employment income. The majority of the laryngectomees were receiving one or more pensions from social security insurances. Only 12% of those interviewed received no pension – hopefully because they were fully integrated employees drawing a working income which excludes insurance payments. The remainder of those employed drew at least a partial pension.

Approximately 80% of those interviewed were drawing a pension from the Swiss Social Security Insurance or from the Insurance for Disabled Persons. For a minority this was supplemented by a pension from a pension fund. The completion of new pension funds (second pillar), will improve the financial status of those drawing pensions.

As we have mentioned, the great majority of the laryngectomees had not yet reached retirement age at the time of operation. It is therefore of interest to look more closely at the financial situation of those drawing disability insurance. The majority of those insured were unsatisfied (29%) or only partly satisfied (27%) with the benefits. This relative dissatisfaction is caused by two main factors: dissatisfaction with the disability insurance procedure and dissatisfaction with the amount of the insurance.

A remarkably large number of those drawing disability insurance complained about the amount of disability insurance (42%) and/or had general financial worries (31%). Furthermore, a considerable discrepancy became visible between the number of those drawing pensions and having financial worries and the number of those drawing benefits supplementary to the social security insurance and the disability insurance. These supplementary benefits are intended to ensure at least a minimal satisfactory standard of living for those drawing a pension. Overall, almost every fifth recipient of disability insurance also draws supplementary benefits; the percentage is considerably lower among laryngectomees.

Summary

It is to be hoped that human aspects have not been forgotten in spite of all these statistics. Behind all these numbers lie the personal fates of approximately 700 laryngectomees in Switzerland. The interview findings reflect their situation in life. In summary, we can say that:

- Half of the laryngectomees lose their job and feel restricted in their daily lives; every third one mentions financial problems.
- A third of the laryngectomees are totally or partly unsatisfied with the speech rehabilitation program.
- There appear to be remarkable differences within the various language regions in Switzerland with regard to preparation for the operation, speech rehabilitation, and the current life situation of laryngectomees.

From our study, we conclude that extensive medical, psychological, and social counseling and assistance for those affected is of great importance. Here we must especially mention the preparation of the patients and their relatives for the operation and its consequences. This should be the task not of one person but of an interdisciplinary team, including a logopedist, a social worker, and also another laryngectomee, with whom contact is often very valuable for the patient. Early speech therapy, reintegration into working life, and improvement of financial status are further factors of great importance.

Spiritual Support and Palliative Cancer Care

C. Odier

Institutions Universitaires de Gériatrie de Genève, Centre de Soins Continus,
1245 Collonge-Bellerive, Switzerland

Imagine for a few minutes that you stand on one of our very high Swiss mountains – the Säntis, for example, very close to St Gallen, and where some of you may go this afternoon. You stand on the summit on a beautiful sunny day and, slowly, you turn in a full circle, 360°: everywhere are mountains. You can see far away to Italy, France, Germany, Austria, the air is so clear, you can only hear silence; some black birds are in majestic flight, and you continue to turn, astonished by the beauty of that wonderful landscape.

You are filled by this beauty, but at the same time you realize that you can't absorb it all: you can only fully appreciate this scene when you have seen it under different conditions of light and weather, and with others who notice details that escaped your attention. . . .

Similarly, to discover the richness, the whole story of each specific patient we take care of in a palliative setting also needs time, needs the care of different people. One will never be able to capture all at once the beauty of that unique person.

Spirituality is part of that landscape. It sustains that deep part of ourselves, that breath of life which blows in us. Spiritual comes from the latin word *spiritus*, *pneuma* in Greek, *ruach* in Hebrew, and means the breath of life, which is given from outside of us. Spiritual support needs team work to allow the variety of life experiences, of ways of expressing our being alive, of ways of witnessing to the life-sustaining energy flowing in ourselves, to manifest themselves.

In this presentation, I draw on the clear distinction made by Phyllis Smyth and Daniel Bellemare of the Pastoral Team of the Royal Victoria Hospital in Montreal, Canada, between Spirituality, Pastoral Care, and Religion. This distinction is a very helpful one, as long as we never forget that we stand in front of a huge landscape, trying to see more clearly by finding the best angle, the best position from which to look. I have found it very useful to me in explaining the various roles in spiritual support. I will then share with you some of my convictions about the care giver's role in this specific support.

Recent Results in Cancer Research, Vol. 121
© Springer-Verlag Berlin · Heidelberg 1991

Spirituality as generally defined, is that deep work that patients are achieving, trying "to interpret their present illness in a way that makes sense within their world view. Terminal illness enforces a time of solitude, which for many becomes a time of reflection, a time to reevaluate priorities, a time to review the accomplishments and the unrealized dreams of their lives. The most poignant questions occur when life itself is threatened". This reflexion is not always expressed in religious language and needs to be taken seriously as the deep expression of a spiritual journey. Caregivers, family, friends, pastoral team, everybody is involved by listening and bringing support to the one who is embarking on this journey. And for me the secret for that support is *awareness*. I will come back to this reality later on.

Religion for many patients who are affiliated with a specific community of people, namely churches, the "big" questions on their minds will be expressed in a specific religious language; they will find the answers linked to their religious *roots*. It is our responsibility to identify the resources in a patient's religious tradition, which will speak to that person. It may require a member of the same faith community who will be indeed able to open them to the presence of their God, to help them to express needs, questions and sometimes provide answers in words or practices to which they can deeply relate.

Pastoral Care. In the palliative team somebody is also needed who is specifically trained to bring spiritual support to dying patients. She or he will be trained to "deal with the increasingly complex ethical and theological issues that arise in the experience of illness, suffering and dying, as well as in the health care strategies that are elaborated to face these clinical situations". This person is used to discern complex philosophical and theological questions that are being raised. She or he won't provide answers (they don't pretend to have them . . .) but helps the patients to "keep on track" with their own questioning in order to find their own answers.

"The pastoral care worker is also a professional who enters into a relationship aimed at helping the patient use spiritual resources and/or traditions to integrate the experience of illness, suffering, dying".

The pastoral care worker is finally able to work in interdisciplinary team, all of whose members understand and speak the same language and who each enrich with his or her own viewpoint, the overall image of the patient's landscape.

Spirituality, Religion, Pastoral Care, this distinction helps us to realize that spiritual support also needs different people, different viewpoints, different expressions of faith even to be supportive to the variety of people whose care is entrusted to us.

This distinction also points to our responsibility to bring spiritual support in a professional way sometimes without regard to our own convictions. And we all know by experience that our convictions are often threatened by those of our patients and their families.

Does it mean that we need to leave our convictions at the door of the hospital?

We know this is impossible, and it is absolutely not what I mean. But aren't we sometimes like Ernest, that big bear, pulled and pushed by the patients?

Listening to their stories, discovering their scale of values, we do not always agree, sometimes we feel that our convictions make it difficult to hear more . . .

And we are sometimes tempted to judge or to ignore . . .

This temptation will especially be there if we think spiritual support is arguing, discussing, sharing ideas.

My conviction is that spiritual support is rather an attitude, a way of being with patients.

Beginning a reflection on "breath", we discovered with a small group of nurses in the Centre de soins continus that spiritual support involves breathing, touching, listening.

Breathing with patients, listening to their different breaths can lead us into a deep communion with them: no necessity to talk; just listening to the spirit of life that flows in us. This is a very moving experience and sometimes a very difficult one but which obliges us to get down deep in ourselves.

Touching the patients, touching their body not as flesh, but as the presence of a person, with memories written in that body: good memories and bad ones. Being then conscious of what happens to a person we touch: when we wash her, when we turn him . . .   What is this body telling us about fears, hopes, peace or anger?

Spiritual support is also being aware of what and how *the patient hears*. They may be afraid by a small noise which brings bad memories or calm by odd noise for us. It is also being aware of the noise we make, the tune of our voice. Spiritual support is finding the just tune of voice to communicate with each different patient, the best sounds of music, songs, silence, birds, water, and so on.

It is indeed by using all our resources that we are present to patients, that we can bring them spiritual support. We become *aware* of that life which runs in us. We discover this breath of life that vivifies our bodies and that won't end as the functions of the body cease.

To be ourselves aware of each breath of life will lead patients to draw their strength from that same breath, which some will identify with the presence of GOD.

It will help them to discover this strength in their present weakness and to realize they are deeply loved as they are, forgiven whatever they went through. They won't only understand the breath of life but they may also experience it in the confines of their world of suffering.

Through our presence they may be able to sew up the pieces of their lives, like patchwork, to finally bring all the pieces together into one integral and lovely quitt.

I was standing last week at the summit of the Säntis. I turned in a full circle several times to appreciate each detail of the mountains surrounding me, and my children helped me to name some of the peaks. Then I closed my eyes and opened them slowly as if it was the last minute of my life, the last time I would ever see those mountains. There were two black birds flying peacefully above us.

I was struck by how they were sustained by the wind, the breath of life . . . by the spirit, the Holy Spirit.

Bringing spiritual support is for me a way of being supported myself by the spirit of life, and I feel priviledged to lead patients to discover that the Breath of life is supporting them also and that they may fly, fly for ever.

Subject Index

academic performance 414
acetaminophene 14
acetylsalicylic acid 13f.
acinetobacter spp. 322, 340
ACTH 94
actinomyces 322
acupuncture 6, 30, 424
acute respiratory distress syndrome 331
acyclovir 220, 383, 353
– resistance 355
addicted person 17
additive analgesic effect 14
aerobic flora 339
affective adjectives 62
– syndrome, organic 379, 381
afterloading 368
AIDS 195, 353
albumin, serum 235
alcoholism, emesis 70
alexithymia 63
algesic substances (see pain mediators)
amino acid imbalances 250
amitriptyline 15, 384
AML (see leukemia, acute myelogenous)
amnestic syndrome 379f.
amphotericin B 220, 347ff., 383
–, toxicity 347
ampicillin 220
anaerobic flora 338
anaesthetics, local 32
analgesic drugs 3, 12ff.
– studies, requirements 403f.
analysis, bioelectrical impedance 235f.

anatomical defects, infections 321f.
anemia 180
–, aplastic, granulocyte-macrophage
    colony-stimulating factor 125
–, chemotherapy 124, 162
–, renal 126
–, tumor 127
anorexia 249ff., 260, 384
–, acute-phase response 250, 252
–, assessment 255
–, causes 250
–, diagnosis 255
–, learned food aversions 253
–, postoperative 253
–, psychogenic 253
–, ratios of protein, fat and carbohy-
    drates 252
–, therapy 256
–, therapy-induced 252
–, tumor-induced 250
anti-inflammatory drugs 11
antianorectics 256
antibiotics 158
–, combination therapy 332
–, empirical 331f.
–, intravenous home therapy 215ff.
–, monotherapy 332
–, non-absorbable 338
anticarcinogens 289
anticholinergics 390f.
anticipatory emesis 68, 80
– fear of pain 63
– fears 61

anticonvulsants 15
–, pain 31f.
antidepressants 15, 256, 384, 390
–, pain 31
antiemetic therapy 68ff., 101
– –, nonpharmacological techniques
    101ff.
– –, – –, conceptual framework 105
antiemetics 68ff., 86ff., 91ff., 384, 390
–, combinations 75ff.
–, corticosteroids 72, 91ff.
– in children 93
antihistamines 384, 390
antimicrobial oral prophylaxis 339
– prophylaxis 339
antiviral drugs 353
anxiety 62ff., 101, 113, 158, 254, 304,
    408, 412, 424, 438
– reduction 295
appetite, depressed 250
–, lack 298
– scores 255
– stimulants 268
– suppression 101
– treatment 256
Aspergillus fumigatus 324f., 327
asphyxia 367
Australia, medical education 414ff.

B-cell function 323
baclofen 15
bacterial contamination 195
– infections 330ff.
Bacteroides fragilis 324
Balint groups 424
barbiturates 391
behavioural therapy 61
benzamides 72f.
benzodiazepines 43, 72, 391
benztropine 384, 389
beta-carotene 288
Betäubungsmittelverschreibungsordnung
    45, 47
biliary sclerosis (see cholangitis,
    sclerosing)
biphosphonates 15, 405
bleomycin, toxicity 326, 373, 375, 383
blood sampling 192
body image, altered 116f.

– language 314
– wasting 249
bone metastases 9
– pain (see pain, bone)
bowel perforation 284
breast cancer 173
– surgery rehabilitation group 307
Bristol diet 293, 424
bromovinyldeoxyuridine 356
bronchoscopy, therapeutic 368
BtMVV (see Betäubungsmittelverschrei-
    bungsordnung)
buprenorphine 14
busulfan 375
butyrophenones 72, 74

cachexia 248ff. (see also anorexia)
– anorexia syndrome 249, 405
calcitonin 15
calcium 289
cancer centers 399ff.
–, chemoprophylaxis 289
– diagnosis 63
– –, psychosocial interventions 303f.
–, interaction with pain 64
– pain (see pain)
–, prevalence 393
– prophylaxis 287, 300
–, terminal phase 63
Candida albicans 324f., 337
cannabinoid 72, 75
carbamazepine 15, 32
carcinoembryonic antigen 199
cardiac tamponade 362
care, competent 320
–, day care 396, 423
– givers 395, 408ff.
–, holistic 115f., 423
–, home (see home care)
–, inpatient 256, 396
–, insufficient 196
–, interdisciplinary 401
–, multi-disciplinary 4
–, outpatient (see home care)
–, palliative (see palliative care)
carotid artery erosion 364
catabolism, protein 243
catheter dislocation 195
– occlusion 200

catheter systems, completely implantable 189ff., 199, 208ff., 223 (see also Port-a-Cath system)
– –, – –, complications 194, 210ff., 327
CEA (see carcinoembryonic antigen)
ceftazidime 332
celiac plexus, neurolytic block 13
cellular defects, infections 323ff.
chemoprophylaxis of cancer 289
chemotherapy, adjuvant 307
–, dose intensification 173ff., 182
–, high-dose 180, 182, 341
–, infections 325f., 341
–, intra-arterial 198ff.
–, malnutrition 252
– c.-related nausea 68ff., 101ff.
chlormezanone 15
chlorpromazine 15, 72, 74, 384, 387
cholangitis, sclerosing 198
cholesterin 289
chronic myelomonocytic leukemia, granulocyte-macrophage colony-stimulating factor 145
ciprofloxacin 339f.
cisplatin 70, 174, 383
–, delayed emesis 80f.
clonazepam 15, 32
clonidine 33
clostridia spp. 322, 339
codeine 13f., 384
cognitive capacity screening 386
colistin 339
colonization, oropharynx 341
colony-stimulating factors (see hemo-poietic growth factors)
colorectal cancer 128
– –, liver metastases 198ff.
colostomy 110, 112, 115, 117
communication 63f., 408, 410, 419f.
– with the family 434
–, nonverbal 313ff., 419
–, verbal 420
complement activation 323
comprehensive cancer center 417
compression of central nervous system 10
computerized ambulatory drug delivery systems 215ff.
confidence 411

constipation 261f.
consultation, employment 310
–, individual 310
–, insurance 310
– service 301ff., 395f., 427
contact, veteran patient 306
control, maintaining 410
coping, ability 319
– behaviors, maladaptive 106
– with cancer 305, 424
– with fear or recurrence 309
– with pain 58ff.
– strategy 65, 307, 409, 427
cordotomy 13, 31
corticosteroids 9, 15, 72, 75, 91ff., 389f.
–, pain 33
–, serotonin antagonists 89, 93
–, side-effects 94, 325, 383f.
cost-minimization analysis 224
counseling services 301ff., 427, 395f.
crisis intervention 296
cyclophosphamide 70f., 129, 185, 326
cyproheptadine 256
cytokines 121ff.
cytomegalovirus 325, 327, 353, 369
cytosine arabinoside 142f.
cytostatic therapy (see chemotherapy)

damage, anatomical, and infections 321f.
–, cellular, infections 323ff.
–, humoral, and infections 323
–, radiation 112
daunorubicin 143
day care 396, 423
death, parental 426ff.
decontamination, selective 338
–, total 338
delirium 378ff.
–, behavioral symptomatology 385
–, etiology 382f.
–, prevalence 381
–, therapy 387ff.
delusional syndrome, organic 379, 381
dementia 378ff.
–, etiology 382f.
–, therapy 387ff.
depression 62, 101, 254, 304
dermatosis, acute neutrophilic 126
desensitization therapy 101

dexamethasone 15, 72, 75, 92
dextropropoxyphene 14
diagnosis of cancer, psychosocial interventions 303f.
diagnostic laparotomy 112
diarrhoea 262
diclofenac 13
–, slow release 14
diet, anticancer 287
–, Bristol 293, 424
–, gastrointestinal cancer 286ff.
–, glutamine-enriched 283ff.
– histories 255
–, improper 296ff.
–, psychological aspects 296ff.
–, wholefood 288, 424
dietary advice 260ff.
– modifications, unorthodox 293fff.
– record 255
– therapy, alternative 293ff.
– –, cognitive dissonance 294
– –, expectancy effects 294
– –, psychological effect 294
diphenhydramine 384, 389
dipyrone 13f.
disseminated intravascular coagulation 364
diversion techniques 61
doxorubicin 156
doxycycline 220
drain tube 110, 112
droperidol 72, 74
drug(s), antiviral 353
–, –, adverse effects 355
– delivery systems 189ff., 198ff., 205ff.
– – –, computerized, ambulatory 215ff.
– – –, direct costs 224
– – –, elastomeric 217
– – –, home care 205ff.
– – –, immunologically compromised patients 219
– – –, implantable 198, 201
– – –, leukemia, acute myelogenous 224
– – –, liver metastasis 224
– – –, maintenance 205ff.
– – –, pain, intractable 224
– – –, portable 199
– – –, –, programmable 53, 218
– – –, socioeconomic aspects 221, 223ff.

– – –, syringe pumps 217
– d.-induced interstitial pneumonitis 373
– stability 220
– use, illicit 4
dying 305, 394, 408, 410, 426ff.
dyspnea 367

early detection, oncological emergencies 360
education, health care workers 6
–, medical in Australia 414ff.
–, palliative care 417ff.
–, postgraduate 420f.
– programmes 309f., 395, 408ff., 415
–, undergraduate 416
electronic voice prosthesis 445
emergence of resistant bacteria 339
emergencies, metabolic 363
–, obstructive 361
–, oncological 360ff.
–, respiratory 366ff.
emesis 101ff., 260f., 347ff.
–, alcoholism 70
–, chemotherapy-related 68ff., 86ff., 101ff.
–, delayed 80f.
employment consultation 310
endoscopic tumor therapy 368
energy requirement 239
enteritis, radiation 283ff.
enterobacteriaceae 322, 339
enterococci 322
environment 313
EORTC (see European Organisation for Research on Treatment of Cancer)
epirubicin 174
EPO (see erythropoietin)
Epstein-Barr virus 353
erythromycin 220
erythropoiesis 147
erythropoietin 123, 126f., 145
Escherichia coli 324, 330, 337
esophageal voice 445
etoposide 156, 174
euphoria 17
European Organisation for Research on Treatment of Cancer 330
experience, surgical 196
experiential learning 319

eye contact 316
– expression 316

failure, bone marrow 162ff.
fear 62, 296, 305, 309, 317
fever 347ff.
fibre, wheat 289
fight-or-flight response 105
financial status, laryngectomee 447f.
flow cytometry 143
floxuridine 198
fluoroiodoaracytosine 356
5-fluorouracil intraarterial 198ff.
–, mental side effects 383
flupirtin 14
flurbiprofen 13f.
folinic acid (see leucovorin)
food presentation 268
– service provision 266ff.
foscarnet 355
frustration 316, 410
fungal infection 322
– –, systemic 347

ganciclovir 355
gastrectomized patients 252
gastrointestinal cancer, diet 286ff.
gastrostomy, percutaneous endoscopi-
    cally guided 269ff.
G-CSF (see granulocyte colony-
    stimulating factor)
germ cell tumor 163
Gerson therapy 293
glutamine-enriched diet 283ff.
GM-CSF (see granulocyte-macrophage
    colony-stimulation factor)
gram-negative bacilli, resistant 339
– rods 322
– –, aerobic 338
gram-positive rods 325
granisetron 79, 87f.
granulocyte colony-stimulating factor
    123, 125f., 141ff., 162, 179, 183
– – –, autologous bone marrow trans-
    plantation 183
granulocyte-macrophage colony-stimu-
    lating factor 122ff., 141ff., 155ff.,
    162, 173ff., 183ff.
– – –, acute lymphoblastic leukemia 143

– – –, – myelogenous leukemia 125, 143
– – –, anemia, aplastic 125
– – –, autologous bone marrow trans-
    plantation 183ff.
– – –, chronic myelomonocytic leukemia
    145
– – –, cytotoxic drugs 142
– – –, myelodysplastic syndrome 124f.,
    145ff.
– – –, toxicity 157f
granulocytes 175f.
granulocytopenia (see neutropenia)
grief 317
group sessions 305f., 310
guided imagery 101

haemoglobin 174
Haemophilus influenzae 322f.
hallucinations, organic 379f.
haloperidol 72, 74, 384, 387, 389, 391
head and neck cancer 269ff.
health care curricula 319
– insurance 301
hematopoiesis 162
hematopoietic (see hemopoietic)
hematopoietins 121ff.
hemopoietic failure 162ff.
hemopoietic growth factors 121ff., 141ff.,
    145ff., 155ff., 162, 173ff., 182ff.
– – –, acute myelogenous leukemias
    141ff.
– – –, autologous bone marrow trans-
    plantation 182ff.
– – –, cell surface receptors 141ff.
– – –, differentiation induction 142
– – –, proliferation induction 142
– progenitor cells 185f.
hemoptysis 369
hemorrhage 364
hemotological malignancies 337
hepatic artery infusion 198ff.
hepatitis, drug-induced 198f.
– virus 327
hernia, strangulated 112
herpes simplex virus 353
– virus infections 331
Hodgkin's lymphoma 173
home care 2, 5, 205, 226, 395, 423ff., 434
– – cancer service 36, 421

hope 402
hospices 2, 396, 423ff.
HPGF (see hemopoietic growth factors)
HPMPA 356
humiliation 316
humoral defects 323
hydromorphine (see morphine)
hydronephrosis 322
5-hydroxytryptamine-3 antagonists 69,
    79, 86ff.
– –, corticosteroids 89, 93
hypercalcemia 363
hypnosis (self-h.) 101
– therapy 65, 424
hypnotic suggestion 61
hypotension 220

ibuprofen 13f.
IFN (see interferons)
ifosfamide 156, 174
IL (see interleukins)
imipenem-cilastatin 220, 332
imipramine 15, 384
immunocompromised patients 321ff.
immunoregulation 122ff.
implantable devices 189ff., 199, 205ff.,
    208ff., 223 (see also Port-a-Cath sys-
    tem)
– –, acute leukemia 208f.
– –, complications 194, 210ff., 327
– drug delivery systems (see drug
    delivery systems, implantable)
index, bioelectrical impedance analysis
    235f.
–, multivariable 235
–, nutritional 235
–, prognostic nutritional 234
indwelling time 194
infection(s) 321ff., 337ff.
–, acquired organisms 337
–, anatomical defects 321f.
–, bacterial 330ff.
–, cellular defects 323ff.
–, chemotherapy 325f.
–, chronic 189
–, combination therapy 332
–, endogenous flora 337
–, fungal 322, 347
–, gram-positive 211f., 333

–, humoral defects 323ff.
–, monotherapy 332
–, nosocomial 326f.
–, prophylaxis 337ff.
–, radiotherapy 326
–, site 330
–, surgery 326
–, venous catheters 327
infusion, hepatic artery 198ff.
– time 347ff.
insurance consultation 310
– costs 301
intensive care monitoring 113
interdisciplinary aftercare 189
interferons 123, 130f
– IFN.-alpha 130
– IFN.-beta 130
– IFN.-gamma 130
interleukins 123, 127ff.
– IL.-1 183, 187
– IL.-2 128
– IL.-3 127f., 145, 162ff., 186
– –, toxicity 168
intervention, preventive 426ff.
–, psychosocial 301ff., 426ff.
intra-arterial hepatic catheter 199
intracranial pressure, increased 361
intrapleural drug administration 371
isolation, protective 338

Klebsiella spp. 330
– pneumoniae 322, 324, 337
Kostmann's syndrome 126
Krebsdiät 287

L-asparaginase 383
laparotomy 112
laryngectomy, preoperative information
    443
–, quality of life 446
–, rehabilitation 442ff.
–, social life 445f.
laxatives 15
Legionella 370
leucovorin 198
leukemia, acute 208, 339
–, – lymphoblastic 143
–, – myelogenous 125, 141ff.
–, chronic granulocytic 131

leukemia, chronic myelomonocytic 145
–, hairy cell 131
leukostasis 364
levomepromazine 15
levorphanol 14
Listeria monocytogenes 325
liver, bacteremia 323
– metastases 198ff.
local anesthesia 11
logopedist 445
lorazepam 72
loss 317
– of a parent 426ff., 435
lung cancer 366ff.
– –, small cell 155ff.
lymphokines 128
lymphokine-activated killer cells 128
lymphoma 112, 208f.

macrobiotics 286, 288, 293
macronutrients 286
macrophage colony-stimulating factor
    123, 128, 183
– – –, autologous bone marrow trans-
    plantation 183
malnutrition 249, 296ff.
M-CSF (see macrophage colony-stimu-
    lating factor)
MDS (see myelodysplastic syndrome)
medical education in Australia 414ff.
medications 62
megakaryopoiesis 147, 162, 165
megestrol acetate 256
melanoma, malignant 128f.
mental illness 304, 378ff.
– stress 254
– suffering 2
– syndromes, organic 378ff.
metabolic emergencies 363
metamizol 13f.
methadone 14, 384
methotrexate 326, 383, 405
methylprednisolone 72, 94
metoclopramide 72f., 86
–, side effects 69, 73, 384
metronidazole 220
micronutrients 286
Mini-Mental State Exam 386
mitomycin-C, intraarterial 198ff.

morphine 14, 384
– infusion 51
–, slow release 14
mourning 427ff., 432
mucosal damage 321f., 325, 342
mucositis 262, 283ff., 331
multi-colony-stimulating factor (see in-
    terleukin-3)
multi-disciplinary care 4
multi-modality therapy 302
multiple myeloma 163
Mycobacteria spp. 325, 369
myelodysplastic syndrome 145ff., 169
– –, combination of low-dose ara-C and
    GM-CSF 147
– –, granulocyte-macrophage colony-
    stimulating factor 124f., 145ff.
myelosuppression 183ff.
myotonolytics 15

nalidixic acid 339
natural killer cells 128f.
nausea 101ff., 260f., 247ff.
–, alcoholism 70
–, chemotherapy-related 68ff., 86ff.,
    101ff.
nefopam 14
Neisseria meningitidis 323
nerve compression 9
neuralgia, postherpetic 15
neuroleptics 15
neurolytic diagnostic nerve block 11
– nerve block 17f.
neutropenia 323f., 330, 337ff.
–, chemotherapy 124f., 155, 173
–, congenital 126
–, cyclic 126
–, idiopathic 126
neutrophil chemiluminescence 159
– chemotaxis 159
Newcastle Medical School 413ff.
nociceptor 14
non-Hodgkin's lymphoma 163
nonpharmacological techniques, antieme-
    tic therapy 101ff.
– –, – –, conceptual framework 105
norfloxacin 340
nosocomial infections 326f.

nursing staff 36, 196, 205, 395, 408ff., 423, 434
nutrient intake 249f., 252
– –, inadequate oral 255
– –, quantification 255
nutrition 233ff., 260ff., 266ff., 286ff., 424
–, economic aspects 262f.
–, enteral 244, 263
–, food service provision 266ff.
–, hypercaloric 241
–, intensified oral 256
–, normocaloric 242
–, oral 263
–, parenteral 192, 244, 264
–, –, duration 239f.
–, percutaneous endoscopically guided gastrostomy 269ff.
–, postoperative complications 233, 235
–, psychological aspects 296ff.
nutritional index 235
– status 233ff., 269ff.
– support 260ff., 266
– therapy 295
– –, postoperative 240f.
– –, preoperative 238f.

obesity 261
obstruction, biliary 110
–, bowel 362
–, bronchial 322
–, central airway 367f.
–, genitourinary 322
–, large bowel 110
–, vascular 322
–, visceral 69, 108ff.
–, –, decompression 112
–, –, palliative surgery 108ff.
–, –, perforation 111
–, –, postoperative complications 113
–, –, sites 108f.
obstructive emergencies 361
OBW (see optimal body weight)
ofloxacin 341
oncological emergencies 360ff.
– –, early detection 360
– –, prophylaxis 360
ondansetron 79, 88f.
opiates (see opioids)
opioid(s) 3, 12, 24ff., 43ff., 396

–, addiction 4, 16, 43
– administration, continuous subcutaneous 51ff.
– –, parenteral 16
– –, subcutaneous 16
– body weight 238
–, dependence 16
– drugs 13
–, euphoria 44
–, factors influencing response 24
–, legal restrictions 45
–, mental performance 45
–, prejudices 43
– prescriptions 3, 48
–, – habits in Germany 46ff.
–, pseudoaddiction 44
– resistance 24ff.
–, respiratory depression 44
–, side effects 26, 390
–, tolerance 16, 25, 44, 56
–, underdosage 17
–, withdrawal symptoms 16
oral absorbable drugs 342
organic mental syndromes 378ff.
osteitis 192
oxygenation 370

P.A.S. Port (see peripheral access system)
Padilla index 275f.
pain 2ff., 8ff., 24ff., 189, 318, 393ff.
–, acute 61
–, anticipatory fear 61, 63
–, anticonvulsants 31f.
–, antidepressants 31
–, assessment 18, 37, 53
– – chart 37ff.
–, bone 11, 13, 405
–, – metastases 9, 15
–, chronic 422
–, constant 62
–, continuous 62f.
– control 36ff., 396, 423
– –, case studies 41ff.
–, coping 58ff.
–, – strategies 59, 61, 63
–, corticosteroids 33
–, course of cancer 61
–, cryoprobe 31
–, diagnosis 58

pain, diagnostic procedures 61
–, – relevance 60
–, distraction 61, 63f.
–, dysregulatory 9
–, fear 63
–, immunization training 61
– impact 59, 61
– intensity 60, 62ff.
–, intractable 17
–, local anaesthetics 32
–, localization 11
–, mediators 9
–, mental factors 58
–, nerve lesion 11
–, neuropathic 9, 15, 26f.
–, –, therapy 29
–, neuropathy 11
–, nociceptive 27
–, nociceptor 9
–, opiate-resistant 24ff.
–, –, management 27ff.
–, palliative chemotherapy 405
–, pathogenesis 8
–, postoperative 60
–, prevalence 2f.
–, prophylaxis 12
–, psychogenic 64
– questionnaire 18
–, rating, terminal phase 17
–, reactive 9
–, self-evaluation 18
–, sensitization of the nociceptors 9
– sites 39
–, somatic nerve block 30
– studies 403f.
–, sympathetic disturbances 11
–, sympatholytic agents 33
–, syndromes 10
–, –, cancer therapy 10
–, –, tumor infiltration 10
–, terminal cancer 65
–, – –, coping strategy 65
–, therapeutic procedures 61
– therapy 3, 11ff., 58, 63, 424
– –, adjuvant medication 15
– –, continuous subcutanous opioids 51ff.
– –, drug therapy 12
– –, guidelines 11ff., 55, 393f.
– –, non-drug therapy 5
– –, psychological methods 30
– tolerance 60, 63
–, tumour stage 60
– types 59
–, visceral 13
palliative care 399ff., 393ff., 408ff., 414ff., 423ff. (–425)
– –, education 417ff.
– chemotherapy 405
– medicine 2ff.
– –, multimodality approach 4f.
– –, prophylaxis 406
– nursing skills 408ff.
–surgery (see surgery, palliative)
pancreatic cancer, pain 13
paracetamol 13f.
parental death 426ff.
pastoral support 423
pentamidine 220
percutaneous endoscopically guided gastrostomy 269ff.
perforation, bowel 284
–, visceral obstruction 111
personal space 315
pethidine 14
phenothiazines 72, 74, 384, 387, 389
phenytoin 32
phlebitis 195
physostigmine 390f.
placebo effect 101, 294
platelets 175f., 209
pleural effusion 371
"PLISSIT" 119
Pneumocystis carinii 325, 369
pneumonia 325
–, pneumococcal 158
pneumonitis, drug-induced interstitial 373
–, radiation 374
pneumothorax 194
polymyxin B 339
polyneuropathy 15
Port-a-Cath systems 189ff., 199, 205ff., 208ff., 223
– –, acute leukemia 208f.
– –, complications 194, 210f., 327
– –, home care 205
– –, implantation technique 189ff.

– –, intraoperative problems 194
– –, maintenance 196
– –, requirements 196
– –, technical problems 194
practitioner, community 414
prednisolone 15
prednisone 72, 92
prevention (see prophylaxis)
procarbazine 383
prochlorperazine 72, 74, 384
professional skills 418
progenitor cells 185f.
prognostic nutritional index 234
prophylaxis, cancer 287, 300
–, infection 337ff.
–, oncological emergencies 360
–, palliative medicine 406
protein catabolism 243
– requirement 239
Pseudomonas spp. 322, 330, 340
– aeruginosa 323f., 327, 332, 337
psychological aspects, alternative diet
    294
– –, improper diet 296ff.
– –, nutrition 296ff.
– distress 254, 303f.
– intervention 65
– methods, pain therapy 30
– support 313, 423ff.
psychophysiological intervention, chemo-
    therapy 105
psychosocial services 301ff., 426ff.
– support 301ff., 394, 423, 426ff.
psychotherapy 295ff., 424
psychovegetative complaints 62
pulmonary emboli 158
– infiltrates, diffuse 369
– toxicity 373
pump, implantable (see drug delivery
    system)
–, portable (see drug delivery system)
psychiatric illness 304, 390
pyonephrosis 322

quality of life 115ff., 196, 249, 252, 254f.,
    275, 319, 396, 423
– –, laryngectomy 446
quinolones 324, 337ff.
–, prophylaxis 331

radiation, abdominal 252
–, head and neck 252
– pneumonitis 374
radioprotective effect, diet 283ff.
radiotherapy, infections 326
–, percutaneous endoscopically guided
    gastrostomy 269ff.
recurrence, fear 311
reexpansion pulmonary edema 372
regulations, bureaucratic 401
rehabilitation 437ff.
relaxation 61, 63
– techniques 65, 307
– therapy 101
relief of suffering 319
renal cell carcinoma 128f.
resilient patients 305
resistance to colonization 338
respiratory distress 366ff.
retinoids 288
retroviruses 357
roxithromycin 340

Salmonella spp. 325
Santé Service 205
sarcoma, osteogenic 173
–, soft tissue 173
satiety, early 250
sclerosing cholangitis 201
Seldinger technique 193
selenium 288
self-directed learning 418
self-esteem 307, 309
sense of touch 318
sensory input 318
sepsis 158, 192
septic shock 331, 364
serotonin antagonists 69, 79, 86ff.
– –, corticosteroids 89, 93
sexuality 115ff.
SIADH (see syndrome of inappropriate
    antidiuretic hormone)
skin graft 112
– lesions 321
slow-release preparations 13f.
social services 301ff., 423, 426ff.
socioeconomic aspects 221, 223
speech rehabilitation 444f.
– therapy 445

spinal cord compression 361
spleen, bacteremia 323
spontaneous pneumothorax 372
stage of illness 63
Staphylococcus spp. 337
–, coagulase-negative 326, 330f.
– St. aureus 321, 324, 327, 330
– St. epidermidis 324, 340
stoma, sexuality 115, 117
Streptococcus spp. 322, 326
–, alpha-hemolytic 330f., 340
–, beta-hemolytic 321
– St. pneumoniae 158, 322f.
–, viridans 330f., 337
stress, psychological 302
stressors 105
study, phase I/II 155ff., 163ff., 173
subclavian vein 189
suffering 317, 394f., 400
sulfamethoxazole-trimethoprim 220
superinfection 194
superior vena cava syndrome 361
supervision, professional 395
support, bereavement 396, 426ff.
–, nutritional 260ff., 266
–, pastoral 423
–, psychosocial 301ff., 394, 423, 426ff.
supportive management 369f.
surgery, curative 111, 112
–, hypercaloric nutrition 242
–, hypocaloric nutrition 242
–, infections 326
–, nutritional support 233ff.
–, palliative 108ff.
–, –, assessment 110, 112
–, –, bypass 112
–, –, colostomy 110
–, –, communication 111, 113
–, –, drain tube 110
–, –, haemostasis 110
–, –, in irradiated areas 111
–, –, nutritional status 110
–, –, principles 108
–, –, psychological status 110
–, –, timing 111
–, postaggression metabolism 240
–, technique 112
surviving cancer, psychological effects
    437

survivors, long-term 437
survivorship 308, 437
suturing 112
Sweet's syndrome 126
sympathetic block 11, 30
– efferent system 11
sympatholytic agents, pain 33
symptom control 394
syndrome of inappropriate antidiuretic
    hormone 363

tactile function 318
taste abnormalities 252
– changes 250, 262
– stimulants 268
teaching 414
–, postgraduate 420f.
–, undergraduate 416
terminal cancer pain 65
– – –, coping strategy 65
– – patients 17
– stage 65
testicular carcinoma 163, 173
theory of self-efficacy 105
therapist effect 295
therapy, antimicrobial 337
–, empirical antibiotic 331f.
–, multimodality 302f.
thio-tepa 174
thioguanine 143
thioridazine 384, 387
threat/appraisal concept 105
thrombocytopenia 175f., 180
–, chemotherapy 124, 162
thrombophlebitis, septic 322
thrombopoiesis 147, 162, 165
thrombosis, hepatic artery 200
–, subclavian vein 195
–, venous 211, 213
tilidine 14
tissue flap 112
tizanidine 15
touch 317
toxicity 157
–, amphotericin B 347
–, haematological 174ff.
–, non-haematological 177
–, pulmonary 373
–reduction, agranulocytosis 155, 173

toxins, tumor 250
Toxoplasma gondii 325
tramadol 14
tranquilizers 256
transcutaneous nerve stimulation 30
transplantation, allogenic bone marrow
    131, 143, 183
–, autologous bone marrow 124f., 182ff.
trimethoprim-sulfamethoxazole, side
    effects 339
tumor lysis syndrome 363
– necrosis factor(s) 123
– – factor-alpha 129, 183

unanticipated bereavement 433
underdosage of nonopioid drugs 17
– of opioid drugs 17
Union Schweizerischer Kehlkopflosenver·
    einigungen 442

valproic acid 32
vancomycin 220, 333
varicella zoster virus 325, 353
VAS (see visual analog scale)

venous access, central 189, 208, 216
– –, peripheral 216
– – system, peripheral 194
– catheters, infections 327
veteran patient contact 306
vinca alkaloids 383
visual analog scale (VAS) 18, 60, 63
vitamin C 288, 293
vitamin E 289, 293
Vollwertkost 288, 424
vomiting (see emesis)
vulnerable patients, psychosocial inter-
    ventions 304

weight changes 252
– control 296ff.
– loss 249, 261, 279
WHO (see World Health Organisation)
working life, laryngectomee 447f.
World Health Organisation 2, 8, 115,
    393, 396
– – –, guidelines for pain therapy 11ff.,
    51, 55, 393f.
wounds, surgical 112